Functional Herbal Therapy

Functional Herbal Therapy

A Modern Paradigm for Clinicians

Kerry Bone

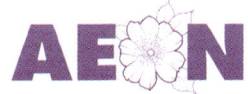

First published in 2021 by
Aeon Books Ltd

Copyright © 2021 by Kerry Bone

The right of Kerry Bone to be identified as the author of this work has been asserted in accordance with §§ 77 and 78 of the Copyright Design and Patents Act 1988.

All rights reserved. No part of this publication may be reproduced, stored in a retrieval system, or transmitted, in any form or by any means, electronic, mechanical, photocopying, recording, or otherwise, without the prior written permission of the publisher.

British Library Cataloguing in Publication Data

A C.I.P. for this book is available from the British Library

ISBN: 978-1-91280-724-6

Printed in Great Britain

www.aeonbooks.co.uk

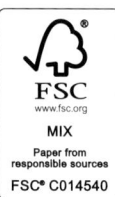

Contents

Foreword by Dr Christopher J. Etheridge   vii
Preface   xi

PART I   FOUNDATIONS OF FUNCTIONAL HERBAL THERAPY

1. An introduction to FHT   **3**
2. The principle architecture of FHT   **23**
3. Game-changing habits of highly effective herbal clinicians   **45**
4. The traditional roots of FHT   *by Simon Mills*   **69**

PART II   EXPANDING THE CORE STRATEGIES OF FUNCTIONAL HERBAL THERAPY

5. Plants and the microcirculation: a powerful new FHT clinical paradigm   **85**
6. Cellular protection and the Nrf2 pathway: a core FHT strategy   **111**
7. FHT strategies to reduce the health impact of environmental toxin exposure   **139**
8. The FHT bowel flora protocol for dysbiosis management   **181**
9. Covert invaders: new FHT herbal defences against old foes   **197**
10. FHT for relieving anxiety and boosting healthy sleep   **233**

PART III   APPLYING FUNCTIONAL HERBAL THERAPY

11. FHT for metabolic syndrome   **263**
12. FHT strategies for atopy, asthma, and allergic rhinitis   **295**
13. FHT for immune and respiratory health: viral infections   **327**
14. FHT strategies for IBS and SIBO   **357**

Acronyms & abbreviations   **389**
Index   **393**

Foreword

Christopher J. Etheridge

My life was profoundly changed when, in 2000, I discovered a copy of *Principles and Practice of Phytotherapy* by Kerry Bone and Simon Mills in a London bookshop. At that time, I was debating whether to leave academia and pursue a new career in complementary medicine. This ground-breaking book was truly inspirational. It talked to me in rigorous but accessible scientific language that modernised and revitalised the practice of herbal medicine. It gave me the courage to consider studying herbal medicine as a science-centred treatment modality and to pursue a sustainable career as a medical herbalist who could support patients in a research-based, holistic way.

While studying herbal medicine at the College of Phytotherapy in East Sussex and, later, as a fledgling herbalist, I was lucky enough to be guided by the books that Kerry published subsequently, on a wide range of herbal medicine subjects, all of which have been fundamental to my growth as a practitioner. I have been even luckier to see Kerry speak on many occasions when he has presented his highly regarded and innovative seminars in the UK.

Kerry originally trained as a chemist and now has more than 35 years of clinical experience as a successful herbalist. This has given him an exceptional ability to identify and interpret key clinical studies in herbal medicine and allied fields. He is then able to concisely pull together all of the different research strands and present them in a form that is highly applicable to, and easily assimilated into, today's herbal medicine practice.

In recent years, I have been particularly inspired by Kerry's lectures, which explore functional medicine and introduce a highly significant new concept: Functional Herbal Therapy (FHT). The time is ripe for such a holistic, multi-disciplinary, multicentred model that equips herbalists to understand and formulate treatment strategies that tackle the complexity of different disease states. Crucially, the time is right for a book exploring this fascinating and rapidly evolving area and bringing the key concepts and understandings together into one place. I was therefore excited – and relieved – when I heard that Kerry was writing this book.

In Part I, Kerry introduces the seven key attributes of FHT. These are a fusion of new research and concepts from the following areas: the Western medicine model for the pathophysiological basis of disease; the understanding of the inherent complexity of different disease states; the need for supportive and sympathetic treatment energetics; the requirement for multi-pharmacological treatments; the use of strategic, targeted therapies; the necessity for modular and pulsed dosing treatments in certain circumstances; and the requirement for a specific tissue-based support approach. Kerry goes on to examine the architecture of FHT, exploring its fundamental principles and introducing the 12 core treatment strategies that target and balance a myriad essential physiological processes. These strategies are of considerable current interest and the focus of pioneering research. They include: support of the endocrine system in its interlocking complexity; eliminating persistent pathogens; aiding the macro- and microcirculation; priming the all-important Nrf2 responses; promoting optimal digestion; and ensuring a healthy microbiome. The use of clinically effective herbs to support the 12 treatment strategies is then explored in detail, providing the modern herbalist with a complete herbal armoury to target diseases both old and new.

Part II gives the reader an in-depth look at some of these core treatment strategies of FHT. We are taken on a fascinating journey, exploring highly topical areas such as cellular protection, targeting covert invaders, limiting the damage from environmental toxins, reducing anxiety, and aiding high-quality rest and sleep. All of these strategies are essential in the modern world, where our health is impacted by environmental damage, global warming, poor lifestyle choices, and persistent viral pandemics.

Part III, the final section, critically examines how the key approaches and treatment strategies discussed in the first two parts can be successfully applied to the modern herbalist's practice. An in-depth consideration of clinically common and important disease states such as metabolic syndrome, atopic conditions, immune and respiratory health imbalances, IBS and SIBO allows the reader to see how specific treatment modules can be easily and effectively integrated into their current treatment regimes.

I am certain that this visionary book will revolutionise the way that medical herbalists and naturopaths understand and treat disease processes. It will also be invaluable to students of herbal medicine, naturopathy and pharmaceutical sciences, both as a standard text and a reference book. It provides them with a framework to examine disease states from a new and more holistic perspective; to learn about exciting lesser-known herbs; to see old, familiar herbs being used in novel ways; and to explore specifically targeted phytotherapeutic treatment regimes. By the end of the book, practitioners and students will be able to view complex disease states with a greatly expanded understanding, and to appreciate the immense potential of FHT to effectively restore the homeostatic balance and self-healing response within our patients' bodies.

I have been greatly inspired by FHT and am already applying its concepts to my own practice. As in all of Kerry's books, his enthusiasm, knowledge and vast experience continues to transform the herbal medicine world. Thank you, Kerry, for producing such an outstanding addition to our herbal medicine libraries.

Dr Christopher J. Etheridge
President of the College of Practitioners of Phytotherapy
President of the European Herbal & Traditional Medicine Practitioners Association
Chair of the British Herbal Medicine Association

Preface

When I was a herbal student in the UK in the early 1980s, a constant theme on the part of both my fellow students and other complementary medicine students I met at the time (osteopaths, homeopaths) was that Western herbal medicine (WHM) had no well-defined philosophy and prescribing system. According to some homeopathy students I enjoyed dinner parties with, it was even worse than that: the use of Western herbs suppressed symptoms the way conventional drugs do, reinforcing the chronicity of disease. All this was seen to contrast with traditional Chinese medicine and Ayurveda, which exhibited sophisticated herbal prescribing systems that were based on a profound understanding of the human condition and our place in the universe (as you can see in Chapter 4 of this book). What seemed to be the norm for WHM was an ad hoc, empirical approach to prescribing that varied from practitioner to practitioner, loosely informed by some of the concepts of twentieth-century naturopathy, but largely using medicinal plants as "green drugs".

However, as I became more informed about the history of WHM (especially after reading the excellent book *Green Pharmacy* by Barbara Griggs, just published at the time) and, in particular, the US herbal movements in the nineteenth century, I began to see that not only was traditional WHM informed by insightful thinking, but its fundamental concepts were still relevant to the modern situation. Gaining valuable experience from herbal practice and reading the biomedical science and herbal research, I realised that this traditional wisdom could be blended with both the latest scientific understanding of diseases and herb properties to develop a robust modernisation of Western herbal therapeutics.

To promote the value of this concept, I first advocated its characterisation under the banner "modern phytotherapy". Eventually I concluded, however, that the term "functional" was a necessary descriptor (as proposed by colleagues Amanda Williams and Billie O'Connor). Slowly my thoughts about what Functional Herbal Therapy should comprise became more consolidated, as they evolved with decades of insights from my clinical practice and some exciting developments in our understanding of the unique characteristics of medicinal plants. Through this evolutionary process, a fully-fledged systematic approach eventually emerged.

In Chapter 1 of this book you will see FHT defined as a system of modern prescribing for Western herbal clinicians that:

- incorporates the defining characteristics of functional medicine and applies these to the unique properties of medicinal plants;
- embraces the concept that contemporary Western herbal therapeutics should draw heavily on its empirical roots, acknowledging that the prescribing systems of key Western herbal movements, especially in the nineteenth and early twentieth century, were essentially a form of functional medicine;
- employs diet as a positive aspect of therapy, especially with the use of phytonutrient-rich plant foods.

This text, in fact, serves two purposes. First, as per the above, it provides a detailed description and discussion of the foundations of FHT and its core strategies. Second, it provides the reader who has not been able to attend all, or even some, of my seminars with an update of the herbal therapeutic guidelines and associated prescribing information found in *Principles and Practice of Phytotherapy*. Due to the pace of research, herbal therapeutics is now a constantly evolving field, so this second objective is only partially fulfilled by this book, and a further volume is anticipated.

For dosage guidelines, please refer to the monographs in *Principles and Practice of Phytotherapy*, or the condensed guide, *The Ultimate Herbal Compendium*.

Finally, the contribution of my long-time teacher, friend, and colleague Simon Mills needs to be gratefully acknowledged. Who better to write about the traditional roots of FHT than this leading thinker in the field of WHM? Simon also contributed to sections of Chapter 1, for which I am also thankful. The input of research assistant Nimisha Singh to some of the technical content of certain chapters is also recognised with thanks.

Further reading

Bone KM. *The Ultimate Herbal Compendium*. Warwick, Queensland: Phytotherapy Press, 2007.

Bone KM, Mills SY. *Principles and Practice of Phytotherapy: Modern Herbal Medicine*, 2nd edition. UK: Elsevier, 2013.

Griggs B. *Green Pharmacy: The History and Evolution of Western Herbal Medicine*, revised edition. Rochester, VT: Healing Arts, 1997.

FOUNDATIONS OF FUNCTIONAL HERBAL THERAPY

1

An introduction to FHT

This chapter introduces the concept of Functional Herbal Therapy (FHT) and gives an overview of its core features. Following a discussion of functional medicine and other relevant movements in modern medicine, the historical roots of FHT are briefly explored (with a fuller exposition in Chapter 4). The basic principles or attributes of FHT are then presented and discussed, together with a brief introduction to the 12 core strategies that form the subject of Chapter 2.

1.1 What is functional medicine?

In 1991, the Institute for Functional Medicine was founded on the basis of the following seven defining characteristics of functional medicine:[1]

1. patient-centred rather than disease-centred
2. systems biology approach: web-like interconnections of physiological factors
3. dynamic balance of gene–environment interactions
4. personalised, based on biochemical individuality
5. promotion of organ reserve and sustained health span
6. health as a positive vitality – not merely the absence of disease
7. function-focused versus pathology-focused

> The functional medicine model for health care is concerned less with what we call the dysfunction or disease, and more about the dynamic processes that resulted in the person's dysfunction.

This quote from Dr Jeffrey Bland underlines that functional medicine is more focused on understanding the causes of a person's health imbalance than with the symptoms that express this imbalance.

Functional medicine aims to address these underlying causes of disease, utilising a systems-orientated approach. It focuses on the whole person rather than just on an isolated set of symptoms. Functional medicine introduces the concept of the "matrix", which explores the patient's history, together with genetic, environmental, and lifestyle factors. It focuses on a patient-centred individualisation of medicine, prescribing remedies to restore the body's physiology (the dynamic interactions that maintain life) to normal functioning.

1.1.1 The P4, precision, and lifestyle medicine movements

There are a few parallel movements in modern medicine that both support and potentially inform the functional medicine approach; specifically, they are P4, precision, and lifestyle medicine.

The vision of a medical approach that is predictive, preventive, personalised, and participatory ("P4") has long been advocated by Leroy Hood and other pioneers of systems medicine.[2] P4 medicine has emerged from the convergence of three major trends:

1. the increasing ability of systems biology and systems medicine to decipher the biological complexity of disease
2. our enhanced capabilities for collecting, integrating, storing, analysing, and communicating data and information, including conventional medical histories, clinical tests, and the results of the tools of systems medicine
3. consumer access to information and consequent interest in managing our own health

Consumers are driving the transformation of healthcare by these megatrends.

According to the Precision Medicine Initiative, precision (or the older term, personalised) medicine is "an emerging approach for disease treatment and prevention that takes into account individual variability in genes, environment, and lifestyle for each person".[3] This approach allows therapists and researchers to predict more accurately which treatment and prevention strategies for a particular disease will work for which groups of people. It contrasts with the one-size-fits-all approach, in which disease treatment and prevention strategies are developed for the average person, with little consideration for the differences between individuals.[4]

Lifestyle medicine has been defined as "the application of environmental, behavioural, medical, and motivational principles to the management (including self-care and self-management) of lifestyle-related health problems in a clinical and/or public health setting".[5] It provides an interdisciplinary, whole-system approach to the prevention and reversal of chronic and lifestyle-related diseases through the modification of the behavioural, social, and environmental drivers. Conditions particularly targeted are those that result from:

- physical inactivity
- poor diet or nutrition
- smoking
- alcohol overconsumption
- chronic stress
- anxiety
- poor or inadequate sleep
- social isolation
- loss of culture and identity
- other influences of society and environment

1.2 Roots of FHT

As Simon Mills writes in Chapter 4 of this book:

> One attraction of functional medicine is that its principles resonate so strongly with ancient wisdoms. Indeed, on looking through the history of medicine around the world, it seems that only in modern times have these principles been forgotten.

In terms of FHT, intimations can be seen in an early mid-West American phenomenon: Thomsonian Medicine. Samuel Thomson was a nineteenth-century herbal clinician who rediscovered ancient principles for the treatment of disease that were, for his time, quite profound and revolutionary. Thomson restored the concept of a vital energy, which he described as the natural, self-restorative healing capacity of the body.

Thomson was horrified by the remedies used in "regular physic", these being dominated by toxic minerals based on mercury, arsenic, antimony, and sulfur. He also saw that there was a fundamental difference in therapeutic approach, with the doctors' objective being to stop the disease (in reality, the symptoms) at all costs. The main conditions of the day were febrile infections, and the regular approach was to use mineral products and bloodletting to stifle the symptoms and bring the temperature down. (This was before germ theory redefined the objective as eliminating pathogens.)

By contrast, Thomson's message was simple. Heat is life; fever is the body mobilising this heat; disease (and death) are degrees of cold. Heating thus provides the fundamental principle of healing. Other measures, principally those improving elimination and digestive performance, were often essential supports to this central measure.

His approach, known as Thomsonian Medicine, became based on the following principles:

1. Health follows from obeying natural laws.
2. Disease is an obstruction or diminution of vital energy.
3. It is caused by violation of natural laws.
4. Symptoms such as fever are caused by the disease and are not the disease itself.
5. Disease has only one basic type of cure: to remove obstructions and restore vital energy using substances that act in harmony with natural laws and the vital energy.
6. In doing so, one or more of the following effects should be achieved:
    a. relaxation
    b. contraction
    c. stimulation
    d. soothing
    e. nourishing
    f. neutralisation

What can be observed within these vitalist concepts is that health is the natural state of the body when all cells are working at their optimum, and disease is caused by a violation of the natural laws. The body does not gravitate towards disease, it gravitates towards health.

There are some obvious and striking parallels between Thomsonian strategies and Ayurveda. In the Charaka Samhita Sutrasthana[6] 1.53 and 22.4 we find: "The goal of Ayurveda is the equilibrium of the tissues" and "One who knows how to reduce excess, nourish deficiency, dry, oleate (lubricate), sweat and astringe is a real Ayurvedic physician." In fact, both the Ayurvedic system and traditional Chinese medicine (see Chapter 4) are very much embedded in concepts that we can employ as part of functional medicine – and, indeed, FHT.

A second significant root of FHT comes from physiomedicalism. The physiomedicalists were neo-Thomsonians – in other words, they took Thomson's principles and elaborated on them. The word "physiomedical" suggests exactly what they were trying to achieve: to develop a medical system that was physiologically informed.

All of these concepts and developments (and more) are fully explored in Chapter 4. The fundamental message is that traditional herbal axioms are still relevant to modern herbal prescribing, especially as embodied by FHT (see Section 1.3).

1.3 The defining attributes of FHT

FHT is a system of modern prescribing for Western herbal clinicians that:

- incorporates the defining characteristics of functional medicine and applies these to the unique properties of medicinal plants
- also embraces the concept that contemporary Western herbal therapeutics should draw heavily on its empirical roots, acknowledging that the prescribing systems of key Western herbal movements, especially in the nineteenth and early twentieth centuries, were essentially a form of functional medicine
- employs diet as a positive aspect of therapy, especially with the use of phytonutrient-rich plant foods

The key defining attributes or principles of the FHT prescribing system are the following:

1. understanding diseases as disordered processes of normal physiology
2. embracing the complexity of mosaic diseases, where the individual story counts most
3. ensuring treatment energetics are compatible with the patient's condition
4. complex interventions (network pharmacology) for multifactorial disorders (mosaic diseases)
5. therapy based on 12 core strategic targets
6. modular treatments and pulsed dosing used as key strategies where appropriate
7. the key overriding consideration: to support the affected tissues

1.3.1 Diseases as disordered processes of normal physiology

To fully appreciate this key attribute of FHT, we must make the reasonable assumption that a normally functioning human body is both free from disease and capable of resisting disease. Therefore, a deeper understanding of the cause and treatment of disease should come largely from a consideration of physiology, the normal functioning of the body, in preference to pathology and pathophysiology.

An excessive focus on pathology inevitably leads to a medical system that is overly interventionist. Its focus will be directed towards compensating for the physiological deficiencies and imbalances that arise in disease (physiological compensation), without seeking a greater understanding of how they arose in the first place. Such a basic strategy will lead to a superficial, short-term approach to treatment. In this model, chronic diseases are viewed as requiring management, rather than cure. (The commercial imperative behind this is obvious.) This is increasingly the conventional drug-based medical system we have today. While it is very useful for advanced pathologies and life-threatening states, it is incomplete and is especially inadequate in the treatment of many modern chronic diseases.

In contrast, most traditional medical systems, which are partially or completely based on herbal medicine, concern themselves more with the underlying physiological imbalances that have led to and sustain the disease. As such, they are focused more on physiology than on pathology. The aim of treatment is, typically, physiological support or enhancement, rather than just compensating for the chemical deficiencies or excesses resulting from an abnormal physiology. Physiological compensation often requires the constant presence of the medicine to achieve the desired effect, whereas providing physiological support can, in time, lead to a permanent correction of an abnormal body biochemistry.

One example of physiological support versus physiological compensation can be seen in the treatment of bacterial infections. The traditional herbal approach (and indeed that of FHT) is to support immunity and to fine-tune the normal mechanisms that protect against infection, such as the physical (anatomical barriers, such as intact skin and mucous membranes) and physiological barriers (such as fever and gastric acidity). In contrast, the conventional approach is to ignore the immune response and barriers and suppress the fever, killing the offending bacteria with antibiotics (thereby compensating for weakened or overloaded bodily defences). The latter approach has life-saving value but will not prevent infections from recurring, and it has a limited life due to the development of bacterial resistance to antibiotics. The traditional herbal approach may see a higher rate of failure in acute situations but can lead to improved immunity and ultimately to a reduced rate of recurrent infections. Clearly, an important complementary role for traditional herbal medicine can be argued from this and other examples.

The FHT approach is not always opposed to employing physiological compensation when needed, although the strategies used are far less interventionist than those possible with modern drugs. FHT recognises that a disease process can often create a vicious cycle, and sometimes only direct intervention to break that cycle can restore health. At a pragmatic level, interventionist treatment gives quicker relief of symptoms, which encourages the patient to persist with the treatment. Sometimes the very concepts treated might require an interventionist approach, because they are orthodox concepts – hypertension and high serum cholesterol, for example. This is not to say that applying the relevant core strategies of FHT will not also be of assistance and ultimately lead to better outcomes.

In general, the goal of physiological enhancement in FHT is to create a state of active, robust health. This is more than just the absence of overt disease, although such a positive state of body and mind would be free of disease and capable of resisting disease. It is the optimum state of body biochemistry and body energy.

Except for "whole-body" medicines such as tonics and adaptogens (see Chapter 2), the general goals of physiological enhancement in FHT are achieved by enhancing the function of individual systems, organs, or even tissues and cells. Such enhancement often involves the correction of imbalances. Deficient function in one physiological compartment can lead to overstimulated function in another, which can, in turn, create a deficiency elsewhere. For this reason, the specific treatment is sometimes not aimed at the problem site: for example, in constipation caused by deficient liver function, liver function would be enhanced instead of — or in conjunction with — enhancing bowel function. In another example, treatment of an excess of female hormones causing a menstrual problem may again be directed at the liver, this time enhancing detoxification processes, since the liver is the organ that breaks down these hormones. In addition, rather than directly manipulating ovarian secretions, the problem may also be corrected by optimising the output from the pituitary, which controls ovarian function.

From the brief examples above, it becomes apparent that fundamental to FHT is the individualisation of the patient (see Section 1.3.2). This is in direct contrast to current medical science, since the double-blind, placebo-controlled clinical trial examines the effect of a treatment only in a group of patients (the more the better, for statistical power) rather than in individuals.

Where appropriate, specific physiological enhancement in FHT might involve the regulation or boosting of digestive function, immunity, circulation, respiratory function, and hormone output. It may also involve the support of specific organs, such as the liver, kidneys, ovaries, and so on. The focus may be on specific tissues, such as the exocrine cells of the pancreas. Specific functions of organs — for example, the bile secretion or the detoxification enzyme systems in the liver — may also be supported. In all cases, this must be assessed on an individual basis and reviewed regularly.

Cells, tissues, organs, and systems will only be capable of optimal function if they are appropriately nourished, protected, and co-ordinated. For example, attempting to stimulate bile flow from a damaged liver will probably fail and might even be counterproductive. For this important reason, the overriding principle of FHT is to first support the tissue (see Section 1.3.7 and Chapter 2).

1.3.2 Embracing the complexity of mosaic diseases

1.3.2.1 What is a mosaic disease?

Mosaic disease as a concept was first suggested by the famous heart specialist Irvine Page in 1950 in the context of hypertension.[7] He proposed that hypertension is a mosaic disease based on eight possible causative factors: genetic, environmental, anatomical, adaptive (stress response), neural, endocrine, humoral, and haemodynamic. Much later, in 1989, immunologist Yehuda Shoenfeld coined the term for autoimmune disease.[8]

Mosaic disease may be described as a "syndrome" or disease that differs in its expression but shares many common factors (these constitute the pieces or tiles in the mosaic). Each piece in the mosaic can be viewed a causative factor in the disease and a potential target for treatment. Therefore, the "matrix" concept of functional medicine is immediately captured by mosaic disease principles. The mosaic disease concept can be readily applied to most modern chronic diseases.

According to mosaic disease principles:

- Every patient presents a unique picture, irrespective of their disease label.
- A chronic disease results from multiple causative factors (pieces in the mosaic).
- Disease occurs in a person due to a random (stochastic) combination of these causative factors.
- Therefore, the patient's story is paramount.

Some specialties of mainstream medicine still struggle with the concept of multiple causative factors, as illustrated by the following quotation from American psychiatrist Kenneth Kendler writing in a journal of the American Medical Association, *JAMA Psychiatry*:[9]

> The search for the causes of medical and psychiatric disorders has gone through 3 historical phases. First, up until the mid-19th century, causes of

illness were anecdotally recorded from individual cases, resulting in long and diverse lists for all disorders. Second, in the latter half of the 19th century, with the use of microbiological methods, single causes were found for many infectious diseases that led to specific diagnostic tests, effective preventions, and, in some cases, treatments. Causal thinking in medicine shifted from the earlier multicausal approaches to monocausal theories of aetiology. Indeed, proving monocausal etiology became a way to establish the legitimacy of a disorder. Through the writings of Kahlbaum and Hecker, psychiatry was deeply influenced by this monocausal perspective, the importance of which was substantially amplified by a twist of fate: the increasing clinical importance of general paresis of the insane throughout the 19th century and the eventual proof that it too was a monocausal condition. However, in the mid-20th century, the third phase began. With decreasing deaths from infectious diseases, epidemiology and clinical medicine shifted to a chronic disease model in which paradigmatic disorders, such as cancer and cardiovascular disease, were shown to be highly multicausal. Biostatistics evolved from deterministic to probabilistic models of disease risk factors. Paradoxically, at this time, biological psychiatry, then rising to dominance in American psychiatry, vigorously pursued monocausal theories, first of neurochemical origin and then of genetic origin. We were trying to establish the legitimacy of our field by pursuing an outmoded model – that "real" diseases are monocausal. Despite ample evidence to the contrary, monocausal thinking continues to influence our field. . . .

1.3.2.2 The three Ps of causation

The question that must be asked at the outset and through all stages of applying FHT is: "What is causing the disease in this individual?" Depending on the causes identified, treatment involving physiological enhancement and/or compensation can be directed at each cause, as informed by the 12 core strategies of FHT.

Using the word "cause" in any medical discussion can ultimately lead to a metaphysical debate, and therefore the word "perceived" becomes an important practical qualification. As the perception and understanding of the patient's problem improve, one gets closer to the "real" cause. Often there is a chain of causal events. Here the FHT approach is to treat as many of the links in the causal chain as are amenable to treatment and are deemed to be active at the time of treatment. This might be done sequentially (the concept of treatment modules). Identification of causes should always be linked to a valid medical diagnosis, although, given the complexity of many clinical conditions and the difficulty that even conventional medicine has in diagnosing some presentations, a more pragmatic "assessment" may be at least as useful.

There are three classes of possible causes that operate in chronic disease. We can list them as the three Ps:

- Predisposing causes: for example, genetics
- Precipitating causes: for example, pathogens
- Perpetuating causes: for example, a maladaptive stress response

Predisposing causes are factors that render the body more liable to disease. They include stress, lowered vitality, poor diet, inherited defects, and so on. **Precipitating causes**, such as infection and trauma, provoke the disease directly. **Perpetuating causes** usually come into play after the initiation of a disease process and hinder the resolution of the disease. In this context, unresolving inflammation can be an important sustaining cause.

In chronic disease, perpetuating causes are the main focus, since they are the factors keeping the disease going. However, if any predisposing or precipitating causes are found to be still relevant, it is important to treat those as well. An example is multiple sclerosis (MS), which some scientists believe to be triggered by the Epstein-Barr virus (EBV), so this is a precipitating factor. However, if one considers that the EBV chronically resides in immune cells, then it might also act as a perpetuating factor in MS.

While targeting perpetuating factors may appear to be a symptomatic approach to treatment, this is actually not the case, because addressing a perpetuating cause might, in fact, resolve the disease and hence be curative. For example: "I'm treating you for inflammation, because your inflammation is stopping you from sleeping properly, and that, in turn, is dysregulating your immune system, and that is feeding your autoimmune disease."

Another way to put this approach to addressing the different classes of causative factors is:

1. elimination/modification of the underlying causes that are still active
2. induction of remission
3. maintenance of remission

1.3.2.3 Applying the OST rule

One of the barriers to effective prescribing in FHT is the reticence and indecision created by the abundance of therapeutic targets it reveals. This can make it difficult to know where to start. The problem can be addressed by applying the OST rule. The basic features of this rule are:

- Overlap therapeutic activity, and use complex treatments: for example, use a single herb, such as Ginkgo, which is anti-inflammatory and neuroprotective and supports microcirculation, to achieve three treatment aims.
- Sequence treatments: for example, in autoimmune disease treatment, everything cannot be addressed at once, so we can sequence treatments to achieve desired clinical outcomes in stages (the concept of treatment modules).
- Triage, and set treatment priorities: for example, set some treatment goals for the first visit and other treatment goals for the future.

As noted above, the OST rule predicates the strategy of modular treatments, which, when appropriate, is a key aspect of FHT (see Section 1.3.6).

1.3.2.4 Case characteristics form the pieces in the mosaic

In terms of selecting the relevant FHT core strategies for a particular disorder, information used to arrive at these (and thereby the individual treatment framework) can be drawn from the following sources:

- the traditional herbal understanding of the disorder
- the clinical experiences of the practitioner in the treatment of the disorder
- a general understanding of the type of the disorder: for example, if it is an infection, what usually leads to this, or if it is an autoimmune disease, the factors that usually precipitate and sustain an autoimmune process
- a scientific understanding of the causes involved in the disorder – information that might be derived from laboratory, clinical, and epidemiological studies that have revealed factors that precipitate and sustain the particular disease process

- a knowledge of scientific studies that have defined the underlying pathological processes for the disorder
- the individual case history

In a sense, the individual case history acts as a filter for all the above information. An obvious example is lung cancer. Smoking is known to cause lung cancer but if a patient has never smoked then this consideration is irrelevant to that patient. In other words, only those known or suspected causative factors that apply to the patient should be incorporated into his or her treatment framework.

1.3.2.5 The critical value of the herbal actions

The herbal actions link the chosen treatment objectives to the choice of herbs. These are often traditional herbal concepts, but more and more, scientific research is now providing information about the actions of a given herb.

It is paramount that herbs chosen to deliver the required actions not only have good evidence to support their use, but also have a good track record in clinical practice. This is typically the biggest mistake made by the herbal novice or dilettante. Often a selected herb will be able to deliver more than one action, which helps to simplify the treatment protocol (see the OST rule above). For example, if anti-inflammatory and antispasmodic actions are required for the gut, chamomile can effectively cover both these requirements. Chosen herbs should be matched to the patient's constitution and general condition, according to the considerations outlined in Section 1.3.3 and in Chapter 4. If a particular action needs to be reinforced, this can be achieved by choosing more than one herb with this action, or by using a very effective herb at a higher dose. Chapter 2 lists the key herbs to deliver each of the actions that underpin the 12 core strategies of FHT.

1.3.3 Treatment energetics

As is plainly apparent (and emphasised in Chapter 4), fundamental to all the traditional herbal systems has been the energetic concept of heat. Both diseases and herbal remedies were viewed through this filter.

Clearly in these systems, heat was equated with vitality. The extreme absence of heat is the striking coldness of the corpse. When Samuel Thomson built his therapeutics around the principle that disease was essentially a cold intrusion and that before all else, remedies should heat the struggling body, he was only highlighting this almost universal therapeutic instinct.

In every tradition there is frequent use of heating remedies: the hot spices, or "pungent" remedies were the strongest for internal use, but there was always a raft of gentler warming remedies as well. Some were applied as aromatic digestives to failing "cold" digestion, others as warming expectorants or mucolytics in treating the effects of cold and damp on the chest and respiratory system. Others gently warmed and thereby supported what we might now call a deficient microcirculation but was, at the time, referred to as blood stasis. There were warming tonics (*yang* tonics in traditional Chinese medicine) and a variety of remedies that brought heat to the head, reproductive system, or kidneys.

Indications for the use of heating agents (apart from fevers) were easily understood: if the patient felt cold, as a whole or in the diseased part, or favoured hot food, hot drinks, hot packs, or hot baths, if there was diminished vitality, if there was pallor (the nail bed was a particularly sensitive guide) or signs of cumulative cold–damp conditions like mucus or gravity-dependent oedema, then heating remedies were indicated. The fact that a headache or arthritic joint or abdominal swelling was relieved by a hot pack was as important in choosing the course of treatment as determining what pathological factor was involved. When the focus of cold was clearly demarcated, then extreme heating, in the form of powerful "counter-irritation" (cayenne, mustard plasters, or stinging nettles, applied topically) sometimes had dramatic beneficial effects.

As mentioned, heat in modern terms also equates with circulation: a rationale that includes improved tissue perfusion, oxygenation, and metabolite removal can easily be drawn, as is delineated in Chapter 5.

Whereas heating was clearly "on the side of the angels" in traditional healthcare, cooling was altogether a more thoughtful matter. Cooling meant reducing vitality. The ultimate cold was death. Inappropriate heat (where cooling is indicated) includes hyperpyrexia in fevers, inflammatory diseases, hypersensitivity or allergic reactions, nervous agitation, and, above all, pain. The respective treatments – diaphoretics, anti-inflammatories, antiallergic remedies, sedatives, hypnotics (and narcotics), and analgesics – would all be classified as cooling in these terms. Indeed, some of the eliminatory treatments often applied for these purposes, especially the laxatives and cholagogues, were also seen as cooling. Almost everything now prescribed by modern doctors would have been classified as cooling.

The one striking exception to the cautions linking cooling to reduced vitality was digestion. Digestion was widely seen as a cooling activity, marked, of course, by a shift of blood flow from the periphery to the core. The archetypal digestive stimulants were the bitters. Of all the herbal strategies in history, these are probably the most respected. (The Chinese even gave them the awesome role in their five-phase classification of tonifying the kidneys – the source of constitutional energies in their system.)

Bitters are universally used before and after eating as appetite stimulants ("aperitifs") and digestives. They were the first resort in digestive difficulties, especially when associated with heat and hepatobiliary ("damp-heat") disorders (bitters are also the most commonly used choleretics). Critically, they were also favourite febrifuges, apparently lowering body temperature in fever. They seemed to correct an apparent design inconsistency in the febrile response, wherein digestion is shut down, leaving undigested material as a source of new toxicity (and even the original source of infection, in the case of gastroenteritis). Bitters seemed to switch on digestive defences, as well as bring the fever down. In many cultural traditions, bitters were seen as primarily cooling. Unlike other cooling agents that counteracted vital functions, bitters appeared to transcend these limitations, to convert heat and vitality into nourishment. However, the cooling effect of bitters may be contraindicated in the failing digestion of the elderly – ageing is a cooling condition – unless they are combined with warming digestive herbs, such as the spices, but especially ginger.

As touched on above, a very important aspect of the best-practice use of treatment energetics in FHT is in the treatment of fever. The significant role of fever management during acute respiratory infections to improve outcomes is flagged in Chapter 13. (See also Simon Mills' exploration of traditional herbal systems in Chapter 4.[10])

1.3.4 Complex interventions for complex disorders

Is there, in fact, any advantage in chemically complex medicines? Life is indeed chemically complex, so much so that science is only beginning to grasp the subtle and varied mechanisms involved in processes such as inflammation and immunity. It does seem logical that, just as our foods are chemically complex, so should our medicines be. But hard proof of this advantage has been difficult to establish to date. There are, however, several examples from the literature of how a distinct advantage might arise from chemical complexity.

The basic considerations supporting complex interventions in complex disorders are the following:

1. Multiple factors (pieces in the mosaic) require multiple interventions.
2. Interventions are determined for each patient via their case history.
3. Targeting just one point in a pathophysiological network and completely shutting it down risks side effects and does not resolve the disease.
4. Network pharmacology achieved by a chemically complex intervention is compatible with functional medicine.

1.3.4.1 Herbal extracts as inherently complex interventions

> The body is not a one-note melody, but a symphony of many interactive components functioning synergistically . . . the active ingredient model does not stem from a strength of the scientific method, as often supposed; rather, it stems from a weakness – from the inability of the reductionist method to deal with complex systems.[11]

It was Gertsch who observed that while herbal extracts might be complex, they are in fact "intelligent mixtures" of secondary plant metabolites shaped by evolutionary pressures.[12] As such, they might represent complex therapeutic mixtures possessing inherent synergy and polyvalence. Polyvalence can be defined in this context as the range of biological activities that a herb may exhibit that contribute to the overall clinical effect. It stems directly from the chemical complexity of medicinal plants.

Gertsch also noted another important concept related to polyvalence: that of "network pharmacology", as originally proposed by Hopkins.[13] In the context of plant extracts – which typically contain hundreds of potentially bioactive natural products with only mild activity – it is possible that different proteins within a particular biochemical signalling network are only weakly targeted. However, because multiple targets are influenced, this is enough to shut down or activate a given biological process by virtue of this network pharmacology. In other words, network pharmacology can explain how the many weakly active plant secondary metabolites in a plant extract may be sufficiently active to exert a potent pharmacological effect. It potentially explains why herbs can deliver surprising therapeutic outcomes without the presence of a highly bioactive compound.

There are, in fact, three layers of complexity that follow from applying the FHT prescribing system to chronic health disorders:

1 complexity due to the multiple core strategic targets for each disorder
2 complexity conferred by using several herbs in combination to address each of those targets
3 the inherent chemical complexity of each plant extract selected

1.3.5 The 12 core strategies of FHT

The following 12 core strategies underpin FHT:

1 supporting key endocrine responses (as appropriate): hypothalamic-pituitary-adrenal (HPA) axis, thyroid, pancreatic beta cells, enteroendocrine cells, male / female
2 eliminating persistent pathogens: stealth pathogens, viruses, bacteria, fungi, parasites
3 lowering danger signals, boosting cellular protection (cytoprotection), enhancing mitochondrial function and biogenesis

4 detoxifying and priming Nrf2 responses
5 improving sleep quality and time asleep and restoring healthy nervous system function
6 boosting macrocirculatory, microcirculatory, and endothelial health, improving blood quality, promoting healing
7 eliminating dysbiosis and promoting a healthy microbiome
8 optimising digestive function
9 optimising and balancing immune function
10 eliminating chronic inflammation, including neuroinflammation
11 improving and enhancing natural barriers: gastric acid, gut, skin, lung
12 addressing metabolic imbalances.

These core strategies are discussed in greater detail, including the appropriate herbs to support these strategies, in Chapter 2.

1.3.6 Modular treatments and pulsed dosing

Early experience with the bowel flora protocol (see Chapters 2 and 8) revealed the value of the use of treatment modules. As mentioned above, in many chronic diseases not every objective can be addressed at once. One way to meet this challenge is to sequence treatments as packaged modules, thereby achieving desired clinical outcomes in stages. Several strategies are well suited to modular treatment, usually applied for a period of a few months each. They include the bowel flora protocol, a detoxification module, a module for addressing the impact of stealth pathogens and one for lowering immunological danger (and hence immune-driven inflammation). This approach is elaborated in subsequent chapters.

Some herbs are safer or have greater impact or more sustained activity when they are not prescribed all the time. This concept of pulsed dosing might have been first introduced for Western herbs by the Soviet scientists working on the development of adaptogenic treatments. The idea was that for maximum benefit adaptogenic herbs were best taken for three weeks every month (or some similar pattern). Several examples of the informed use of pulsed dosing are provided in subsequent chapters.

1.3.7 Support and protect the affected tissues

The physiomedicalist Thurston (see Chapter 4) stressed the distinction between functional symptoms and those arising from organic ("trophic") origins. I can still remember from my childhood being fascinated by the television series *Ben Casey*. One of the regular issues that brain surgeon Ben Casey pondered with his mentor, Dr Zorba, was whether a patient's condition was functional or organic. This overriding principle of FHT acknowledges that the state of a tissue – the "organic" reference in the above anecdote – can determine health just as much as its function. With herbs, we are uniquely placed to support and restore a range of tissues in the body. Failing that, there are also herbal agents that can help to protect a tissue under attack, leaving the natural physiology free and unencumbered to do the healing (see the examples provided in Chapter 2). Also, many of the 12 core strategies above, such as strategies 3, 4, 6, and 11, are tissue-supportive, especially via protection.

References

1. Bland J. Defining function in the functional medicine model. *Integr Med (Encinitas).* 2017 Feb; **16**(1): 22–25. PMID: 28223904. [p 22]
2. Flores M, Glusman G, Brogaard K, et al. P4 medicine: how systems medicine will transform the healthcare sector and society. *Per Med.* 2013; **10**(6): 565–576. PMID: 25342952.
3. https://rushu.libguides.com/precision_medicine
4. https://ghr.nlm.nih.gov/primer/precisionmedicine/definition
5. https://www.lifestylemedicine.org.au/lifestyle-medicine
6. Ray P, Gupta HN. *Charaka Samhita: A Scientific Synopsis.* New Delhi, National Institute of Sciences of India, 1965.
7. Page IH. The mosaic theory 32 years later. *Hypertension.* 1982 Mar–Apr; **4**(2): 177. PMID: 7068177.
8. Shoenfeld Y, Isenberg DA. The mosaic of autoimmunity. *Immunol Today.* 1989; **10**(4): 123–126.
9. Kendler KS. From many to one to many: the search for causes of psychiatric illness. *JAMA Psychiatry.* 2019 Jun 19. doi:10.1001/jamapsychiatry.2019.1200. PMID: 31215968. [p 1085]

10. A full exposition of fever management can be found in Chapter 8 in Bone KM, Mills SY. *Principles and Practice of Phytotherapy: Modern Herbal Medicine*, 2nd edition. Elsevier, UK, 2013.
11. Sharma HM. Phytochemical synergism: beyond the active ingredient model. *Altern Ther Clin Pract*. 1997; **4**: 91–96.
12. Gertsch J. Botanical drugs, synergy, and network pharmacology: forth and back to intelligent mixtures. *Planta Med*. 2011; **77**(11): 1086–1098. PMID: 21412698.
13. Hopkins AL. Network pharmacology. *Nature Biotechnol*. 2007; **25**(10): 1110–1111.

2

The principle architecture of FHT

Constructing herbal protocols using the systematic approach of Functional Herbal Therapy is based on seven fundamental principles (as discussed in Chapter 1) and 12 core strategies. The 12 strategies, and the associated herbs that can deliver these desired outcomes, are discussed in this chapter.

2.1 Fundamental principles of FHT

FHT is based on the following seven fundamental principles:

1. understanding diseases as disordered processes of normal physiology
2. embracing the complexity of mosaic diseases, where the individual story counts most
3. ensuring treatment energetics are compatible with the patient's condition
4. complex interventions (network pharmacology) for multifactorial disorders (mosaic diseases)
5. therapy based on 12 core strategic targets (this chapter)
6. modular treatments and pulsed dosing engaged as key strategies where appropriate
7. the key over-riding consideration: to support the affected tissues

2.2 The 12 core strategies of FHT

Box 2.1 shows the core strategies that underpin the system of FHT, introduced in Chapter 1.

The information provided in Sections 2.2.1–2.2.12 expands on each of these FHT core strategies and provides a therapeutic overview in terms of recommended herbs. (Several of these strategies are the subject of individual chapters in this book, as noted.)

Box 2.1   The 12 core strategies of FHT

1. **Support** key endocrine responses (as appropriate): HPA axis, thyroid, pancreatic beta cells, enteroendocrine cells, male/female
2. **Eliminate** persistent pathogens: stealth pathogens, viruses, bacteria, fungi, parasites
3. **Lower** danger signals, boost cellular protection (cytoprotection), enhance mitochondrial function and biogenesis
4. **Detoxify** and prime Nrf2 responses
5. **Improve** sleep quality and time asleep and restore healthy nervous system function
6. **Boost** macrocirculatory, microcirculatory, and endothelial health; improve blood quality; promote healing
7. **Eliminate** dysbiosis and promote a healthy microbiome
8. **Optimise** digestive function
9. **Optimise** and balance immune function
10. **Resolve** and eliminate chronic inflammation, including neuroinflammation
11. **Improve** and enhance natural barriers: gastric acid, gut, skin, lung
12. **Address** metabolic imbalances

2.2.1 Core strategy 1: Support key endocrine responses

Key HPA axis herbal actions

Adaptogens *conserve* adaptation energy	▷ Eleutherococcus ▷ Withania (ashwagandha) ▷ Rhodiola ▷ Schisandra ▷ Tinospora
Tonics increase or *release* adaptation energy	▷ Korean ginseng ▷ Gynostemma
Adrenal herbs *support* and *restore* the adrenal cortex under stress	▷ licorice ▷ Rehmannia

Male endocrine support

▷ Tribulus
▷ Withania (ashwagandha)
▷ saw palmetto
▷ fenugreek
▷ Korean ginseng

Pancreatic support

Endocrine	▷ Gymnema
Endocrine and exocrine	▷ bitter herbs

Female endocrine support

Balancing/Prolactin excess	▷ chaste tree
Oestrogen modulation	▷ shatavari ▷ false unicorn root ▷ wild yam
Female androgen excess	▷ paeony ▷ licorice
Female androgen deficiency	▷ Withania (ashwagandha) ▷ Korean ginseng

Thyroid

Boost function
- bladderwrack
- Coleus
- Withania (ashwagandha)
- Rhodiola
- Nigella
- Bacopa
- Rehmannia

For supporting the HPA axis response and increasing resilience to stress, consider adaptogens such as Rhodiola and Withania (ashwagandha), and tonic herbs such as Korean ginseng and the newer herb, Gynostemma. In cases featuring adrenal fatigue or adrenal dysfunction, the adrenal cortex should be supported with licorice and Rehmannia. If blood sugar dysregulation is present, pancreatic function can be primed using Gymnema and the bitter herbs. Note that bitter herbs work on both endocrine and exocrine aspects of the pancreas.

For male endocrine support, a number of herbs – Tribulus, Withania (ashwagandha), saw palmetto, fenugreek, and Korean ginseng – have value.

For female hormone issues, chaste tree is a balancer; oestrogen modulation can be achieved with shatavari, false unicorn, or wild yam. White peony and licorice are useful for androgen excess, whereas Withania and Korean ginseng are valuable if there is androgen deficiency.

2.2.2 Core strategy 2: Eliminate persistent pathogens

Support immunity
- building: Eleutherococcus, Astragalus, medicinal mushrooms
- support white blood cell count: Withania, Astragalus, Tinospora
- innate immunity, natural killer (NK) cells, preventative: Echinacea root
- acute and preventative: Andrographis, Pelargonium, diaphoretic herbs
- stealth pathogens: cat's claw

Bacterial and fungal infection
- berberine herbs, oregano oil, garlic (allicin-releasing)
- myrrh, propolis, sage, tannin herbs

Viral infection	▹ St John's wort, licorice (enveloped viruses) ▹ Thuja, bioavailable curcumin, Qing Hao (*Artemisia annua*) (all viruses) ▹ Pelargonium (respiratory viruses) ▹ with immune support (e.g., Echinacea root, Andrographis)
Parasites	▹ unicellular: berberine herbs, oregano oil, garlic (allicin-releasing), myrrh ▹ for complex organisms: wormwood, myrrh, Qing Hao, clove oil, Stemona, Andrographis, black walnut hulls

This strategy is fully explored in Chapter 9. For persistent pathogens, it is vital to commensurately support immunity while treating with appropriate antimicrobial herbs. Berberine-containing herbs are useful for bacteria, fungi, and protozoa. An important herb to consider here is Phellodendron, which, by virtue of its berberine content, is good as a metabolic balancer, but also valuable for killing microorganisms. Pelargonium was a traditionally used remedy in South Africa for tuberculosis, so might have significant antibacterial properties as well (at higher doses). But all of its effects in infection might be via immune modulation, and it might possess no direct antiviral or antibacterial activity.

2.2.3 Core strategy 3: Protect and re-energise cells

Cytoprotection	Boost cytoprotection to reduce "danger" and lower inflammation ▹ ⇩ oxidative stress via Nrf2 herbs (see Section 2.2.4) ▹ ⇧ heat shock proteins (HSPs): adaptogens? Echinacea root? ▹ ⇧ SIRT1 (sirtuins): Polygonum (resveratrol), milk thistle (silymarin) ▹ for neuroprotection: add Ginkgo and saffron ▹ ⇧ microcirculation protection: gotu kola, grape seed, Ginkgo, and 5-point phytonutrient dietary plan (Chapter 5)

Energise cells mitochondrial support
▹ key herbs: hawthorn, Polygonum (resveratrol), Ginkgo, Korean ginseng, Rhodiola
▹ all Nrf2 herbs

We can propose the four Rs of cellular protection: **R**esist, **R**esolve, **R**epair, and **R**estore. This can also apply at the tissue level, and even for organ, system, and whole-body effects. Boosting cytoprotection will reduce the release of immune danger molecules (alarmins) by reducing necrotic cell death, thereby lowering inflammation. This will help to resolve inflammation and improve general health.

Lowering oxidative stress helps cells survive better under stressful conditions, and priming Nrf2 (nuclear factor erythroid 2-related factor 2) responses is the key strategy here. Indeed, priming a cell's Nrf2 response can help to achieve all four Rs of cytoprotection, as discussed in Chapter 6.

While priming Nrf2 is an excellent strategy for cancer prevention, it is not advisable during chemotherapy. In fact, as a rule it is best not to use any cytoprotective strategies during actual chemotherapy, because the aim is to kill the cancer cells. We can then follow up to protect the healthy cells once the chemotherapy is completed. Nrf2 herbs should only be used at least a day or two after chemotherapy, or maybe even a fraction later.

Herbs that boost heat shock proteins are also important, because when a cell is stressed, its proteins begin to unfold and can become non-functional. Heat shock proteins act as chaperones to protect against this (a process known as proteostasis). We are yet to definitively understand the role that herbs can play to support this vital cytoprotective process of proteostasis, but some suggestions are made above.

The Australian scientist David Sinclair developed the understanding of resveratrol as a cellular protector by activating sirtuin 1, leading to intense scrutiny of its potential as an anti-ageing phytochemical. He is currently working on mitochondrial factors, the next big step in antiageing.

For cytoprotection for nerve cells (neuroprotection), we can add Ginkgo and saffron. A healthy microcirculation is also vital for optimal cellular health and can be supported with gotu kola, grape seed, and Ginkgo, and by using the 5-point diet (see Chapter 5).

Herbs can play a vital contribution to re-energising cells via mitochondrial support. Important herbs in this regard include hawthorn, Polygonum/

Fallopia/Reynoutria (resveratrol), Rhodiola, Korean ginseng, and Ginkgo, as well as the Nrf2 herbs. The key aspects of a comprehensive mitochondrial therapy strategy are as follows:

- boosting substrates – nutrient cofactors
- enhancing mitochondrial biogenesis and dynamics – major targets are 5′ AMPK (adenosine monophosphate-activated protein kinase); SIRT3 to 5 (and sirtuins in general); Nrf2
- boosting mitochondrial protection – with Nrf2 herbs and targeted antioxidants, especially phytomelatonin
- lowering toxin exposure that impairs mitochondrial function.

Herbs/phytochemicals targeting AMPK include berberine, resveratrol, and Gynostemma. Resveratrol mainly acts via SIRT1 but has also been shown to activate SIRT3, which is in mitochondria. The Nrf2 priming herbs are listed in Section 2.2.4.

2.2.4 Core strategy 4: Detoxify and prime Nrf2 responses

Detoxify

- Heavy metals
  - Nrf2 herbs
  - garlic, hawthorn, milk thistle (silymarin)
- Organic pollutants
  - Nrf2 herbs
  - Schisandra
  - choleretic herbs (such as globe artichoke, milk thistle)

Nrf2

- Using key Nrf2 primers
  - turmeric
  - rosemary
  - green tea
  - grape seed
  - garlic
  - Ginkgo
  - resveratrol (Polygonum/Fallopia)
  - broccoli sprouts

(For a more detailed study of the Nrf2 pathway, see Chapter 6. The role of FHT in addressing the impact of environmental toxins is explored more fully in Chapter 7.)

2.2.5 Core strategy 5: Enhance nervous system function and sleep

Enhance nervous system function

- Calm anxiety
  - ▹ kava, valerian, Mexican valerian
  - ▹ passionflower, Zizyphus, Withania, St John's wort
  - ▹ skullcap for frustration, anger, and aggression
  - ▹ adrenal support

- Boost mood
  - ▹ St John's wort, Rhodiola, saffron
  - ▹ Schisandra, kava (comorbid with anxiety)
  - ▹ HPA axis supporting herbs

- Relax smooth muscle
  - ▹ cramp bark, Corydalis, chamomile, kava
  - ▹ ginger, fennel, wild yam, valerian

- Manage pain
  - ▹ Corydalis, Californian poppy, Jamaica dogwood, willow bark
  - ▹ St John's wort, turmeric (curcumin)

- Reduce sympathetic dominance
  - ▹ hawthorn
  - ▹ anxiolytic herbs
  - ▹ HPA axis supporting herbs

- Boost cognition
  - ▹ Bacopa, Ginkgo, saffron
  - ▹ St John's wort, Schisandra, Korean ginseng, Rhodiola, Withania, rosemary, bilberry, sage
  - ▹ with microcirculation support

- Enhance neuroprotection
  - ▹ Ginkgo, saffron
  - ▹ Nrf2 herbs and other cytoprotectants
  - ▹ with microcirculation support

Promote healing sleep

Sleep onset problems	▹ valerian, kava, passionflower, Zizyphus, Corydalis, chaste tree, Mexican valerian, Californian poppy, chamomile, Magnolia, lavender
Sleep maintenance problems	▹ St John's wort, chaste tree, valerian, kava, licorice, Rehmannia, Magnolia, Mexican valerian
Restorative sleep problems	▹ Withania, Rhodiola, Korean ginseng, licorice, Rehmannia

Note that for the management of mood disorders it is desirable to also support the HPA axis. For managing pain, it is important to know when to use willow bark rather than, say, Californian poppy. (Willow bark also features in the discussion on inflammation.) Essentially, if there is tissue-driven pain and inflammation, then willow bark and Boswellia would be appropriate. Where there is nerve-driven pain, Californian poppy, Jamaica dogwood, and Corydalis are often more useful.

One aspect of balancing the nervous system is to address sympathetic dominance (or even parasympathetic dominance, if need be, but what occurs more commonly in clinical practice is sympathetic dominance). Hawthorn and anxiolytic and HPA-axis-supporting herbs play the major role in assisting with this. When working on boosting cognition or enhancing neuroprotection, the importance of strengthening the microcirculation (see Chapter 5) should be emphasised, as it enables blood to adequately perfuse the brain tissue.

Three types of sleep difficulties can occur in patients, and the relevant herbs for each are listed in Section 2.2.6 (see also Chapter 10). With sleep onset insomnia, the person has trouble falling asleep. In the case of sleep maintenance insomnia, the person wakes up after sleep onset has been achieved and then has difficulty getting back to sleep. This might occur several times throughout the night. In non-restorative sleep, the quality of sleep is subjectively poor, and the person awakes unrefreshed.

2.2.6 Core strategy 6: Improve circulatory flow

Macrocirculation

- Heart
  - ▷ hawthorn
  - ▷ dan shen
  - ▷ Astragalus
  - ▷ Korean ginseng
  - ▷ Ginkgo
  - ▷ arjuna
- Veins
  - ▷ horse chestnut
  - ▷ butcher's broom
  - ▷ gotu kola
  - ▷ bilberry
- Arteries
  - ▷ Ginkgo
  - ▷ garlic
  - ▷ gotu kola
  - ▷ turmeric

Blood quality
- ▷ ginger
- ▷ turmeric
- ▷ garlic
- ▷ Coleus
- ▷ dan shen
- ▷ Ginkgo

Endothelial function
- ▷ green tea
- ▷ garlic
- ▷ Korean ginseng
- ▷ Turmeric (curcumin)
- ▷ grape seed

Microvascular integrity
- ▷ grape seed
- ▷ bilberry
- ▷ gotu kola

Microvascular flow
- ▷ Ginkgo
- ▷ ginger
- ▷ garlic
- ▷ dan shen
- ▷ turmeric (curcumin)
- ▷ Coleus

The key herbs in this list support all aspects of the circulation. Strengthening the lining of blood vessels, especially the arteries, is important in determining a healthy circulation, and the herbs listed for supporting endothelial health will assist with this aim. Another focus is ensuring that fine blood vessels are tight and strong, so they can resist damage: this is microvascular integrity. Grape seed, bilberry, and gotu kola are recommended for this purpose. Some herbs can be used both to promote microvascular flow and to improve blood quality; these include ginger, garlic, and dan shen (see Chapter 5).

2.2.7 Core strategy 7: Eliminate dysbiosis

Bowel flora protocol outline
- novel protocol employing a weed, feed, and seed strategy.
- based on a weekend/weekday cycle, but can be varied as desired.
- weekend is weeding, weekdays are feeding and seeding.
- carry out 6–10 cycles for best results.

Bowel flora protocol herbs
- antimicrobial herbs, such as oregano and anise oils, Phellodendron (berberine), and (optionally) garlic or myrrh provide the weeding.
- slippery elm provides the feeding treatment, done in conjunction with grape seed and green tea to depress pathogenic bacteria.
- combine with appropriate diet, depending on the pattern of dysbiosis.
- optionally, use an evidence-based probiotic (twice a day in the feeding phase) to enhance clinical results.

My teacher, Hein Zeylstra, developed a bowel flora protocol (BFP) based on a treatment he found in an old naturopathic textbook, for use with patients with Crohn's disease and ulcerative colitis. The original protocol predated the current concept of dysbiosis and involved fasting for one day and then fasting with high doses of garlic for 2 days, followed by normal eating plus abundant slippery elm for 11 days (see Chapter 8). This was repeated for several cycles. In terms of patient compliance, it proved difficult to encourage patients to fast and eat huge amounts of garlic at the same time.

It is for this reason that the current BFP was developed using other herbs and essential oils for the weeding. Garlic can still be used, either in addition or as an alternative. With a stronger killing option, the fasting is not as necessary, but if the patient can eat less on weeding days, it will help to starve the pathogenic bacteria, making them more vulnerable.

The other reason that drove the elaboration of this protocol was the recognition that conventional probiotics are not a permanent fix for gut dysbiosis, because they do not survive for more than a few days. They only work while you take them. The BFP is designed to act as an "endogenous faecal transplant". It starts with the person's own gut bacteria and manipulates them towards a healthier profile. It is not a strategy for eliminating gut pathogens. For that, different and more aggressive strategies are needed.

The BFP gradually manipulates the microbiome over 6–10 cycles. It can then be stopped and reintroduced a few months later, if needed. An appropriate diet is also essential, including a variety of fibre and plenty of it, because that feeds the healthy bacteria. (See Chapter 8 for a detailed discussion of the BFP.)

2.2.8 Core strategy 8: Optimise digestive function

General functional support	▷ bitter herbs, ginger, Coleus, chen pi
Liver support	choleretic herbs such as: ▷ globe artichoke ▷ milk thistle ▷ dandelion root
Gallbladder support	cholagogue herbs, such as: ▷ globe artichoke ▷ peppermint
Mucoprotection and healing	▷ slippery elm ▷ licorice ▷ meadowsweet ▷ chamomile ▷ gotu kola ▷ golden seal
Correct dysbiosis	see Section 2.2.7
Reduce inflammation	▷ chamomile ▷ licorice ▷ Calendula

Correct smooth muscle function	▹ carminatives and spasmolytics: ▹ peppermint ▹ chamomile ▹ chen pi ▹ fennel ▹ cinnamon ▹ cramp bark ▹ ginger
Improve transit	▹ ginger ▹ slippery elm ▹ choleretic herbs

Note that gut anti-inflammatory herbs are different from those used for general inflammation, and this is because they mainly act locally – although we could add curcumin (turmeric) to this list. Chamomile, licorice, and Calendula are good choices for eliminating gut inflammation; their advantage is that they can have direct contact with the site of the inflammation.

Improving gastrointestinal transit time (GTT) is desirable in many cases: in general, a slow transit time is detrimental. GTT can be increased by using fibre, like slippery elm, but also with ginger and many of the spices that will have a warming effect on the digestive processes. Choleretic herbs increase the amount of bile reaching the distal ileum, and this can also accelerate GTT. If it is desired to slow GTT, then reducing the inflammation driving the faster GTT is essential, and bitter and tannin herbs can be useful here as well.

2.2.9 Core strategy 9: Optimise and balance immune function

Support immunity	▹ Eleutherococcus, Astragalus, Tinospora (building) ▹ Withania, Astragalus (boosting white cell count) ▹ Echinacea root (innate immunity, NK cells, preventative) ▹ Andrographis (acute, preventative) ▹ cat's claw (stealth pathogens) ▹ medicinal mushrooms (innate immunity, immune surveillance)

Support HPA axis function	▸ Eleutherococcus ▸ Korean ginseng ▸ Gynostemma ▸ Rhodiola ▸ Withania
Modulate the febrile response in acute and subacute infections	▸ peppermint ▸ chamomile ▸ yarrow ▸ pleurisy root ▸ lime flowers ▸ elder flowers ▸ ginger ▸ cinnamon ▸ cayenne ▸ bitter herbs
Modulate inappropriate immune responses	▸ Hemidesmus ▸ anti-inflammatory herbs for immune-driven inflammation: Rehmannia, Bupleurum, feverfew, turmeric (curcumin), Boswellia ▸ antiallergic herbs: Baical skullcap, Albizia, feverfew, Nigella, Tinospora
Reduce danger signals	▸ Boost detoxification and cytoprotection. ▸ Address causes of excessive tissue necrosis.

Many of the immune herbs featured in Core Strategy 9 are also listed in Core Strategy 2, to eliminate persistent pathogens (see Section 2.2.2). Supporting the HPA axis with herbs such as Eleutherococcus, Korean ginseng, Rhodiola, and Withania is particularly beneficial in the long term for immune function. In a clinical trial I was involved in several years ago at the then Natural College of Naturopathic Medicine in Portland, Oregon, one group were given Echinacea root, one group were given placebo, and a third group were given a tonic herb formula comprising Eleutherococcus, Korean ginseng, and Withania. Respiratory infection rates were studied over the ensuing three months, and in the group given Echinacea root, infections dropped dramatically. But infections also fell equally as much in the group given the tonic formula.

For treatment during fevers, diaphoretic herbs are best provided in the form of hot aqueous infusions or decoctions. They include yarrow, elder flowers, chamomile, and lime flowers. Their effect in the hot form, seen only in a febrile state, is subjectively to reduce chill and encourage cooling perspiration; but they also have a variety of other useful benefits for the digestion, mucous membranes, and the neuromuscular system. They may be combined with peppermint tea for a more accelerated cooling effect. For a gentle but stronger reduction in febrile temperature, the cooling bitters, such as dandelion root and gentian, are favoured.

In addition to containing excessive body temperature, there may be a need to encourage it to rise. If it is clear that the fever is not adequately materialising and that there is no serious infection or underlying pathology, warming remedies might be chosen. This is a common scenario in affluent societies. Here, after childhood, fevers are rare, but unresolved low-grade chronic infections are not. In a case of persistent catarrh, for example, it is often useful to take advantage of a partial attempt by the body to raise the stakes and set a "therapeutic fever" in train. It is then possible to use the many circulatory stimulants, such as cinnamon, ginger, or even cayenne (as per Thomson, see Chapter 4), together with diaphoretic herbs taken in hot water. A modest febrile process can then be encouraged into existence, often to considerable advantage. (These issues regarding the best use of diaphoretic and immune herbs are explored more fully in Chapter 13.)

2.2.10 Core strategy 10: Eliminate chronic inflammation

Address any identified drivers of inflammation	▹ dysbiosis ▹ toxins ▹ metabolic imbalances ▹ pathogens
Reduce immune-driven inflammation	▹ Bupleurum ▹ Baical skullcap ▹ feverfew ▹ Ginkgo ▹ Boswellia ▹ bioavailable curcumin ▹ Hemidesmus ▹ Rehmannia ▹ willow bark

Reduce neuroinflammation	▹ Boswellia ▹ bioavailable curcumin ▹ address any inflammation drivers ▹ neuroprotective herbs
Reduce tissue-driven inflammation	▹ Boswellia ▹ willow bark ▹ Baical skullcap ▹ celery seed ▹ ginger ▹ turmeric and bioavailable curcumin ▹ devil's claw
Reduce tissue-driven inflammation with swelling	▹ horse chestnut ▹ butcher's broom ▹ microcirculation dietary protocol

Some examples of the drivers of chronic inflammation are included here, but this list is not comprehensive. For tissue-driven inflammation (e.g., osteoarthritis), Boswellia, willow bark, celery seed, or ginger are particularly indicated. A very powerful strategy for tissue-driven inflammation with swelling (when that swelling subsequently causes a secondary problem, such as a ruptured disc pressing on a nerve) is the use of horse chestnut and butcher's broom. Together with the microcirculation protocol, these can reduce the local oedema, increase healing, and thereby alleviate the impact of secondary problems, such as sciatic pain.

2.2.11 Core strategy 11: Enhance natural barriers

Gastric acid barrier	▹ bitter herbs ▹ ginger ▹ Coleus ▹ chen pi
Gut-wall barrier	▹ licorice ▹ meadowsweet ▹ chamomile ▹ golden seal ▹ slippery elm

Upper respiratory barrier	▹ eyebright ▹ ribwort ▹ golden seal
Lower respiratory barrier	▹ golden seal ▹ mullein ▹ Adhatoda ▹ key expectorant herbs (such as fennel, Grindelia, thyme)
Any mucous membrane barrier	▹ golden seal
Skin barrier	▹ gotu kola ▹ grape seed ▹ depurative herbs?
Eye surface barrier	▹ eyebright
Blood–brain barrier	▹ bioavailable curcumin ▹ Polygonum (resveratrol) ▹ Boswellia ▹ microcirculation protocol
General	▹ cytoprotection ▹ boost microcirculation

Enhancing natural barriers, such as the gastric acid barrier, is a capability that is unique to natural treatments. The gut wall barrier can be improved with herbs like licorice, meadowsweet, chamomile, golden seal, and slippery elm. Slippery elm does not actually restore the barrier: it supplements it because of its mucilaginous quality.

With respect to hay fever, if there is an effective barrier in the upper respiratory tract, an allergen will not reach the mast cells to cause a reaction. Allergies generally only happen in disrupted barriers, where an allergen can access vulnerable areas and trigger an allergic reaction (see Chapter 12).

Agents to help restore the blood/brain barrier include curcumin and resveratrol. Boswellia is relevant here because it inhibits metalloproteinases that break down such barriers – there is clinical data to support this. Finally, in general, for any barrier, the health of the cellular components and their resistance to damage can be improved by cytoprotection and boosting the microcirculation that supplies them. These two strategies can improve the strength of any barrier in the body.

2.2.12 Core strategy 12: Address metabolic imbalances

Enhance AMPK responses	▹ berberine-containing herbs (plus silymarin to improve bioavailability) ▹ Gynostemma ▹ Polygonum/Fallopia/Reynoutria (resveratrol)
Enhance sirtuin-related responses	▹ Polygonum/Fallopia/Reynoutria (resveratrol) ▹ milk thistle (silymarin)
Reduce insulin resistance	▹ Nigella ▹ cinnamon ▹ fenugreek ▹ Korean ginseng ▹ green tea ▹ bitter herbs ▹ *and see* AMPK and sirtuin herbs above
Improve lipid handling	▹ garlic ▹ berberine-containing herbs (plus silymarin) ▹ Gymnema ▹ cholagogue and choleretic herbs
Lower excessive uric acid	▹ celery seed ▹ sarsaparilla ▹ dandelion leaf ▹ herbs for insulin resistance
General considerations	▹ detoxify endocrine disruptors ▹ boost sleep quality ▹ boost mitochondrial function

AMPK is the switch that determines whether a cell will burn up or store energy. In insulin resistance (IR), type 2 diabetes, and metabolic syndrome, fine-tuning the AMPK response with berberine (and silymarin to help the berberine become more bioavailable), resveratrol, and Gynostemma will help improve clinical parameters.

Polygonum and milk thistle (silymarin) are key to improving sirtuin-related responses. Reducing IR can be achieved with Nigella, cinnamon, fenugreek, or Korean ginseng, but the AMPK herbs and berberine are also quite important here (see Chapter 11). For correcting blood lipids, again the berberine herbs, garlic, milk thistle (silymarin), Gymnema, and choleretic herbs are indicated.

Endocrine disruptors are a modern problem leading to metabolic imbalances. There is even a school of thought that the rising incidence of type 2 diabetes is not just lifestyle-related, but is also due to environmental toxins acting as endocrine disruptors (see Chapter 7). Helping sleep quality is essential, because poor sleep can create metabolic imbalances. It is also important to support mitochondrial function. (See Chapter 11 for a fuller exploration of these topics.)

2.3 The overriding consideration in FHT

There is one overriding consideration in FHT, and that is to always support the tissues involved in the disease process (see **Table 2.1**).

Along with the specific strategies, the four Rs of cytoprotection are also relevant in supporting any target tissue (see Core Strategy 3).

2.4 Applying the core FHT strategies to chronic diseases

Table 2.2 provides a few examples of how the 12 core strategies, plus tissue support, can be applied to the treatment of various chronic diseases (in the form of a list of the relevant strategies). (The application of FHT to additional chronic diseases is examined in other chapters.)

Table 2.1 The overriding consideration at the tissue level: always support the tissue

Tissue	
Endocrine pancreas	▷ Gymnema
Liver	▷ milk thistle (silymarin)
Kidneys	▷ Bupleurum ▷ Rehmannia ▷ Astragalus ▷ mitochondrial therapy ▷ microcirculation protocol
Prostate	▷ saw palmetto
Male or female gonads	▷ Tribulus
Connective tissues	▷ gotu kola
Mucous membranes	▷ golden seal
Heart	▷ hawthorn ▷ arjuna ▷ dan shen
Bladder lining	▷ licorice
Bladder muscle	▷ Crataeva

Table 2.2 Examples of applying FHT strategies to chronic diseases

Disease	FHT strategy
Osteoarthritis	▷ Reduce both immune and tissue-driven inflammation ▷ Boost microcirculation and promote healing ▷ Address metabolic imbalances ▷ Support the tissue (more nutritional)
Autoimmune disease	▷ Support the HPA axis ▷ Eliminate persistent pathogens ▷ Lower danger signals (including those via diet) and boost cytoprotection ▷ Eliminate dysbiosis and promote a healthy microbiome ▷ Optimise and balance immune function ▷ Detoxify and prime Nrf2 responses ▷ Improve barriers and support the attacked tissue

Table 2.2 Examples of applying FHT strategies to chronic diseases *(continued)*

Disease	FHT strategy
Depression	▸ Enhance nervous system function, especially mood, sleep, and cognition; address any co-morbid anxiety ▸ Support the HPA axis ▸ Eliminate chronic inflammation and neuroinflammation ▸ Support the blood–brain barrier ▸ Support the tissue with neuroprotective herbs
Type 2 diabetes	▸ Support pancreatic endocrine responses (Gymnema) ▸ Address the key metabolic imbalance of insulin resistance ▸ Detoxify and prime Nrf2 responses ▸ Reduce chronic inflammation ▸ Boost microcirculation ▸ Correct dysbiosis (if relevant to the case)
Sinus allergy	▸ Improve upper respiratory barrier ▸ Support immunity and modulate inappropriate allergic response ▸ Reduce chronic inflammation ▸ Support mucous membranes ▸ Support the HPA axis, reduce stress, and improve sleep, as appropriate to the case ▸ Correct dysbiosis (if relevant to the case)
Disc prolapse with nerve compression	▸ Reduce tissue-driven inflammation with swelling ▸ Reduce tissue-driven inflammation ▸ Manage pain ▸ Improve healing responses and microcirculation ▸ Support the nerve tissue with St John's wort
Autism spectrum disorder	▸ Detoxify and prime Nrf2 responses ▸ Support mitochondrial function ▸ Support immunity and modulate inappropriate allergic responses ▸ Reduce chronic inflammation, especially neuroinflammation ▸ Correct dysbiosis (if relevant to the case) ▸ Enhance nervous system function, especially mood, sleep, anxiety, cognition, and autonomic balance ▸ Support the HPA axis ▸ Support the blood–brain barrier ▸ Eliminate persistent pathogens ▸ Address metabolic imbalances; support thyroid function ▸ Optimise digestive function ▸ Support the tissue with neuroprotective herbs
Neuroplastic brain healing	▸ Boost brain mitochondrial function ▸ Downregulate neuroinflammation ▸ Repair the blood–brain barrier ▸ Promote healing sleep ▸ Boost neuroprotection and Nrf2

Table 2.2 Examples of applying FHT strategies to chronic diseases *(continued)*

Disease	FHT strategy
Cancer prevention	▹ Lower general inflammation ▹ Improve immune surveillance and general resistance to infection ▹ Boost Nrf2 ▹ Maintain a healthy microbiome ▹ Correct metabolism, especially lower insulin resistance/blood sugar and related growth factors, such as insulin-like growth factor 1 (IGF-1) ▹ Boost cytoprotection to delay cellular ageing and encourage a tissue state that is hostile to tumour growth ▹ Encourage "thinner" blood, healthy vascular endothelial responses, and improved tissue perfusion ▹ Boost mitochondrial function
Ischaemic heart disease	▹ Correct metabolism (especially lipids, insulin resistance) ▹ Improve microcirculation and blood quality ▹ Boost mitochondrial function ▹ Lower general inflammation ▹ Detoxify and prime Nrf2 responses ▹ Support the heart tissue, including lowering hypertension ▹ Boost arterial healing ▹ Modulate HPA axis responses ▹ Enhance nervous system function and sleep
Acne	▹ Support the skin with depurative herbs ▹ Support key endocrine responses (decrease excess androgens and effects) ▹ Eliminate persistent pathogens: *C. acnes* ▹ Optimise immune function ▹ Eliminate chronic and skin inflammation ▹ Address metabolic imbalances – reduce insulin resistance, lower mammalian (or mechanistic) target of rapamycin complex 1 (mTORC1) ▹ Address skin and gut dysbiosis

Further reading

Further information and references to support the choice of herbs in the strategies described in this chapter can be found in the following texts:

Bone KM. *A Clinical Guide to Blending Liquid Herbs*. UK: Elsevier, 2003.
Bone KM, Mills SY. *Principles and Practice of Phytotherapy: Modern Herbal Medicine*, 2nd edition. UK: Elsevier, 2013.

3

Game-changing habits of highly effective herbal clinicians

Good health throughout life is a valuable and rare gift these days, and more than ever there is a pressing need to help people with chronic health problems by offering viable, safe, and effective health treatments. This can be a highly rewarding experience and one that drives us to learn more to obtain the best outcomes for our patients with herbal prescribing. Understanding the attributes needed to become more successful as a herbal clinician is an important part of this growth. In fact, prescribing herbs effectively does not have to be a complicated process. Six herbal game-changing practices have the capacity to transform a herbal practice:

1. **right dosing and frequency**
2. **right quality:** clinical results are only good as the quality of the herbs we use
3. **right products:** including the right selection and combination of herbs
4. **right protocol for treatment:** which ties in with the FHT system discussed in Chapters 1 and 2
5. **right resources:** what we draw on to inform our prescribing choices
6. **right practice:** how we can best interact with patients, from a herbal clinician's perspective

3.1 Right dosing and frequency

The subject of appropriate dosage is probably the most controversial aspect of contemporary Western herbal practice. Many different dosage approaches are found among Western herbal clinicians, from country to country and even within countries. Underlying these different approaches are contrasting philosophies about the therapeutic action of medicinal plants.

At one extreme is the assumption that the therapeutic effect relies on a specific dose of the active phytochemicals contained in each particular plant, which is essentially a pharmacological model. At the other extreme, emphasis is placed on the assumption that a herbal medicine, being derived from a living organism, carries a certain energy or vital force. The quality of this energy is thought to confer the therapeutic effect, and hence the amount of actual herb is not as important (as long as some is present). Others in the middle feel that the active components act as catalysts to restore health and do not need to be present in pharmacologically relevant quantities.

In the modern context, the clinical trial is arguably the best way to determine the effective dose of either a single herb or a formulation. It does not necessarily determine the optimum dose. However, replicating the dose used in a positive trial does confer a greater certainty for clinical results in practice. Generally, the doses used in herbal clinical trials are at the higher end of the spectrum mentioned above. The physiomedicalists and other nineteenth-century herbalists also used doses that would be considered high by some today. Ayurveda and traditional Chinese medicine also use high doses – sometimes what might be construed to be very high.

Based on the above discussion, we can advance the proposition that adequate dosing is a critical consideration for successful herbal practice. Indeed, the biggest mistake often made in Western herbal practice is to prescribe subtherapeutic doses. There are several clinical trials showing clear dose-response curves, tending to argue against the widespread value of the lower dosage approaches mentioned above.

Information about appropriate dosing can be found in reliable texts and on the labels of products from good manufacturers. Should the recommended dose on the label always be strictly adhered to within our clinical practice? The answer is no, because the label dose may not always be appropriate for different types of patients. Some may be frail, elderly people who may not actually be able to metabolise herbs as efficiently. Some patients are extremely sensitive, in which case it is important to begin with a sub-clinical dose and build up to the full dosage over time. On the other hand, the label dose may be exceeded in certain situations – for example, in acute disorders for a short period. The higher the acuteness of the condition being treated, the higher the dose required.

Another important consideration is that the dose recommended on a label assumes an average-weight person with average metabolism and with a chronic condition. All of the doses specified, even in textbooks, assume these circumstances.

3.1.1 Dosage frequency

Different dosing frequency may apply to different clinical scenarios. Some protocols – such as the bowel flora protocol (see Chapter 8) – involve different dosing regimens for weekdays and weekends, using different herbs. There are other examples. For instance, with parasite treatment, the patient is dosed heavily for 3–6 days and then has a break. This is, first, because the treatments being given are fairly robust, and, second, in order to monitor or observe the degree of parasite elimination, and then dose again if necessary.

It is not always necessary to keep to the conventional one tablet three times a day or 5 mL three times a day. Even though most herbal schools teach that the dose for liquid herbal combinations is 5 mL three times a day, most practitioners actually use 7.5 mL or 8 mL twice a day, because of poorer patient compliance with the third dose. In certain circumstances, however, it is critical that the patient takes the herbs at 5 mL three times daily – and will, therefore, have to remember to take that third dose. One example is for digestive conditions. When bitters are administered to a patient, it is important to have one dose of herbs before each meal, so in this case frequency becomes critical. Dosing before each meal is also optimal for many of the herbs that can assist in blood sugar control – Gymnema and green tea, for example.

3.1.2 Dosing for children

For children's dosages, there are several rules that can be used in clinical practice to work out an appropriate dose according to the child's weight or age. Some of the commonly used rules include Clark's, Young's, and Fried's rules. However, the rule recommended as the most appropriate is the Salisbury rule:

> - **For a child up to 30 kg, the percentage of the adult dose equals double the weight of the child in kg.**
> - **If the child is 30 kg or more, then their weight in kg plus 30 equals the percentage of the adult dose.**

The reasons why the Salisbury rule is preferable include both its simplicity and its accurate approximation of the complex algorithms normally used to calculate doses based on body surface area.

There is one important exception to the Salisbury rule, which is when determining the dose for a small child up to about 18 months. It is advisable here to use Fried's rule as the starting point (but only as the starting point) and then cautiously increase from there:

> - **The dose for a child is calculated by dividing the child's age in months by 150 and multiplying the result by the adult dose.**

This is because very young infants can have unpredictable metabolisms and we need to be extra cautious, especially when using alcohol-based liquids.

3.1.3 Doses for synergistic prescribing

Usually, say when prescribing three herbs that might be good for promoting gastric acid, the doses for each herb do not all need to be at the high end of the dosage range. This is because they are all working on the same clinical objective. They might even be prescribed at the lower end of the dosage range, or sometimes below the dosage range, since there are other herbs reinforcing their action.

3.1.4 Loading doses

A loading dose is where a much higher dose is administered initially, in order to quickly achieve a therapeutic effect. It is effectively the same dosing approach as for an acute situation, but applied to chronic situations.

An example is Boswellia for arthritis; because Boswellia is slow to exert its therapeutic effect, a loading dose can be used to accelerate the time to a clinical response. For example, a patient with osteoarthritis could be given double the normal amount as a loading dose, but when they start to improve, the dose is reduced to the normal level.

There are many other clinical scenarios in which loading doses are appropriate. When someone has a semi-acute exacerbation of a condition, a loading dose can be used, and then the dose is reduced when the symptoms subside. Another example is feverfew, which usually takes several months to have an effect in patients with migraine. Most patients (despite the word!) cannot wait that long. In this case, a loading dose assists in helping the feverfew to take effect faster.

3.1.5 Dried herb equivalent calculations

When considering doses, it is important to be able to translate doses across different dosage forms, from tablets to capsules to liquids to powders. This is especially important when comparing doses across different companies' products. It is also imperative for interpreting doses used in a successful clinical trial. We must be able to work out and replicate the trial dose in terms of whatever product we are prescribing.

The mechanism to achieve this is called the "dried herb equivalent" (DHE). It converts all doses to a common basis: the amount of raw material used to make the extract used in the product, be it a liquid or a solid extract. Surprisingly, even some experienced herbal clinicians are not readily adept at these calculations.

One of the problems on tablets and capsules (with Australian labels especially) is statements like: "Contains extract equivalent to 5,000 mg of herb dried". Unfortunately, it is impossible to know from this statement how the product was manufactured. Was it 500 mg of a 10:1 extract, or 50 mg of 100:1 extract? This would be useful to know, because a 10:1 extract might be more desirable. An extract ratio as high as 100:1 means there have probably been enrichment steps to achieve such a high degree of concentration from the starting raw herbal material. That information is not necessarily provided on labels.

The 10:1 and a 100:1 ratios in the example above represent what is known as the drug extract ratio or herb extract ratio. This is the information needed to calculate the DHE. It represents the ratio of the quantity of the starting herbal material used with the final quantity of the resulting preparation. In other words, 10 kg or 100 kg of herb was used to make 1 kg of extract, respectively. Because the first number in the ratio is higher than the second, it reflects that the product is more concentrated than the original crude herbal material. For liquid herbal products, which are typically more dilute than the starting herbal material, the second number is higher than the first. So, for a 1:2 liquid extract, 1 kg of herb was used to make 2 L of product.

How are doses calculated in terms of DHE? For example, if the dose of a 1:2 liquid is 20–40 mL per week, as normally shown on labels, what does that convert to as a DHE dose per day? This 20–40 mL per week represents around 3–6 mL/day. Since the product is a 1:2, this converts to 1.5–3 g/day DHE (divide the liquid dose by 2). If switching over to a tablet, in order to make sure that the same therapeutic effect is achieved from the tablet form, the equivalent dose must also be 1.5–3 g/day.

For a DHE of 1 g, the various doses of herbal preparations could be:

- 2 mL of a 1:2 liquid
- 1 mL of 1:1 liquid
- 250 mg of 4:1 soft extract
- 200 mg of a 5:1 dried powder extract

A good example of the pitfalls of not understanding DHE issues in dosing can be seen in interpreting the doses used in clinical trials. Here is one example with the herb Gymnema. In a positive clinical trial in type 2 diabetes patients, the dose of Gymnema used was described as 400 mg/day of the water-soluble acidic fraction of an ethanol extract of the leaves.[1] Delving deeper into the information provided in the paper and its references, this extract turned out, in fact, to be a 33:1 concentrate from the original dried leaf starting material.

Hence, the daily DHE of the dose used in the trial was $0.4 \times 33 = 13.2$ g – quite a high dose. Yet a colleague once had a lengthy debate with a well-regarded herbal educator who insisted that the DHE dose in the trial was in fact just the 400 mg. Such misunderstanding will result in serious underdosing and little chance of a therapeutic effect.

3.2 Right quality

3.2.1 Correct species and correct plant part

Even though the intention is always to use the right species of a herb, nowadays herbs are still being substituted with other (usually inferior) species. Examples include Rhodiola and Echinacea.

In addition, although it is acknowledged that the correct plant part is always important, there is considerable debate for some herbs over which plant part is desirable. Take the example of Echinacea: is it the root, or the leaf, or even the whole plant that is preferred? Another subtler example is for Korean ginseng, where the fine root hairs or the leaf are substituted for the main or lateral roots. There are, indeed, companies selling ginseng extracts containing the root hairs and the leaf, and these are definitely not the right plant parts to use.

Plant part is fundamental, yet it can be overlooked as a practice issue. If one looks at websites, there are various monographs on herbs discussing their many virtues, but they make no mention of the plant part to use. I have even peer-reviewed clinical trial manuscripts that do not specify the plant part for the herbs tested in the trial. These are such basic omissions that they encourage any informed reader to question the credentials and training of the authors. Likewise, patients sometimes come in with products purchased online, and the herbal labels do not state the plant part used. It is important to explain to the patient that, although the product might be suitable, since it does not mention the plant part, there can be little certainty about its benefit.

This basic issue can represent the difference between something that is safe and something that is toxic. A good example is the common rhubarb.

Someone who eats the leaves of the rhubarb may become very ill and might even die. But the same person can safely consume the rhubarb stalks with no symptoms and a great deal of pleasure.

3.2.2 Right marker compounds at desired levels

There are several relevant examples to discuss here, but first some definitions.

3.2.2.1 Marker compounds or constituents

Marker compounds are the characteristic phytochemicals found in a plant that are chosen to represent a quality standard for the plant and its products, for example, for a standardised extract. So, in the case of, say, passionflower (*Passiflora incarnata*), the marker compound often chosen is the flavonoid isovitexin. A standardised extract of passionflower can then be fixed to contain a consistent level of this compound (usually a few per cent). Marker compounds are not necessarily active compounds (see Section 3.2.2.2.); however, if well chosen, they do serve a useful function in terms of quality, such as for the purposes of identification and ensuring appropriate drying, handling, and extraction of the herbal starting material.

Usually, to achieve a consistent level of a marker compound (or compounds) in a standardised extract, the starting herbal raw material will need to contain a minimum acceptable level. This implies consistent quality practices in terms of harvesting, drying, and storage of the herb to achieve this. Also, the way in which the herb is processed, such as extraction conditions and choice of solvent, will need to be carefully controlled. Because of this, it is likely that fixing an extract to a consistent level of marker compound(s) will also render the extract more or less consistent in terms of other phytochemical components, at least for that particular manufacturer. This aspect underpins much of the utility of standardised extracts as consistent products.

However, the difficulty arises when a different manufacturer then attempts to produce the same standardised extract. Although this "imitation" extract will typically be made to contain the same level of marker compound(s), it is not necessarily true that it will be identical to that produced by the original manufacturer (see the concept of phytoequivalence in Section 3.2.2.3).

3.2.2.2 Active compounds or constituents

Active constituents are phytochemicals that are important for a given therapeutic effect of a herbal extract. This is a highly complex issue, but one proposition is simple and clear: marker compounds are not necessarily active compounds. Hence, when *Ginkgo biloba* leaf standardised extract (GBE) was originally manufactured to contain 24% Ginkgo flavone glycosides, there was no unequivocal evidence that these compounds conferred the various and exciting therapeutic activities that had been discovered for the extract. Later research suggested that a different group of phytochemicals – the ginkgolides and bilobalide – were more important, and GBE is now standardised for these as well. But in terms of, say, its effects in Alzheimer's disease, the active compounds in GBE are not known. Even if the ginkgolides and bilobalide were found to be important (this could be achieved by a clinical trial comparing two Ginkgo extracts with high and low levels of these compounds which were otherwise identical), it would be unlikely that they were the only compounds important for activity. This observation is also well illustrated by the example of St John's wort, where several of its phytochemical components have been shown to have antidepressant activity.

Such a dilemma supports the basic premise of herbalists: that the true active component is the herbal extract itself. Nonetheless, it is also likely that an extract will be less likely to confer a therapeutic effect when it is low in marker compounds that have some relevant activity (from pharmacological experiments).

This last issue underlies an important point regarding marker compound selection: they should be chosen carefully. Preference must be given to phytochemicals that – based on current knowledge – are likely to have some pharmacological activity that is relevant to the proposed use of the extract. On the other hand, if a marker compound that has no known useful pharmacological activity is chosen, it should not be optimised in the extract at the expense of other phytochemicals – for example, selecting for and optimising echinacoside levels in *Echinacea angustifolia* root at the expense of the alkylamides. Where the marker compound is inactive (on current knowledge), the safest approach to take is to produce a normal galenical extract (just extracted with ethanol and water) standardised to the marker.

3.2.2.3 Phytoequivalence

When positive clinical trial data for a herbal product using a specific extract are made public, as there are usually no protective patents, other manufacturers will produce and sell copies of this product. Typically, such copies will contain extracts that have the same level of marker compound(s), but are they really the same as the extract used in the clinical trial? Can the other manufacturers legitimately claim that their extract will produce the same clinical results as seen with the original extract?

To answer this question (a real regulatory conundrum in countries such as Germany, where prescribed herbal products were rebated under a type of pharmaceutical benefits scheme) the concept of phytoequivalence was initiated. The above questions can only be answered in the affirmative if the two extracts are phytoequivalent.

But what does phytoequivalence mean? First, the second extract should closely match the **full** phytochemical spectrum of the original extract. In other words, it is not just the level of marker compounds that should be the same; all other measurable compounds in the extract should be present at similar levels. Some authorities suggest that a second criterion must also be met: the levels of marker compounds (or their derivatives) achieved in the bloodstream of humans after oral doses of the two products should be similar. This, however, is a much more challenging criterion to meet and is often not attempted because of the experimental difficulties involved.

3.2.2.4 Some examples of active/marker compound issues

It is known that for authentic-quality *Rhodiola rosea*, the ratio of rosavins to salidroside is around 3:1. There are about 30 Rhodiola species, and if the ratio is different, it is probably a species that is different from this desirable one.

The kava story is wonderful, because kava has been used in the Pacific Islands for centuries. After a kava ceremony, if the locals had a good experience with the kava, it would be selected and cultivated. These kava "noble cultivars" have been bred via constant human interaction and selection over centuries. In other words, humans have been the guinea pigs over hundreds of years to develop the noble cultivars. And they are thought to deliver superior clinical results and have fewer side effects.

Another issue in terms of herbal quality is the preservation of activity across different dosage forms. Pictured in **Figure 3.1** are HPLC (high-performance liquid chromatography) traces of *Echinacea angustifolia* root.

The top image is a dried version of a 60% ethanol–water extract put into a tablet. The second image displays the same 60% ethanolic extract in its original form, and the third represents the root itself, which has been extracted in the lab with organic solvents, such as chloroform and methanol, for analysis. The blue arrow represents the direction of increasing processing.

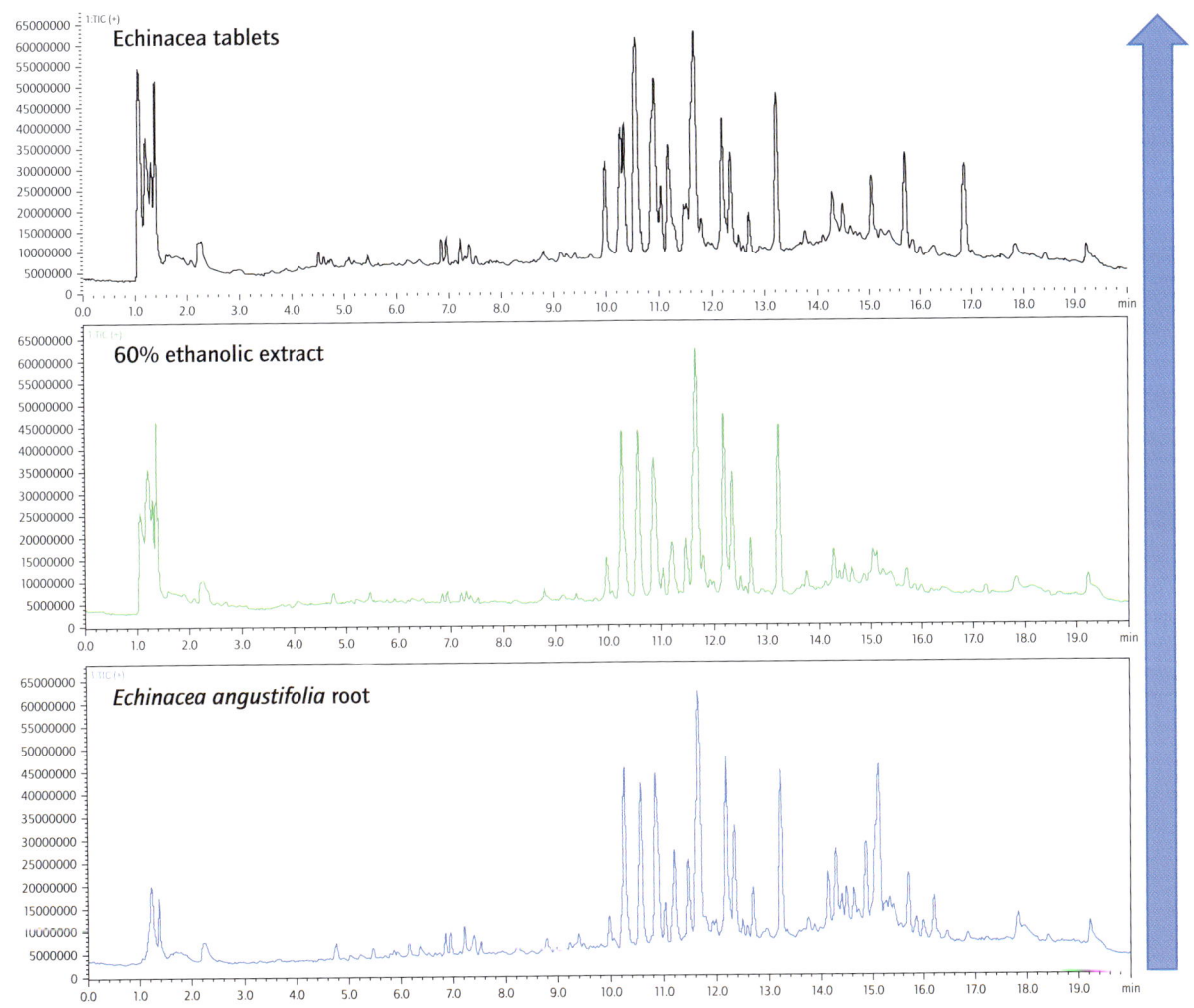

Figure 3.1   High-performance liquid chromatography traces of *Echinacea angustifolia* root.

Looking at these profiles, where each peak represents a different alkylamide in the Echinacea, the key observation is that activity appears preserved across the three dosage forms. Some constituents are lost purely because of the effect of the solvent. This is because the 60% ethanol-water will extract some constituents (at the more polar end of the spectrum, as ethanol-water is quite a polar solvent) and not others. This might invite the suggestion that the dried herb as a capsule is preferable; but we must recognise that the digestive system is a solvent too, and so the fact that a solvent will not extract everything from the root cannot be avoided. (*Note:* there are some extra peaks visible in the tablet. This is because the tablets also contain *Echinacea purpurea* root, and those extra peaks come from the *E. purpurea*.)

3.2.3 Avoiding adulterated products

The two keys issues of herbal adulteration are substitution and contamination.

3.2.3.1 Substitution problems in herbal medicine

Substitution of one herbal raw material with another can pose a considerable problem for the herbal clinician. This has already been mentioned in Section 3.2.1, on having the correct species and plant part. Substitution can in fact occur at several different levels:

- within a species, by a less active chemical race or subspecies
- by the wrong or less active plant part
- within a genus of a related plant
- by a completely different genus

Many problems associated with herbal safety and quality have been caused by substitution, particularly the last example. This especially applies to herbs that have suddenly become so popular that demand exceeds supply, such as substitution of Echinacea with *Parthenium integrifolium* and the replacement of Arnica species with Mexican arnica (*Heterotheca inuloides*). It is very serious where safety is compromised by substitution, for example the substitution of *Teucrium species* (germander) for *Scutellaria lateriflora* (skullcap).[2]

Some substitution practices may avoid detection at manufacture, even under pharmaceutical good manufacturing practice (GMP), and are occasionally detected in over-the-counter products in some countries. However, the knowledge of a specific substitution, and the application of an appropriate test method to detect it, can and does expose such practices. On the other hand, despite the substitution of Stephania by Aristolochia being implicated in renal disease and carcinoma, reportedly this practice does still commonly occur.[3]

3.2.3.2 Contamination issues in herbal medicine

Herbal products can sometimes be contaminated with other agents, and a few isolated instances have raised public health concerns. For example:

- Products made in China and India might be contaminated with heavy metals (sometimes added intentionally) or potentially pathogenic microorganisms.[4]
- Products made in China may be contaminated with conventional drugs.[5]
- A safe herb may be contaminated with a toxic herb – for example, belladonna root found among *Arctium lappa* (burdock) root.[6]
- A range of herbs may be contaminated with species containing toxic pyrrolizidine alkaloids (usually as weeds co-harvested with the herb).[7]

The practice of pharmaceutical GMP in a well-regulated environment should eliminate the possibility of these types of contamination, especially if the manufacturer has a comprehensive testing regime in place.

3.3 Right product selection (including selecting the right herbs and combinations)

In selecting products and protocols for patients, it is imperative that we view herbs functionally, and the linking concepts for this are the herbal actions. A good example is whether a clinician views cramp bark as just good for period pain and cramping (dysmenorrhoea), or whether it as seen as a smooth muscle relaxant. If we think of the herb as being of use just for period pains, that limits the way it will be prescribed. But if cramp bark is regarded as a smooth muscle relaxant, then, thinking functionally around actions, its uses become wider and might encompass hypertension, tension headache, asthma, gastrointestinal cramping, and various other conditions.

Do you know how many plant (and hence potential herb) species exist? The answer is: approximately 400,000. Therefore, as Western herbal clinicians, we are really only scratching the surface, since on average we use fewer than 150 herbs in clinical practice. It is vital, then, especially for this core of favourites, that they are well understood by the clinician in terms of their versatility and how they can be best used in a range of situations. It is also important in this context to remember the concept of therapeutic overlap (discussed in Section 1.3.2.3), where the prescriber can select herbs with dual or multiple actions, thereby addressing several of the patient's issues at once.

Understanding prescribing differentials is also an important skill. For someone who has pain, when would it be appropriate to use Californian poppy versus willow bark? It depends on the type of pain (as outlined in Chapter 2). When would a practitioner use kava in preference to valerian? In this example, kava might be selected over valerian when a stronger effect is desired. For example, if the patient is an anxious child, kava might be too strong and therefore not suitable. Valerian, which is mild and gentle, would be the preferred choice, or even passionflower. For an adult who is experiencing panic attacks, the stronger kava would most likely achieve more effective clinical outcomes. However, the rider here is that individual patient responses vary, and some patients might find valerian much more effective than kava in the above example.

Another question is: when would a clinician use a single herb, versus herbs in combination? St John's wort is a good example. St John's wort is very effective on its own in strong doses for neuralgic pain. However, because depression is such a complex mosaic disease, it is usually better to use St John's wort in combination in this case. And the advantage of using St John's wort in combination for depression is that the dose can be lowered, allaying any concerns about herb–drug interactions (because the dose will be lower than those implicated in the interactions).

Now one big question is: "How many herbs do I prescribe?" In this context, is important to be open to working with liquid herbs as well as tablets and capsules (and even herbal teas). Liquids allow practitioners to be targeted and versatile in their prescription. Depending on the complexity of the problem and the other pathologies and issues presenting, a liquid formulation in addition to tablets and capsules may be appropriate. If a liquid is not prescribed, then generally it is best to prescribe three or four herbal tablet or capsule formulations, depending on the condition. Simple conditions may only need one or two products; complex conditions like chronic fatigue syndrome or fibromyalgia may require many more than three or four.

It is important to select products that are backed by a level of clinical evidence. Preference should be given to products directly supported by either primary or secondary clinical evidence. What is meant by primary clinical evidence? The product is the original source of the evidence – in other words, the product you are prescribing is exactly the one used in the clinical trial that generated the positive evidence.

What, then, is secondary evidence? Ginkgo is a good example, because most Ginkgo products have only secondary evidence supporting their use. Let us say, someone has published a clinical trial on Ginkgo demonstrating benefits for memory. Another unrelated manufacturer has examined the characteristics of the product used in the trial. They may have even analysed it and tried to develop a phytoequivalent product (one that closely matches it in terms of its phytochemical composition and dosage; see Section 3.2.2.3). Use of that copy product is then underpinned by secondary evidence.

The best clinical evidence exists at two main levels. The first is the gold standard, where a systematic review and meta-analysis of several trials provides proof of efficacy for the herbal product. (Meta-analysis is where results of several trials are pooled together to make one synthetic large trial.) An example would be horse chestnut for vein problems, which has a positive review and meta-analysis from the independent Cochrane collaboration. Meta-analyses are good to have, but if that meta-analysis was done by the Cochrane group, this is even better, because they are considered to be independent and free of any bias.

For the next level of evidence, one or several good trials might show that a herb is beneficial for treating a specified condition. For example, there is the positive trial published for chamomile in generalised anxiety disorder (GAD).[8] The *Diagnostic and Statistical Manual of Mental Disorders* (*DSM-5*) criteria were used to confirm that the trial participants suffered from GAD, helping to make this a high-level trial, together with the six-month duration.

In addition to information supporting herb selection from well-designed trials, there is also the important consideration of traditional evidence. The herbs eyebright and meadowsweet are largely backed only by traditional evidence. But it is good, widespread, consensus-based traditional evidence, and many writers agree that these herbs have these properties.

Animal and test tube studies are aimed more at understanding mechanisms and what might be important in the plant in terms of delivering an activity, but they do not generally provide evidence for clinical choices (see Sections 3.5, 9.5.3, and 9.5.4).

Having evidence backing a herbal treatment is desirable for any disease, and especially for chronic disease. But it is often unavailable: there is no direct research for the use of herbs for several of the conditions that patients might present with. However, this does not mean that the clinician cannot adopt an evidence-based approach. It can be constructed by using a two-step process, which also allows the individualisation of treatments. This process is, in fact, the core thinking that underlies all the FHT treatment recommendations in this book.

For Step 1, we choose those therapeutic targets that have good evidence supporting their relevance for the disease in question. This is drawn from a comprehensive review of the biomedical understanding of that particular disease, as well as any relevant traditional herbal considerations. These therapeutic targets are next reviewed against the framework of the 12 core strategies of FHT, including the key herbal actions required. But the most important step is Step 2: we examine the herbal evidence and select those herbs that are most likely to deliver favourable outcomes in terms of these strategic targets and required actions. This two-step process is actually a progressive, forward-thinking, cutting-edge methodology sometimes used, knowingly or unwittingly, by conventional medical practitioners.

When prescribing preformulated products, it is imperative to choose the ones that have been put together by trained practitioners with clinical experience. In this way, many years of clinical experience and insight can be built into the product. In contrast, some products are formulated based on: "Let's throw in every herb that's known to be good for condition X." In order to achieve this, several of the herbal ingredients are included in amounts well below therapeutic levels. This is sometimes referred to as "fairy dusting" the product. Needless to say, such products should be avoided, and they cast doubt on the clinical understanding and ethics of the companies selling them.

3.4 Right protocols

For the development of treatment protocols consistent with the precepts of FHT, see all the other chapters in this book. Other key considerations are discussed in this section.

Important factors to keep in mind are budget, patient sensitivity, and patient compliance. With respect to budget, for example, in the case of a chronic fatigue syndrome patient, I might say to them, "You could walk out here with six or eight products or three or four. What would you prefer according to your budget?" Some will say, "I don't care how much it costs, give me the lot." And yet others will say, "No. Give me three or four." To those who have selected to have three or four, I might respond: "Don't worry, you'll get the others, we'll just stage it. We will put you on these products now and then introduce the others later, pulling others out, so that it meets your budget."

What do you do when the patient is sensitive to your treatments? Sometimes this is because of impaired detoxification capacity. Milk thistle extract (silymarin) for 1–2 months to condition the person's liver can be a useful strategy. Other treatments are then introduced gradually.

In the following case even that strategy failed, possibly because the patient could not tolerate tablet excipients. A 55-year-old woman was suffering from insulin resistance, an elevated androgen level, high body fat mass (weight more than 100 kg), and a lack of well-being. She had seen several practitioners, but in all instances was unable to continue with the prescribed herbal treatments due to a range of adverse reactions.

The following was initially prescribed: milk thistle extract (silymarin) tablets (1 per day, building up to 3 per day) and Gymnema (1 tablet per day). Neither treatment was tolerated. The patient experienced nausea, reflux, and general malaise. This was changed to a phase II liver formula powder (with broccoli sprouts and turmeric) at 2 scoops a day and a Schisandra 1:2 liquid at 2.5 mL twice a day with water. The patient was advised to start low and build up to these doses, and it took a few months until this was achieved. Six months after her first consultation she was doing well, feeling good, taking full doses of these herbs. We increased the Schisandra target to 4 mL twice a day. Two months later the Gymnema was started again as a 1:1 liquid extract at 2.5 mL twice a day. Her words were that the Gymnema was "working an absolute treat", and with exercise and improved diet she had lost 6 kg. Three months later her TSH (thyroid-stimulating hormone) level was high normal, so Withania 2:1 at 5 mL/day was added, and the Gymnema was increased to 4 mL 3 times a day. Two months after that she was doing very well, had lost another 5 kg, had more energy, and could tolerate food she could not have before. Monitoring her blood glucose readings showed that it could rise to more than 10 mmol/L (180 mg/dL) after a meal. But if she were then to take Gymnema, the reading would drop below 10 mmol/L within 15 minutes, where otherwise it would take hours.

It is critical to check the compliance of patients. This can be readily done by asking them how much they have left of what had been prescribed. A simple calculation will reveal if they have been consistent with taking their herbs. As I observed one senior naturopath say to his patient when I was doing clinical observation as a student: "It won't do you any good if it is still in the bottle!" If a patient has not been very compliant, consider reducing the number of treatments that are being prescribed, then encourage them to comply. You might say: "Please make sure you take just this one thing."

3.5 Right resources

The selection of the best resources to inform clinical practice is critical and includes catalogues, textbooks, and charts. Here the successful herbal clinician exercises great caution and considerable scrutiny. In addition to having accurate clinical indications for a herb, it is important to access reliable information for contraindications and cautions. Potential herb–drug interactions and pregnancy and lactation issues are also highly relevant. In summary, we need well-researched

- product catalogues
- contraindication and caution charts
- herb–drug interaction charts
- pregnancy and lactation charts
- above all, accurate texts and compendia

Having the right resources also relates to the third of the herbal game changers listed at the start of the chapter, as it is good practice to favour products with primary and secondary clinical evidence.

As noted in Section 3.3, animal and test tube studies are more for understanding mechanisms and active components and should not, generally, inform clinical decisions. This is a significant issue concerning herbal information today across the internet, in lectures, in seminars, and even in textbooks. There is an abundance of misinformation (herbal fake news) arising from misunderstood, careless, and sometimes naïve or amateur extrapolations or interpretations of herbal research. This applies especially for misinterpretations of test tube research, but it can include other misunderstandings or examples of simplistic logic (see example below). These issues are not confined to information relevant to clinical choices: they also include safety concerns. Detractors or sceptics of herb use are indeed promoting *in vivo* and *in vitro* studies to impute spurious dangers.

The following recommendations were found in a recent high-level textbook (which will remain unnamed) from a major academic publisher:

> Astragalus should be avoided in patients with autoimmune disease or receiving immunosuppressive therapy due to its immunostimulatory effects. As Astragalus may contain selenium, ingestion of large amounts may lead to selenosis. Astragalus may potentiate the effects of antithrombotic and anticoagulant medications.

The species of herb referred to above was *Astragalus membranaceus*. Bone and Mills give the following information:[9]

> Although many species are used as forage for livestock and wild animals, some (including the locoweeds) are known to cause intoxication in livestock, which can be passed to humans through milk and meat. *Astragalus membranaceus* is **not** one of these selenium-accumulating species. . . .
>
> A US group of doctors described two separate cases (published 3 years apart) of remission of idiopathic membranous nephropathy (IMN, probably autoimmune in origin) after therapy with Astragalus. . . .
>
> *In vivo* studies suggest that Astragalus may reduce the efficacy of cyclophosphamide (an immunosuppressive agent). However, the clinical relevance of this is uncertain. In principle, immune-enhancing herbs should not be given long-term to transplant recipients receiving immune-suppressing drugs.

Furthermore, there is no credible suggestion from any research at the time of writing that Astragalus will adversely affect autoimmunity (see the case studies above noting benefit) or interact with antithrombotic and anticoagulant medications. Hence, of the four pieces of safety advice from the unnamed text only one was partially accurate (avoid in transplant recipients on immunosuppressive medication).

Misinformation derived from *in vitro* research applies especially to the issue of herb–drug interactions. When a herb is mixed with liver cells in a test tube, it might influence several cytochrome p450 enzymes. This is then taken to mean that the herb will interact with the metabolism of all the drugs that are processed by these p450 enzymes. What results is a list of interaction concerns that goes on for several pages. Such extrapolation is unfounded and does not have any clinical relevance, as can be seen from the many studies where the *in vitro* findings for the herb (in terms of its influence on drug metabolism) do not even translate to animal studies, much less to human trials.

3.6 Right practice

Managing patient responses, their expectations, and their adverse responses can be a critical part of ensuring that good clinical outcomes are achieved. Major adverse reactions to herbs are extremely uncommon; minor reactions may, however, occur. The patient might say: "I've started taking the herbs, and I feel nauseous" or "It's caused diarrhoea" or "It's giving me headaches." It is possible to have sensitive patients who are highly somatised and so quite prone to adverse effects (see the case history in Section 3.4). How is this best managed?

If a patient feels they have experienced an adverse reaction to a prescribed herb, it is best that they first stop taking it. Unless the reaction has been severe or unpleasant, the advice should be to wait a few days and then recommence at about a third of the dose. Monitor the patient's progress, and then, after a week, if there is no reaction, gradually increase back to the original dose. In more than 9 out of 10 cases the patient will then be fine taking that herb (or herb combination). If the patient continues to react adversely, the treatment should be promptly changed.

In one of her lectures entitled "The Follow-up Appointment", naturopath Ruth Trickey made the point that practitioners' training and seminars usually focus on the first appointment and rarely address the follow-up appointment.

The follow-up appointment is actually as critical as the first. At this time, the therapist can assess how the patient is feeling and check if they are responding to the treatment. It is helpful to check for indicators that treatment is on the right track. The patient might even say – and I have heard this or similar a few times – "Well, my pain levels haven't changed, but I'm sleeping better, and I feel better in myself, and I know that the rest will follow." The response to this is to stay on track.

Other patients may say, if you ask, "Oh I'm no good. I'm just the same, maybe a bit worse." In these circumstances it is good to conduct a brief audit of the patient's progress. For example, I might say: "Oh, well, last time you came in, you were complaining of headaches, how have your headaches been?" The surprised response might be: "Well, no, I haven't had any of them since." I might also ask: "And what about that other thing (poor sleep, reflux etc.)?" "Oh no, that's gone too." Hence, we should not necessarily rely on a broad, overall self-assessment.

It may be a good idea to ask some patients to rate how they are feeling. Say, they have three core problems. We can ask them to rate each out of ten each day, and record the numbers. From this, both the patient and the clinician can see if there is progress or not.

But we should keep our options open and know when to switch products or treatments. If patients have not been helped in four weeks, it would be advisable to change at least some aspects of the treatment, in terms of either herbs and/or targets. The main exception to this 4-week guideline is a case of a really depleted condition, like chronic fatigue syndrome or fibromyalgia, in which case there may not be a substantial change for months.

One more aspect relating to the follow-up appointment is to pre-empt it at the first consultation. I typically mention what I plan to do as a follow-up at the next appointment. We need to give the patient a good reason to come back, something to look forward to. This can be in terms of: "When you come in next week (or month), we will be looking at this particular aspect, and I will give you a protocol for . . . but we're not doing that right now." As therapists, we may not necessarily be able to do everything at once, and this is not a bad thing, because otherwise the patient might think, if nothing happens, "Oh, I haven't been helped, so I won't go back." Always leave it open that you have other possibilities and other areas to explore with that patient at the following appointment.

There are a few prescribing tips related to right practice:

- Herbs for gastro-oesophageal reflux should be given after meals.
- For bronchial herbs, and indeed cold and influenza herbs, if there are diaphoretic herbs in the liquid mixture, it should be taken in hot water and consumed like a tea.
- Boswellia should be taken with fat and oil, because that helps its absorption (this might apply for quite a few other herbs that have mainly fat-soluble constituents).
- Willow bark and other herbs containing tannins may cause stomach irritation, so ensure that the patient takes them with a protein meal. The protein in the meal will tie up the tannins and reduce the irritation. It is just like drinking strong black tea on an empty stomach: it can irritate because of the tannins it contains.

The final thing is to be unfailingly professional. This is a significant challenge these days, because there are patients who come to see us who, thanks to Dr Google, know more than we do. Or at least they think they do. This can be both challenging and frustrating. It is important to remind ourselves constantly that our role is that of a facilitator to help the person to get well and to put our ego aside and not react.

References

1. Baskaran K, Kizar Ahamath B, Radha Shanmugasundaram K, Shanmugasundaram ER. Antidiabetic effect of a leaf extract from Gymnema sylvestre in non-insulin-dependent diabetes mellitus patients. *J Ethnopharmacol.* 1990 Oct; **30**(3): 295–300. PMID: 2259217.
2. Sandasi M, Vermaak I, Chen W, Viljoen AM. Skullcap and germander: preventing potential toxicity through the application of hyperspectral imaging and multivariate image analysis as a novel quality control method. *Planta Med.* 2014 Oct; **80**(15): 1329–1339. doi:10.1055/s-0034-1383037. PMID: 25184892.
3. Tankeu S, Vermaak I, Chen W, Sandasi M, Viljoen A. Differentiation between two "fang ji" herbal medicines, *Stephania tetrandra* and the nephrotoxic *Aristolochia fangchi*, using hyperspectral imaging. *Phytochemistry.* 2016 Feb; **122**: 213–222. doi:10.1016/j.phytochem.2015.11.008. PMID: 26632529.
4. Efferth T, Kaina B. Toxicities by herbal medicines with emphasis to traditional Chinese medicine. *Curr Drug Metab.* 2011 Dec; **12**(10): 989–996. PMID: 21892916.
5. Wang XB, Zheng J, Li JJ, et al. Simultaneous analysis of 23 illegal adulterated aphrodisiac chemical ingredients in health foods and Chinese traditional patent medicines by ultrahigh performance liquid chromatography coupled with quadrupole time-of-

flight mass spectrometry. *J Food Drug Anal.* 2018 Jul; **26**(3): 1138–1153. doi:10.1016/j.jfda.2018.02.003. PMID: 29976406.
6. Bryson PD, Watanabe AS, Rumack BH, et al. Burdock root tea poisoning. Case report involving a commercial preparation. *JAMA.* 1978; **239**: 2157.
7. Kaltner F, Rychlik M, Gareis M, Gottschalk C. Occurrence and risk assessment of pyrrolizidine alkaloids in spices and culinary herbs from various geographical origins. *Toxins (Basel).* 2020 Mar 1; **12**(3): E155. doi:10.3390/toxins12030155. PMID: 32121600.
8. Mao JJ, Xie SX, Keefe JR, Soeller I, Li QS, Amsterdam JD. Long-term chamomile (*Matricaria chamomilla* L.) treatment for generalized anxiety disorder: a randomized clinical trial. *Phytomedicine.* 2016 Dec 15; **23**(14): 1735–1742. doi:10.1016/j.phymed.2016.10.012. PMID: 27912875.
9. Bone KM, Mills SY. *Principles and Practice of Phytotherapy: Modern Herbal Medicine*, 2nd ed. Elsevier, UK, 2013, pp 381–392. [pp 381, 388, 389]

4

The traditional roots of FHT

Simon Mills

One attraction of functional medicine is that its principles resonate so strongly with ancient wisdoms. Indeed, on looking through the history of medicine around the world, it seems that only in modern times have these principles been forgotten. As most early medicines were herbal, a brief review of traditional approaches will provide a solid bedrock for the application of FHT.

In this chapter we look briefly for key functional medical principles in the earlier traditions of healthcare and can note that they are generally central in each case. In particular, we see recurring the first four principles developed in this book: the way these traditions

- understood diseases as disorders of normal function
- embraced the complexity of diseases, where the individual story counts most
- matched treatment with each patient's individual energetics
- applied complex interventions for complex disorders

There is much overlap among the world's medical traditions, as well as similarities between them. We look at three major healthcare systems that all began some two millennia ago and then at two that marked the herbal-specific renewal of these principles in the nineteenth century:

1. Ayurvedic medicine
2. Chinese medicine
3. Graeco–Roman and Islamic medicine

4   nineteenth-century North American herbal medicine

   5   Middle-European herbal medicine and naturopathy

We finish by extracting common principles from them all.

4.1 Ayurvedic medicine

It is clear that the Ayurvedic tradition from India has involved a significant systematising of earlier folk practices and is the earliest developed health culture in history still in use today.[1,2] Although the living tradition was obscured over the last four centuries by the dominance of the British Raj and later Western medical cultures, it is clear that this was extraordinarily rich. Over almost 3,000 years, medicines and illnesses were classified and sophisticated treatment modalities were described.

Like its later contemporary in Graeco–Roman Europe, the application of medicines in Ayurveda was essentially based on humoral principles. The workings of the body in health and disease were understood by the observation of its "humours" or fluids, most often as excretions. In Europe there were four humours, in India three, known as the *doshas*. These three – *kapha*, *pitta*, and *vāta* – provide the primary orientation in Ayurvedic medicine.

The word *dosha* derives from the same root as the English "dys-", as in "dysfunction": *doshas* are essentially faults in the healthy state of the body. Each is a condensation of a pair of five elements (earth, water, fire, air, and ether) – waste products produced when the body replenishes its elements. The *doshas* support the body only as long as they continually flow out of it, as proper eliminations of urine, faeces, and sweat.

Kapha is a condensation of water and earth (the damp and dry elements of matter) and projects itself into the production of lubricant fluids in the body. It is the stabilising influence in the body and generally concentrates in the thorax (to steady rising *vāta*) and is associated with mucus. Illnesses of excessive *kapha* are marked by symptoms of cold, damp, and heaviness (e.g. catarrh, oedema, abdominal congestion) and are relieved by warming, drying, stimulating remedies such as pungent spices, warming diaphoretics and expectorants, emetics, aromatic and bitter digestives and carminatives, and to a lesser extent, perhaps combined with the above, diuretics, laxatives, and astringents.

Pitta collects fire and water elements into the production of bile and is associated more generally with digestive juices: it is in charge of transformation and processing and concentrates in the mid-abdomen. Illnesses of excessive or obstructed *pitta* are marked by biliary disturbances and may include symptoms of heat, damp, and excessive activity (e.g. fever, inflammation, infection, blood toxicities, bleeding). They are relieved, as appropriate and perhaps in combination, by cooling, drying, nutritive, or calming remedies, such as the bitters, purgatives, sweet tonic remedies, astringents, cooling diaphoretics, alteratives, and diuretics.

Vāta arises from condensation of air and ether and is the – often unstable – windy form of *prāṇa*, linked to the functions of the respiratory system. It is in charge of all movement in the body; it concentrates in the lower abdomen to help lift *kapha*. Illnesses of the *vāta* type, marked by cold, dryness, and excessive – especially nervous – activity, are of two types. Deficient *vāta* (e.g. emaciation and constitutional dehydration) is treated with sweet and nutritive tonics, bulking laxatives, demulcents, and salty remedies. Accumulated or obstructed *vāta* is a congestive version that may include abdominal distension and gas, constipation, and rheumatic and arthritic conditions. This is treated with modest pungent herbs in the short term only, moderate warming diaphoretics, carminatives and antispasmodics, and temporary laxatives. All *vāta* conditions are indications for traditional Ayurvedic enema therapy.

Ayurvedic medicine also sees many conditions as combinations of the *doshas* with toxicity, "damp", or *āma*, a common orientation among early traditions that presaged the modern definitions of infection and inflammatory disease. This is a *kapha*-like influence, being generally cold, slimy, heavy, and dense, with phlegm and mucus, loss of taste and appetite, indigestion, depression, and irritability as common symptoms; it may arise from emotional difficulties as well as physical ones. It lies at the root of much chronic disease and immune disturbance. Where there is evidence of *āma*, improving eliminations is the first priority of treatment. This is a universal theme in traditional herbal therapeutics. The prime herbal influences in the elimination of *āma* are the bitter and pungent herbs, often in that sequential order, perhaps after a fast. (This is very like the strategy in Galenic traditions for the elimination of "damp".) Sweet, salty, and sour herbs can increase *āma*.

The treatment of *āma* is, however, complicated by its combinations with the *doshas* (in which case it has the suffix *sāma*). Combined with *kapha* (*kapha sāma*), it is marked by severe mucus conditions and is a clear indication for pungent with bitter herbs. *Pitta sāma* is like "damp-heat" in the Galenic tradition, with yellow tongue coating, urine and faeces, congestive anorexia, loss of thirst, and biliousness. Bitter herbs lead the treatment, with modest amounts of pungent herbs, as appropriate. *Vāta sāma* is associated with constipation, painful abdominal congestion and flatulence, anorexia, and bad breath; it is treated with pungent herbs, warming aromatic digestives, and carminatives combined with laxatives, as required.

If hygienic and other observances are insufficient to deal with the accumulations, a range of therapeutic measures is indicated. These may include an elaborate programme called *panchakarma*, designed to purify the body from the accumulations and pacify associated disturbances. Herbal or other remedies would be applied at any stage, with the most active tactics being those that lead to the most vigorous eliminations (emetics for accumulated *vāta* and *kapha*, purgatives for *pitta*), but because of the risks of depletion there are many approaches to consider, some being particularly gentle. The physician respects the relative strength of the patient in relation to the disease and adopts only those treatments that do not disturb or debilitate. (There is little attraction to the modern concept of "healing crisis".) For every purification treatment successfully completed, there would be a mandatory convalescence to allow recovery, perhaps augmented by appropriate rejuvenating remedies.

As with the Chinese view (see Section 4.2), the effects of foods and the pharmacology of medicines are classified in terms of their immediate impact on the body. Tastes, or *rasas*, are not only subjective impressions, but attributes of the body itself in its relationship with its environment: everyone craves the taste most lacking within. The choice of both medicines and foods is thus often determined by such assessments, the distinction between them again being a function of their effects on the body: foods nourish, medicines balance, and poisons disturb.

The effects of *rasas* on the body are complex and rarely isolated. For example, the sweet, sour, and salty tastes decrease *vāta* and increase *kapha*, but sour, salty, and pungent tastes increase *pitta*. Bitter, pungent, and astringent tastes increase *vāta* and decrease *kapha*.

Ayurvedic texts provide considerable detail in their therapeutic recommendations. According to a recent seminal English text,[3] Ayurvedic treatment is based on:

- correct diagnosis
- defined treatment principles
- understanding the disease process and the cause
- defined treatment strategies with an emphasis on the above
- developing a unique prescription

Preparation of herbal remedies, for example, is elaborate, with a wide range of methods designed to transform the original plant material to match the typology of the disturbance. The remedies are also applied to the body in many forms and at various times in the treatment.

As well as using the pulse, tongue, and other traditional diagnostic methods, Ayurveda also invokes the 10 assessments: constitution, habits (lifestyle), state of balance in the body, mental state, quality of the tissues, digestive power, quality of the body, energy levels, body type, and age.

According to the same text,[4] the fundamental Ayurvedic treatment principles are:

- reducing excess: excess pathologies are treated either by purification or palliation
- tonifying deficiency with tonics (*rasayanas*)
- drying therapy for excess dampness; diuretic and anticatarrhal herbs are Western examples
- lubricating dryness with oily or demulcent herbs
- fomentation or sweating therapy for reducing coldness, heaviness, stiffness, or trapped heat – using steam and diaphoretic herbs (analogous to Thomsonian medicine -see Sections 1.2 and 4.4)
- astringent herbs for excess flow of bodily fluids

Whatever the sophistication in Ayurvedic texts, it is clear, however, that they were meant to be enabling rather than formulaic prescriptions: they encouraged a respect for diversity and complexity, for the individuality of the patient. Empiricism and pragmatism are essential features of any survival strategy, and the repeated emphasis in the texts on judging a remedy or tactic by its effects on the ill body rather than in theory, and the transparency of the therapeutic tactics, all point to the value of the individual in the treatment plan.

4.2 Chinese medicine

Chinese medicine has survived without colonial intrusions as a major part of healthcare provision for well over two millennia, to the present day. Through this extraordinary continuity it also constitutes the most comprehensive clinical strategy for the use of herbal medicines anywhere. Over its long history, seminal texts and systems have been developed, each incorporating the developments of its predecessors.[5,6] These were often very intricate systems, reflecting initially perhaps the priorities of scholarship and portent lore (much theorising at the early stages was for the Imperial court[7]).

It is important to emphasise that whereas the West diverged from a subjective view of the world (a divergence already apparent in Graeco–Roman culture, and that arguably led to the major achievements of modern medicine), the traditions of medicine that developed in Asia from prehistoric times elaborated instead on what we might now call a "science of qualities".[8] This cultural distinction has important lessons for the study of functional medicine and is particularly well articulated in the medicine of China.

In Chinese origins, everything moves (the seminal classic, the *I Ching*, is translated as the "Book of Changes"), and there are five "elements" (more accurately, phases) that are seasonal and cyclical transitions through which all the universe moves: they are constantly in flux. Events are automatically described by their transient qualities in relation to other events and are manifestations of energies in ways that the West understood only after Einstein.[9] The generic term for these energies is *qi*, but in the case of the living body there are many forms of varying density, from *wei qi* as the most rarefied on the body surface, manifest in acute defensive reactions like fever and colds, through *ying qi*, the nourishing *qi* flowing through meridians, to *xue* or blood, the most substantial aspect of *qi*, manifest in many somatic events. *Qi* is also manifest in *jing* (essence) and the body fluids. The comparison with modern physics is even more apposite as *qi* is, simultaneously, energy, movement, and fluid (reminiscent of attempts to define light as waves and/or particles).

In Chinese medicine there is little regard for anatomy, and the main entities upon which pathogenic or therapeutic forces act are essentially functional and physiological. There are six pairs of functions, often confusingly translated in the West as "organs". (They should not be confused: for example, the Chinese spleen is the function responsible for nourishment and assimilation – rather like the Western liver – and all the other functions are different from their Western namesakes.) These, like all phenomena in the Chinese world, are ascribed to points on the five-phase cycle that further illuminate their qualities. They have a multitude of dynamic relationships with each other and an array of more or less consistent qualities. The five phases, their attributes, and their relationship with the six pairs of functions are illustrated in **Table 4.1**. There is also a specific quality of medicines – their "tastes", like the Ayurvedic *rasas*, as an early, and astonishingly predictive, pharmacology – that can also be understood in terms of these dynamic relationships.

However, Chinese concepts were not entirely fluid. Like the Graeco-Roman and later Western model, there were polarities and counterpoints, the division of the world into opposites. Originally there was the energetic duality *yin* and *yang*, the concrete and dynamic poles, respectively (in Anglo Saxon and other early European cosmologies the concepts of Ice and Fire had similar energetic meanings), but these were not yet static – rather, endlessly flowing back and forth.

A more static framework soon did emerge, and after the Communist Revolution of 1948 one ancient strand became the mainstream "Traditional Chinese Medicine". This was applied particularly to the prescription of – mostly herbal – medicines. In this framework, diseases are addressed in part as four sets of polar opposites: the "eight conditions".

Each of the four pairs denotes a spectrum of qualities onto which any illness can be placed; each implies that the aim of any therapeutic measure is

Table 4.1 Properties of the Five Phases

Phase	Quality	Function Yin	Yang	Taste
Fire	hot, ascending	heart	small intestine	bitter
		heart protector	three heater	
Earth	nourishing, stable	spleen	stomach	sweet
Metal	strong, protective	lungs	large intestine	acrid
Water	cold, still, deep	kidneys	bladder	salty
Wood	growing, spreading	liver	gallbladder	sour

compensatory, like the Galenic *antidotos* (see Section 4.5), to move extremes back towards a healthy mean. Accordingly, herbs are ascribed temperaments or tendencies: they may be *yin* or *yang*, tonic or dispersive, cooling or heating, eliminative or constructive. These manifestations are, in turn, aspects of fundamental properties of the remedies.

4.3 Graeco–Roman medicine

The founding traditions of European medicine were adapted from the works of Hippocrates in Greece in the fifth and fourth centuries BCE by Roman physicians such as Galen and by Dioscorides 500 years later. These all introduced new standards of empiricism, logic, and rigour into the delivery of health care, challenging the view that disease was caused by malevolent forces and could be reduced by appeasing the gods (and paying the priests to do so!). These pioneers asked not "*who causes this disease?*" but "*by what process does this disease occur?*" They set the framework both for the flowering of Islamic medicine 700 years later and for our modern Western medical culture. Moreover Graeco–Roman–Islamic traditions were founded on the Hippocratic foundations of dietary, lifestyle, environmental, and psychotherapeutic approaches to encouraging health,[10] with more specific strategies to deal with disease developed later by Galen[11] and Dioscorides.[12]

These authors understood nature as an expression of dynamic forces and phenomena that were normally held in balance (in modern systems theory this is understood as the self-organisation of ecological systems). Ill health was a manifestation of imbalance that indicated corrective measures, in Galen's terms, either, in the case of drugs, through their own dynamic "qualities" or, in the case of foods, by the qualities of their substance. A key example of the natural dynamic forces were the temperaments hot, cold, dampness, and dryness, reflecting the paired impacts of the four elements that were understood to make up nature: earth, water, fire, and air. The elements were, in turn, associated with the four fluids ("humours"): black bile, phlegm, yellow bile, and blood (their more everyday manifestations being faeces, mucus, vomit, and bleeding). They are most often recognised today by their associated personality types: respectively melancholic, phlegmatic, choleric, and sanguine.

Therapeutically, the humours were the cornerstone, and physicians moved to counteract excess (*plethora*) or deficiency (*kenos*) in any of them:

- For excess or toxic conditions the aim was to provide *antidotos*, primarily heating, cooling, drying, and moistening, as needed; remedies in the "first degree" were milder than those in the third or fourth degree, which became increasingly dangerous.
- For deficiency conditions, *physic* remedies (from the Greek *phusikē*, or Nature) were replenishing or supportive.

The works of the Graeco–Roman writers were extensively remodelled by the medical writers of the Islamic era. Up to 100 authors on pharmaceutics and *materia medica* are identifiable in the Arabic bibliographies, most of them copying and adapting directly from Dioscorides and Galen. There were, however, notable developments, including the work of the Persians al-Majusi (Ali Abbas), ar-Rhazi (Rhazes), and Ibn-Sina (Avicenna), the Jew Maimonides and the Christian Hunayn ibn-Ishaq.[13]

It is apparent that in Islamic pharmaceutics considerable respect was paid to the qualities of individual herbs. Formulating was seen as reflecting a secondary skill – unlike traditions further East. Physicians were expected to understand intimately the nature of each remedy, its natural habitat, its specific energy pattern, actions, indications, specific relationships to the organs, duration of action, toxicity and contraindications, types of preparation, dosage, administration, and antidotes.[14] These principles anticipated modern pharmaceutical medicine.

Islamic medicine is still taught at universities and medical schools through the Middle East and, as Unani medicine, is widely practised around the world in Pakistani and Bangladeshi communities.

4.4 Nineteenth-century North American herbal medicine

The majority of the early immigrants to North America were Europeans looking for a fresh start in the vast spaces of the "New World", so it is not surprising that this was also a time of enterprise. In the case of health care, this involved transposing cultural traditions to a new landscape. Although there were new towns and cities, significant numbers of people lived remotely from any organised services – for example, often hundreds of miles from a doctor (who was often poorly qualified). These were hardy, self-reliant people who had to find all resources on their doorstep. They also had to rediscover their self-sufficiency in health terms, combining their (imported) old European home remedies with native North American flora and a considerable amount of native American lore as well.

A new group of practitioners emerged, now sometimes referred to as "travelling medicine shows", more often contemporarily as "white Indian doctors", often peripatetic, exploiting their claimed skills and usually their own patent herbal nostrums. One such nineteenth-century herbal tonic was to become, as Coca-Cola, the most massively consumed product of all time. Among a motley crew there were also true pioneers, passionately keen to develop a self-reliant healthcare system based on what they knew of plant remedies.

One "white Indian doctor" went into print. Samuel Thomson (1769–1843), was a shepherd boy from New Hampshire who, with the early help of a "wise woman", Mrs Benton, became adept at treating his neighbours. He substituted indigenous herbs for the prevailing but intermittent service of a "regular physic", generally involving disease-attacking medications often based on minerals like mercury, arsenic, antimony, and sulfur, and on practices like bloodletting (which had hastened the demise of George Washington). Thomson saw all these as depleting strategies that weakened the patient.

The main presentation in those days was fever. Unlike physicians who saw this as a threat, Thomson maintained and supported the process. He saw fever as a sign of healthy resistance: it was possible for damage to follow if it got out of hand, but the main risk was failure of the febrile defence. Thus Thomson used *Capsicum spp.* (cayenne) as a powerful support to the febrile mechanism, along with a range of other native remedies, including *Lobelia inflata* (lobelia), *Myrica cerifera* (bayberry), *Viburnum opulus* (cramp bark), and *Zanthoxylum* (prickly ash) to modulate and support various aspects of the febrile response.

Thomson was sufficiently enthused by the distinction between his and the "regular physic" approaches to learn to read and write, so that he could pass on his message. He set out a principle that at once encapsulated this tradition and fired the public imagination. The book in which he promoted his views[15] was a runaway publishing success across the East and Mid-West, and at the time it was calculated that over half the population of Ohio were adherents of Thomsonian medicine.

Thomson's language was simple, even simplistic, and aimed at a God-fearing readership. However, he seemed to have touched a gut instinct that life and health are positive virtues, to be protected or recovered through personal self-sufficiency using medicines provided by the Maker. In one key passage he adopted the language of Graeco–Roman medicine:

> I found that all animal bodies were formed of four elements. The Earth and Water constitute the solid; and the Air and Fire (or heat) are the cause of life and motion; that the cold, or the lessening of the power of heat, is the cause of all disease; that to restore heat to its natural state was the only way health could be produced, and that, after restoring the natural heat, by clearing the system of all obstruction and causing a natural perspiration, the stomach would digest the food taken into it, and the heat (or nature) be enabled to hold her supremacy.[16]

To a readership versed in the Book of Genesis, the fact that earth and water (or clay) were the stuff of life – the dry and wet principles, respectively – would have been readily appreciated. For those spending all their lives in the open, Air would have been easily equated with its original meaning, wind, a persistent metaphor for movement. The important vital principle was, of course, Fire or Heat, the obvious difference between a living body and a corpse, the universal metaphor for life. Thomson's message was simple. Heat is life. Disease (and death) are degrees of cold. Heating thus provides the fundamental principle of healing. Other measures, principally in improving eliminations and digestive performance, are often essential supports to this central measure. Cayenne is literally a life promoter.

Some of Thomson's followers diverged from his simple messages. There were different emphases on the need to control excess heat (in fact, circulation) and variations in the mechanisms for keeping the blood "clean". In the later part of the nineteenth-century, Thomsonian approaches inspired both Eclecticism and physiomedicalism, these emerging at same time and in the same mid-west locations as Osteopathy and Chiropractic.

Physiomedicalism in particular anticipated functional medicine. Among key authors, T.J. Lyle produced a superb herbal *materia medica*,[17] concentrating on the observed influence of each remedy on the human being rather than listing its symptomatic indications. J.M. Thurston posed operational definitions of the vital force, health, and disease and the distinctions between functional symptoms and those arising from organic ("trophic") origins and elaborated on the need to use only such remedies as supported vitality.[18] W.H. Cook developed the theme that the living body is essentially a functional entity, and disease starts as a disturbance of normal functional rhythms – for example:

> Regularity in periods of alternate labor and rest is characteristic of all vital action . . .
>
> . . . the earliest departure of the tissues from under the full control of the vital force will be in the lack of ability either to relax or to contract some of the tissues as readily as in the healthy state.[19]

Like other physiomedicalists, Cook started with the principle that the ideal medicine should support recuperative functions, but he added considerably to the view that thereafter they should have a gentle dynamism, helping to correct distorted functions, either "relaxing" overstimulated tissues or functions or "contracting" those that are sluggish.

The Eclectics, as their name suggests, embraced a wide range of remedies with a less than overall cohesive philosophy. Their wealth of clinical experience, however, was outstanding, and they made substantial contributions to Anglo–American medicine through their developments of the *materia medica.*

4.5 Middle-European herbal and naturopathic medicine

Much of Western herbal therapeutics is imbued with the values of a healthcare tradition that arose in central Europe from the eighteenth century on. Built on the philosophical foundations of Goethe and Schiller, a cultural view arose of health as a refinement, a separation of the pure from the greater impure.

In Germany, this culture inspired the homoeopathy of Samuel Hahnemann, the biochemic tissue salts of Schuessler, and, in the twentieth century, the anthroposophical medicine of Rudolph Steiner – and, indirectly, in the flower remedies of Edward Bach in England. It also provided the founding principles of a variety of practices that have been grouped under the heading of "naturopathy". The use of dietary changes (and, in later years, dietary supplements), hydrotherapy, and a range of physical therapies in order to allow a "nature cure" has one of its strongest cultural roots in this tradition.

The European naturopathic tradition also developed Galenic concepts of heat and cold and, notably, that of damp. The concept of "catarrh" and "mucus" became a cornerstone of naturopathic treatment, as might be expected in northern Europe. Following the Graeco–Roman lead, many infectious and inflammatory diseases were seen as congestive toxicities to be warmed and dried. When germ theory established the role of bacteria in infections, these were seen as "saprophytes" rather than pathogens: in other words, essentially beneficial cleansing organisms, like forest fungi breaking down dead wood, taking advantage of the catarrhal nutrients to effect extraordinary healing responses like inflammation and fever. As in earlier traditions, herbal remedies were seen as important contributions to detoxifying damp conditions, although these were closely interwoven with dietary techniques in ways that have permeated much herbal practice in the West to this day.

The Middle-European tradition also shifted the emphasis on dosage, moving from simple high "heroic" doses for acute conditions to more nuanced complex mixes for chronic conditions. Led by the subtleties of homoeopathy this morphed perhaps too far into minute ("nano") doses that have become less plausible, but it did presage the modern focus on managing complex diseases. At lower doses, hawthorn adapted from being a fever remedy to managing long-term heart conditions, valerian moved from being a strong convalescent tonic to a gentle sedative, and garlic moved from being an antiseptic to managing high plasma cholesterol.

4.6 Common elements

Several themes emerge from these reviews of traditional therapeutic systems.

1. Medicines, most of which were herbal, were seen as correcting internal disharmonies ("dis-eases") rather than targeting symptoms.
2. In the absence of modern instrumentation, internal disharmonies were understood subjectively, first seen as body fluids or excretions (the humours, the *doshas, qi, xue* and *jing*) and then often described in climatic or emotional metaphors, in language that was readily understood among the general population.

3 By definition, the humours suffused equally the body and the mind (and even the spirit), so that one internal disharmony could affect all levels of experience. There was no Cartesian body/mind split in traditional medicine, and medicines worked equally across all levels.

Herbal remedies were usually classified by the internal disharmony they affected. As the modern "allopathic" shift took hold, these classifications were replaced and new powerful treatments sought to target pathologies. A "cooling", "drying", or "moistening" remedy might be converted to an anti-inflammatory, antibiotic, or proton pump inhibitor. Some of the old "true physic" involving "heating" or "tonic" remedies and convalescent recovery were almost entirely lost to modern medicine.

References

1. Wujastyk D, Meulenbeld GJ (Eds). *Studies in Indian Medical History*. Forsten, Groningen, 1987.
2. Leslie C (Ed). *Asian Medical Systems: A Comparative Study*. University of California Press, Berkeley, 1976.
3. Pole S. *Ayurvedic Medicine: The Principles of Traditional Practice*. Elsevier Health Sciences, Philadelphia, 2006.
4. *Ibid*.
5. Wiseman N. *Fundamentals of Chinese Medicine*. Paradigm Publications, Massachusetts, 1994.
6. Unschuld PU. *Medicine in China: A History of Pharmaceutics*. University of California Press, Berkeley, 1986.
7. Needham J. *Science and Civilisation in China, Vol 2: History of Scientific Thought*. University of Cambridge, Cambridge, 1956.
8. Goodwin, BC. *How the Leopard Changed Its Spots: The Evolution of Complexity*. Weidenfeld & Nicolson, London, 1996.
9. Capra F. *The Turning Point: Science, Society, and the Rising Culture*. Wildwood House, London, 1982.
10. Lloyd GER (Ed). *Hippocratic Writings*. Pelican, London, 1978.
11. *Galen: Selected Works* (trans. PN Singer). Oxford University Press, Oxford, 1997.
12. Scarborough J. Drugs and medicines in the Roman world. *Expedition*. 1996; **38**(2): 38–51.
13. Ullmann M. *Islamic Medicine*. Edinburgh University Press, Edinburgh, 1978.
14. Pormann PE, Savage-Smith E. *Medieval Islamic Medicine*. Edinburgh University Press, Edinburgh, 2007.
15. Thomson S. *New Guide to Health; Or the Botanic Family Physician*. Boston, 1835.
16. *Ibid.* [p 150]
17. Lyle TJ. *Physio-medical Therapeutics, Materia Medica and Pharmacy*. Ohio, 1897.
18. Thurston JM. *The Philosophy of Physiomedicalism*. Nicholson, Indiana, 1900.
19. Cook WH. *The Science and Practice of Medicine*. Cincinnati, 1893. [p 86]

II

EXPANDING THE CORE STRATEGIES OF FUNCTIONAL HERBAL THERAPY

5

Plants and the microcirculation: a powerful new FHT clinical paradigm

This chapter reviews the supporting evidence and clinical ramifications of the core FHT strategy of supporting and enhancing endothelial health and the microcirculation. This is a powerful clinical paradigm that can deliver surprising results, even in problematical cases. A key aspect of the chapter is the design and use of a 5-point microcirculation phytonutrient dietary plan, which can be applied on its own or in conjunction with any prescribed herbs.

We receive nearly all our tissue nourishment and oxygen via the circulation of our blood. The common view is that the circulatory or cardiovascular system consists of veins, arteries, and the heart. Hence, all circulatory health problems are seen to arise from malfunctions of these key structures of the macrocirculation. Missing from this perspective is any consideration for the largest, and most neglected, part of our circulatory system. This is the microcirculation: the part that actually does the job of tissue nourishment. Allied to, and intimately connected to, the microcirculation is the concept of healthy vascular endothelial function. If the vascular endothelial cells of the human body were aligned end to end, they would go around the world four times.[1]

Gaining new insights into this overlooked topic can transform the way many patients are treated, including not only those with just circulatory problems, but those with an extraordinarily wide range of other common diseases. There is abundant clinical evidence that herbs and plant foods can play a key role in maintaining microcirculatory and endothelial health. In fact, at present there is much more comprehension of the benefits of plants in this context than for drugs.

In support of this contention, a scientific review of the role of the microcirculation in health and disease observed:[2]

> The difficulty of accessing microcirculation in view of the extremely small dimensions of these vessels has been by far the principal reason why this enormous anatomical entity has been essentially neglected for decades. . . . With very few exceptions, pentoxifylline and the antidiabetic metformin, no specific treatments have been developed for treating disorders at the microcirculatory level.

5.1 What is the microcirculation?

The microvascular bed is an anatomical entity comprising countless small arterioles, capillaries, and venules. Tissues such as the retina of the eye and the glomeruli of the kidney are particularly rich in microcirculation, because of their specific functions. The health of the microcirculation determines the blood supply and nutrient flow to all our vital tissues, but especially to vulnerable structures such as the long nerves that flow out of our spinal column to our limbs. Hence, with diabetes, which damages the microcirculation (diabetic microangiopathy, the best-known expression of microvascular disease: see Section 5.9), the above-mentioned tissues are specifically affected as, respectively, retinopathy, nephropathy, and neuropathy.

5.2 The vascular endothelium

The vascular endothelium is the delicate monolayer of cells lining all blood vessels. It regulates the contractile and proliferative state of underlying smooth muscle cells and the interaction of the blood vessel wall with the circulating blood (e.g., as the gateway for immune cells and the interactions that trigger haemostasis). The multitude of tiny vessels throughout the body means the microcirculation contains the most significant proportion of the endothelial surface of the vascular bed. Hence, much of the understanding and implications of endothelial dysfunction are relevant to a consideration of microcirculatory health and vice versa.

5.3 Microvascular physiology

The small arteries and arterioles dilate or contract to maintain a constant flow of blood to the microvascular bed. Capillaries are also able to regulate their flow by transmitting signals to upstream controlling arterioles. A multitude of factors influence the contraction or relaxation of arterioles (such as innervation, insulin, melatonin, blood viscosity, and metabolites), but a key factor is nitric oxide (NO). In addition to this arteriolar control of capillary blood flow, other considerations are at play in determining the effective flow of blood through the capillaries. These include the haematocrit, blood viscosity, and red blood cell deformability/aggregation.

In terms of the last point, erythrocytes are biconcave-shaped cells with an axial diameter that is usually greater than the internal diameter of capillaries. They must therefore elongate to cross the capillary. Hence, red cell deformability is a crucial parameter for normal capillary flow, as illustrated by the vascular pain crisis in sickle cell anaemia patients.

5.4 Microvascular function and disease

According to the key review mentioned above:[3]

> The fundamental role of microvessels is to supply target tissues with oxygen and nutrients; therefore it appears logical that microvascular disorders will impact on tissue function, given the close coupling between flow and metabolism.[4]

This review then goes on to list a large range of diseases linked to microvascular dysfunction. These include overweight/obesity, diabetes, hypertension, low birth weight, sleep disorders, Alzheimer's disease (AD), gout, erythromelalgia, venous insufficiency, lupus, haemochromatosis, high serum ferritin, cardiometabolic syndrome, non-alcoholic steatotic hepatitis, polycystic ovary syndrome, gestational diabetes, acromegaly, rheumatoid arthritis, scleroderma, Bechet's disease, hyperdynamic circulation, myocardial infarction, stroke, beta-thalassaemia, and HIV. But even this extensive list is incomplete. Based on the current literature we can credibly add the following diseases or applications: liver disease in general, kidney disease, neuropathies/neuralgias, restless legs syndrome, osteoarthritis (OA), retinal diseases, poor healing of any tissue, intervertebral disc damage, recovery from ischaemic damage, anti-ageing, athletic performance, and cancer (especially to mitigate the damage caused by conventional treatments).

5.5 What damages the microcirculation?

Smoking is a key factor. A single cigarette has an immediate effect on microcirculatory control. Passive smoking (second-hand smoke) for 10 minutes from two cigarettes decreased capillary blood flow by more than 50%.[5] Based on assessment of dental surgical procedures, current smoking status was observed to adversely affect healing capacity, most likely reflecting on microvascular health.[6]

Other factors shown to damage vascular endothelial and microcirculatory integrity include poor glycaemic control (see Section 5.12.10), hypertension, increased oxidative stress, elevated homocysteine, obesity (see Section 5.9) and a high-fat meal.[7,8,9]

Surgical wound repair is a challenge in the elderly patient, with complications including dehiscence and infection. One proposed reason is that surgery disrupts the microvasculature of the aged skin, which already has diminished microcirculatory support. Most anaesthetics are also thought to adversely affect the microcirculation.[10]

5.6 Osteoarthritis and the microcirculation

One review has suggested that there is mounting evidence that a microvascular pathology plays a key role in the initiation and/or progression of OA.[11] Disruption of microvascular blood flow in subchondral bone may reduce nutrient diffusion to the articular cartilage. Specifically, ischaemia in subchondral bone due to microthrombi may produce osteocyte death, bone resorption, and articular damage. Another earlier review suggested that vascular disease in subchondral bone might accelerate the OA process.[12] This is either via reduced cartilage nutrition or, as per above, due to direct ischaemic effects on bone, depending on whether cartilage damage is the primary or secondary inflammatory event in OA. Bone marrow lesions, linked to a poorer prognosis for knee OA, could be secondary to such vascular events. Hence, regardless of its role in initiating OA (more relevant for prevention), microvascular disease is suggested to be highly relevant to its progression.

5.7 Heart disease and microcirculation

Coronary microvascular dysfunction (CMD) is under intense investigation because of a growing awareness of its importance. For example, in 354 patients with angina or angina-like chest pain with a normal angiogram, coronary flow reserve (a measure of heart microvascular health) was a comprehensive indicator of cardiovascular risk.[13]

More than half of women suffering from angina have no significant coronary artery obstruction. This is thought to be due to CMD.[14] In other words, CMD both is a predictor of cardiovascular events and contributes to the pathophysiology of angina.

Another interesting and related phenomenon is coronary slow flow. Coronary slow flow phenomenon (CSFP) is an important angiographic entity characterised by delayed progression of an injected contrast medium through the coronary tree. It is a frequent finding, typically observed in patients presenting with acute coronary syndromes.[15] Although well known to interventional cardiologists for approximately four decades, the exact pathogenic mechanisms remain unclear, but the microcirculation is clearly involved. The clinical implications are significant, with over 80% of patients experiencing recurrent chest pain, resulting in considerable impairment in quality of life. Studies have shown that small blood vessel disease, endothelial dysfunction, subclinical atherosclerosis, inflammation, and the anatomic properties of the coronary arteries are related to its occurrence. CSFP has been linked to smoking and elevated plasma homocysteine.[16]

5.8 The liver and microcirculation

There are major changes in the microcirculation of the liver with ageing. These include increased endothelial cell thickness and reduced numbers of pores (fenestrations). Such changes are thought to contribute to dyslipidaemia, vascular disease, liver degeneration, and poor drug metabolism.[17,18]

An article in the newspaper *The Australian* in 2006 by journalist Jill Margo noted the following about this research:

> Australian researchers have made a discovery that could prove beneficial to millions of older people. Through identifying how an ageing liver is starved of oxygen, they believe they may have uncovered an important factor in susceptibility to age-related diseases, including coronary artery diseases and nervous system disorders such as Parkinson's. . . . What they found had never been described before. They discovered that with age, tiny blood vessels in the liver undergo microscopic changes that can potentially translate into major diseases. Associate Professor David Le Couteur, a geriatrician and clinical pharmacologist at the Canberra school, says a young, healthy liver has unique blood vessels. Unlike vessels anywhere else in the body, they are very thin and full of holes and look rather like the wire mesh in flyscreen. This mesh allows oxygen being carried in the blood to pass effortlessly into the liver cells where it is used to fuel metabolic processes. With age, Le Couteur says this fine mesh-like structure changes dramatically. The vessels thicken, the holes close off and an underlying basement membrane develops. This means less oxygen can get through and that the liver cells have less oxygen to do their metabolic work (including processing toxins). The researcher's theory suggests that in old age these substances (toxins) can bypass the liver and deposit themselves elsewhere in the body where they can cause harm. Some fats may, for example, accumulate in coronary artery while a particular family of toxins might travel to the brain where they congregate and later manifest, perhaps as Parkinson's disease.[19]

5.9 Diabetic microangiopathy

Diabetic microangiopathy is directly linked to hyperglycaemia and can be detected in people with only marginally raised blood glucose levels. A popular theory focuses on postprandial hyperglycaemia: the rise in blood sugar after meals can interfere with normal blood vessel function even in healthy people. Poor eating (fat and/or sugar-rich meals) can, over time, damage the endothelial cells lining the microcirculation.[20]

As noted above, type 2 diabetes (T2D) causes microvascular disease. But there is a growing school of thought that microvascular dysfunction might actually be a fundamental cause of insulin resistance (IR), eventually leading to T2D. For example, retinal vascular calibre is one of several surrogate measures of microvascular dysfunction. A meta-analysis including more than 44,000 individuals found obesity to be significantly linked to narrower arteriolar and wider venular calibres.[21] We also know that obesity is a risk factor for IR.[22] Another study concluded that the data[23]

> indicate that various estimates of microvascular dysfunction were associated with incident T2DM and, possibly, impaired fasting glucose, suggesting a role for the microcirculation in the pathogenesis of T2DM.

5.10 Alzheimer's disease, brain health, and the brain microcirculation

One theory gaining increasing credibility is that the cause of AD lies in the cardiovascular system. Important aspects of the research focus are the roles of subcortical white matter lesions (WMLs) of the brain that appear to result from cerebral small vessel disease (see Section 5.10.5) and brain microbleeds (see Section 5.10.2).

5.10.1 White matter lesions

WMLs are indicated by areas of rarefaction or low attenuation on brain computed tomography (CT) scans. They are also described as white matter hyperintensities, because on magnetic resonance imaging (MRI) they show up as a more intense signal. The vulnerability of the white matter to ischaemia is due to it being supplied by long penetrating end arterioles from the surface and base of the brain, that travel for a long distance with very few interconnections.

CT of the brain shows that 30% of people aged 85 years have evidence of low attenuation of white matter. In contrast, MRI shows an incidence approaching 100% at age 85. Studies demonstrate that normal people with white matter ischaemia might have subtle neuropsychological deficits, such as a slower rate of mental processing and impaired attention and concentration.[24] For example, a meta-analysis of 27 published studies examined investigations in older adults who had a clinical diagnosis of cognitive impairment due to a vascular cause (WMLs), but not serious enough to impair their ability to function (no dementia).[25] Results demonstrated that those individuals had weaknesses across all cognitive domains relative to healthy controls, with the greatest impairment in the domain of processing speed, and the least affected being working memory and visuospatial construction. The authors concluded that disruption to subcortical white matter impairs more cognitive processes than typically thought. White matter ischaemia is also closely associated with vascular or so-called multi-infarct dementia. The key difference is that a patient need not show a history of strokes to have a cognitive impairment brought about by this ischaemia.[26] Hence it is appropriate to describe it as a quiet saboteur of the brain.[27]

5.10.2 Brain microbleeds

Another related concept is the origin of Alzheimer-like dementias (ALDs) from capillary haemorrhages.[28] The theory elevates the role of the microcirculation to a high importance in the aetiology of AD. To quote from a paper from Jonathon Stone, an Australian scientist championing this line of thinking:

> This paper proposes that the formation of each plaque is initiated by bleeding from a cerebral capillary, which creates the conditions for formation of an amyloid-rich plaque. Specifically, it is argued that ischaemia caused by the haemorrhage upregulates the expression of beta-amyloid by local neural cells, and that haemoglobin released into the neuropil binds to the beta-amyloid and promotes its oligomerisation. The premise that the event that initiates plaque formation is vascular explains why the risk factors for ALDs and cardiovascular diseases overlap; why drugs and lifestyle changes with vaso-protective effects protect against dementia; and why oxidative stress

is prominent early in the genesis of Alzheimer-like dementias. The vascular premise also suggests that the anatomical substrate for the spread of plaque formation is the capillary bed of the cerebral cortex, and provides an explanation of why plaque formation is age-related, occurring as the capillary bed becomes fragile with age. The more specific premise, that haemorrhage creates the conditions for plaque formation, explains many of the features of plaques: their small and relatively uniform size, each being at the site of a capillary bleed; why plaques form around capillaries; why haem is found in every plaque; why an inflammatory response is prominent where plaques form; why plaque formation and haemorrhagic stroke commonly co-occur in both sporadic and familial dementias; why plaques form around vessels in mouse models of plaque formation induced by transgenes that mimic the mutations that cause familial disease; why the acute petechial bleeding caused by brain trauma can lead to the formation of plaques. The hypothesis also suggests an explanation of how ALD's can occur without plaque formation, as when the cerebral capillaries become blocked or constricted in flow, without haemorrhage. Advances in the prevention of dementia will be gained, it is argued, from understanding of why the cerebral capillary bed becomes unstable with age, and how that instability can be prevented, delayed, or slowed. Advances in the treatment of dementia will be gained from techniques that minimise the neural damage caused by a multitude of tiny strokes.[20]

To quote further from Dr Stone in an Australian ABC radio interview:

> The beat of our heart is symbolic of life, of energy, of courage and determination. Yet . . . if we live to old age, the heart destroys us. And it does so in a terrible way, pummelling the brain beat after beat until its small blood vessels burst, and lesions, tens of thousands of them, erode its circuitry, until the brain shrinks around the debris, its function failing. Slowly, relentlessly – this evidence goes – the beat of the heart destroys the memory, the intellect and the personality of the person it had so long served to keep alive.[30]

In other words, brain microbleeds result from pulse-induced damage to the small cerebral vessels. The pulse becomes increasingly destructive with age because of the age-related stiffening of the aorta and great arteries, which causes an increase in the intensity of the pulse pressure.[31] This hypothesis highlights the dementia-preventing role of agents that maintain arterial elasticity, lower blood pressure, improve microvascular integrity, and protect the brain from microscopic ischaemic damage.

5.10.3 The role of arterial stiffness

Stiffening of the large arteries places extra pressure on the heart and increases the vascular load and stress on the microvasculature within the brain and the kidneys. Arterial stiffness describes a reduction in the ability of large arteries to easily accommodate the increase in blood volume following left ventricular ejection during systole and the correspondent increase in pulsatile force.[32] Arterial stiffness might also be considered an indirect measure of the level of microcirculatory damage within the brain and is a strong predictor of adverse cardiovascular outcomes, vascular morbidity, and mortality.[33] Pulse wave velocity (PWV) is used frequently as a measure of arterial stiffness and may be considered reflective of the overall "cardiovascular burden".

The link between arterial stiffness and AD has been explored in several research studies. One review article investigating the role arterial stiffness plays in AD pathogenesis proposed that arterial stiffness connects the pulsatile force of the heart to the brain.[34] Symptoms of AD were observed to be related to microvascular damage in the brain, which may be why the use of antihypertensive medications or natural treatments that preserve the integrity of the microvasculature can delay onset or slow progression of AD.[35]

One study explored diastolic function and aortic stiffness in 29 AD patients versus 24 healthy controls with normal cognitive function. Altered diastolic function was evident in the AD group.[36] Aortic distensibility and pressure-strain elastic modulus were used as measures of aortic stiffness and correlated with the presence of AD. Atrial conduction times were also associated with aortic stiffness and observed to be increased in the group of patients with AD.

Arterial stiffness leads to structural changes in the brain, as shown in the Second Manifestations of Arterial Disease–Magnetic Resonance (SMART-MR) study, where 526 participants underwent brain MRI and carotid artery distension measurements.[37] Increased arterial stiffness was linked with larger areas of atrophy within the brain and a higher density of vascular brain lesions. Stronger associations were observed in older patients with unaddressed hypertension and in those with a greater carotid intima media thickness. These factors suggest the presence of atherosclerosis and endothelial dysfunction. This study demonstrated that arterial stiffness, coupled with β-amyloid plaque deposition, induces brain atrophy and degenerative brain changes, producing observable cognitive deficits.

5.10.4 Pulse wave velocity and endothelial and cognitive functions

Carotid to femoral and carotid to radial PWVs are commonly used measures to detect arterial stiffness. The interrelationship between arterial stiffness (as indicated by pulse wave velocity), endothelial function, and cognition is also significant. This was explored through an assessment of stroke and dementia-free Framingham Offspring Study participants in a study of the relationship of tonometric arterial stiffness and endothelial function with brain MRI and cognition.[38] Greater arterial stiffness and pressure pulsatility were associated with brain ageing, MRI vascular insults, and the memory deficits typically seen in Alzheimer dementia.

A population-based study featuring 1,433 older adults measured PWV from carotid to femoral and carotid to radial arteries.[39] High arterial stiffness was associated with poorer cognitive function across several areas, including executive function, psychomotor speed, and memory. In this study, carotid to femoral PWV seemed to have a stronger link to decreased cognitive function than carotid to radial. These results also support the idea that arterial stiffness in large vessels is linked with poorer cognitive function.

As shown consistently across various research studies, PWV and cognitive function share an inverse relationship. The peripheral microcirculation consists of high-resistance vessels with a diameter of 300 µm that work towards maintaining steady blood flow.[40] With the ageing process, increased arterial stiffness leads to higher pulsatility, the impact of which ultimately results in an inward remodelling and rarefaction of the microvasculature in the cerebral arteries. This eventually leads to cognitive impairment and explains the increasing prevalence of dementia and AD with advancing age. Clinical utilisation of routine PWV measurement in the elderly is important and can help in the detection of AD and dementia symptoms, progression of these conditions, as well as targeting treatment measures aimed at improving the microcirculation and lowering arterial stiffness.

5.10.5 Cerebral small vessel disease

Cerebral small vessel disease (CSVD) is a collective term for several diseases affecting the small arteries, arterioles, venules, and capillaries of the brain, and refers to several pathological processes and aetiologies. Neuroimaging features of CSVD include recent small subcortical infarcts, lacunes (small deep infarcts resulting from occlusion of penetrating branches of larger cerebral arteries), white matter hyperintensities, perivascular spaces, microbleeds, and brain atrophy. It describes various pathophysiological processes that decrease the functionality of the microcirculation of the brain.[41] Although it remains contentious as to whether CSVD is a cause or sequela of AD, it is not far-fetched to suggest that effective therapeutic measures to ameliorate or prevent CSVD would mitigate the overall burden of dementia.

There are several classifications of CSVD; however, the most prevalent forms of are amyloidal CSVD (sporadic and hereditary cerebral amyloid angiopathy) and non-amyloidal CSVD (age-related and vascular risk-factor-related small vessel disease). Cerebral non-amyloid small vessel disease (NA-SVD) leads to narrowing of the arteriolar lumen, which decreases vascular conductance, along with the thickening of the vessel walls and loss of smooth muscle cells.[42] Vascular mild cognitive impairment (VMCI) precedes vascular dementia (VD) in more than half the patients who develop VD, and about two thirds of VMCI patients have NA-CSVD without the presence of infarcts.[43] Cerebral NA-SVD risk may be attributed to a variety of factors, some of which include genetics, lifestyle, environment, cigarette smoking, hypertension, diabetes, and age.[44] Significantly, the integrity of the blood–brain barrier may be lost in NA-SVD, leading to white and grey matter damage via neuroinflammation, leakage of fibrinogen and other neurotoxic proteins, and inadequate removal of toxic brain metabolites such as amyloid β.[45]

A measure reflecting capillary density is the level of von Willebrand factor, which correlates closely with a conventional quantification of capillary density.[46] The level of von Willebrand factor was found to be reduced markedly in the frontal white matter of people with severe NA-SVD. This could mean that NA-SVD eventually leads to cerebral hypoperfusion via capillary loss in the white matter, as well as to structural and non-structural changes in vessel quality.[47]

5.11 Endothelial function and disease

Closely allied to microcirculatory dysfunction is poor endothelial health. It is now thought that the key initiating event in the development of atherosclerosis is endothelial damage, followed by an inflammatory response. In support of this, endothelial dysfunction appears to predict arterial (large vessel) disease and the risk of a hard cardiovascular event (heart attack or stroke). Endothelial function can be measured by a number of techniques, including flow-mediated dilatation (FMD) and peripheral arterial tonometry (PAT). The latter is also known as the reactive hyperaemia index (RHI) (and sometimes called RH-PAT).[48] The former (FMD) tests endothelial function in large conduit blood vessels, while the latter tests such function in small arteries and the microcirculation.

A review concluded that traditional cardiovascular (CV) risk factors based on the Framingham study do not adequately predict future CV events. As per above, RHI, a non-invasive measurement of endothelial function, is emerging as a promising tool in CV risk prediction. Improvements in endothelial function have recently been linked to lower CV morbidity and mortality. A poor RHI has also been associated with the presence of vulnerable plaque, which is more likely to rupture and cause an acute CV event.

Erectile dysfunction (ED) in an otherwise healthy man is a warning sign of poor vascular endothelial health. In particular, endothelial NO production is typically impaired.[49]

5.12 Herbs and plant foods that benefit microcirculatory and endothelial health

5.12.1 Bilberry and other berry anthocyanins

The bilberry (*Vaccinium myrtillus*) contains blue-red plant pigments known as anthocyanins. These phytochemicals are also found in other berries.

Bilberry has a long-held reputation for benefitting vision, and a significant part of this probably arises from its support of the microcirculation. For example, in open trials, bilberry extract improved symptoms caused by decreased capillary resistance (microvascular bleeding, bruising, and faecal occult blood),[50] reduced the microcirculatory changes induced by cortisone therapy in patients with asthma and chronic bronchitis,[51] and improved diabetic retinopathy with a marked reduction or even disappearance of haemorrhages.[52] Post-operative complications from surgery of the nose were reduced in patients who received bilberry extract administered for 7 days before and 10 days after surgery. This was probably because of its benefits for the microcirculation.[53] In placebo-controlled trials, bilberry extract improved early-phase diabetic retinopathy.[54]

We could also add the blueberry (*Vaccinium corymbosum*), as a less active alternative. Indeed, a controlled clinical study involving 21 healthy men found that blueberry polyphenol intake improved FMD, with significant increases at 1–2 hours and then 6 hours after consumption (possibly reflecting the differing pharmacokinetics of the various polyphenolic metabolites).[55] Relevant to the previously noted vascular theory of AD, an 8-week, randomised, double blind, placebo-controlled clinical trial ($n = 40$) found that daily blueberry consumption (22 g freeze-dried powder) improved blood pressure, plasma NO, and arterial stiffness in postmenopausal women with early hypertension.[56]

In a randomised controlled trial of 51 metabolic syndrome patients, 750 mg of black raspberry extract (*Rubus occidentalis*) daily for 12 weeks significantly decreased arterial stiffness and increased circulating endothelial progenitor cells, thereby reducing overall cardiovascular risk.[57] The augmentation index is the percentage of central pulse pressure attributed to reflected wave overlap in systole and is associated with negative cardiovascular outcomes. Decreases in the radial artery augmentation index in contrast to placebo were also observed in the black raspberry group, possibly due to its anti-inflammatory and vasodilating actions.

5.12.2   Garlic

Garlic (*Allium sativum*, particularly as the fresh-crushed raw clove or as an allicin-releasing powder) is good for both the microcirculation and microcirculatory flow. For example, in a controlled clinical trial, a single 900 mg dose of garlic powder significantly increased capillary skin perfusion by 55%.[58] Another study found that garlic powder (600 mg/day) administered for 7 days increased calf blood flow by approximately 15%.[59]

These favourable effects of garlic on the microcirculation are probably mediated by its capacity to increase the production of the gas hydrogen sulfide (H_2S). In a remarkable scientific breakthrough, research on garlic revealed that it generates this significant gaseous signalling molecule. H_2S, also known as rotten egg gas, is toxic in high amounts. But it appears that the small quantities induced in the body by the ingestion of garlic could exert considerable cardiovascular benefits, as well as the characteristic garlic breath. Scientists were able to demonstrate that garlic-derived organic polysulphides, such as diallyl disulphide and diallyl trisulphide, act as H_2S donors: human red blood cells were able to convert these molecules into H_2S. The authors of the study suggested that the major beneficial effects of garlic intake on overall health might be mediated mainly by the biological production of H_2S.[60]

5.12.3 Gotu kola

Two controlled trials investigated the activity of gotu kola (*Centella asiatica*) actives (triterpenoids) in patients with microvascular damage due to diabetes. The largest trial involved 100 patients with or without neuropathy and 40 healthy controls and compared the extract with placebo over 12 months.[61] The herbal actives were significantly more effective at improving microcirculatory measures and oedema. A smaller trial in 50 patients compared a similar dose of gotu kola actives to placebo or no treatment over 6 months.[62] There was significant improvement in the active treated group in measures linked to microscopic vascular damage, including capillary permeability.

5.12.4 Ginkgo

Clinical studies of Ginkgo (*Ginkgo biloba*) in retinal problems best illustrate its positive effect on the microcirculation. For example, improved retinal artery and capillary flow rates have been observed,[63,64] which probably would explain its beneficial effect on vision in patients with glaucoma,[65] since glaucoma results in poor blood flow to the retina. In earlier research, a single dose of standardised Ginkgo extract (112.5 mg) resulted in a significant increase in blood flow in the nail capillaries of healthy volunteers.[66] Another study demonstrated increased blood flow to the forearms of volunteers.[67] These studies confirm the ability of Ginkgo to enhance microcirculatory flow, and one aspect of its activity might be the improvement of erythrocyte deformability.[68]

5.12.5 Grape seed

Several clinical trials using doses of 100–150 mg/day of oligomeric procyanidins (OPCs) from grape seed (*Vitis vinifera*) have demonstrated a beneficial effect on capillary resistance and capillary permeability.[69] For example, 100 mg/day of OPCs was administered to elderly patients with capillary fragility. Very good results were achieved in 67% of patients, good in 17%, and moderate in 13%. More recently, grape seed extract (GSE) at 133 mg/day for 14 days reduced leg swelling in healthy women during prolonged sitting (6 hours).[70]

In a small open trial, GSE supplementation at 300 mg/day for 4 weeks reduced systolic blood pressure ($p < 0.05$) and increased FMD ($p < 0.001$) in postmenopausal women.[71] Oral GSE therapy (150 mg/day) for one year improved hard exudates (HEs) in patients with non-proliferative diabetic retinopathy. The efficacy of GSE for HEs was higher than that of oral calcium dobesilate in the study patients.[72]

5.12.6 Cocoa

There are several studies suggestive of the positive effect of cocoa (*Theobroma cacao*) on the microcirculation and endothelium. In one clinical trial, the impairment of endothelial function caused by a glucose challenge was reduced by dark chocolate, but not by white chocolate.[73] Dark chocolate also reduced endothelial dysfunction in breath-hold divers.[74] A single dose of a flavanol-rich cocoa improved cerebral perfusion in 18 healthy older adults (placebo-controlled, crossover trial).[75]

A randomised controlled trial in 60 healthy young volunteers found that 10 g of dark chocolate a day (75% cocoa) for one month improved pulse wave velocity, arterial stiffness index and FMD.[76] A double blind, randomised controlled trial of 20 sedentary people found that 20 g of epicatechin rich dark chocolate daily for 3 months increased exercise capacity (VO_2 max output and maximum work in watts), which may have resulted from increased skeletal muscle mitochondrial efficiency.[77] Reduced glutathione levels and decreased protein carbonylation were also observed in the dark chocolate group.

Habitual cocoa consumption decreased arterial stiffness in a randomised, parallel-group study conducted on 26 post-menopausal women, who ingested 17 g of cocoa once daily over 12 weeks.[78] Cocoa flavanols have also stimulated NO production in endothelial cells.[79]

5.12.7 Beetroot

The beetroot (*Beta vulgaris*) is one of the richest sources of dietary nitrate. It is now realised that a specific pathway in the body can make NO from dietary nitrate: the nitrate–nitrite–NO pathway.[80] This has profound implications for microcirculatory and endothelial health and for regulating blood pressure, as many clinical studies have already demonstrated.

Several studies also support the use of beetroot juice high in nitrate for improving athletic performance and endurance. In a study with 32 well-trained male soccer players, supplementation with nitrate-enriched beetroot juice (equivalent to 800 mg nitrate daily) for 6 days resulted in a 3.4% improvement in performance of high-intensity intermittent-type exercises, when compared to a nitrate-depleted beetroot juice.[81] This is probably due to the ability of nitrate to increase blood flow and enhance the contractile capacity of type II muscle fibres. Another study in 2017 demonstrated the effect of nitrate in beetroot juice on physiological performance and functioning in trained runners and triathletes.[82] Acute beetroot juice supplementation (140 mL) significantly enhanced the 1500 m, but not 10,000 m time-trial performance.

5.12.8 Coffee and green tea

With the changes in microcirculation affecting the liver due to ageing in mind, it is interesting to note that coffee plays a role in reducing liver stiffness, as discovered through the ongoing prospective population-based study known as the Rotterdam Study.[83] As part of this study, 2,424 people participated in transient elastography and ultrasound and completed a food frequency questionnaire. The researchers discovered that liver stiffness measurements were decreased with higher coffee consumption. Participants consuming herbal teas also exhibited lower liver stiffness. It was concluded that three or more cups of coffee daily or herbal tea was linked to lower liver stiffness.

Green tea (*Camellia sinensis*) for two weeks improved forearm endothelial dysfunction in smokers.[84] There was also a significant increase in plasma NO. Green tea (4 weeks) also improved FMD (from $5.7 \pm 2.7\%$ to $8.7 \pm 3.5\%$) in patients with chronic kidney disease.[85] Another clinical study in healthy volunteers found epigallocatechin gallate (EGCG) is most likely not involved in the observed improvement of FMD by green tea. Instead, other tea compounds and/or metabolites may play a role.[86]

5.12.9 Korean ginseng

Outcomes of some clinical trials suggest that Korean red ginseng (KRG, *Panax ginseng*) also improves microcirculation. For example, a randomised, placebo-controlled trial in 80 women found that 6 g/day of KRG for 8 weeks significantly increased the skin temperature of the hands and feet.[87] Another trial found 1.5 g/day of KRG extract for 8 weeks decreased the imbalance in local thermal distribution of the body (as assessed by digital infrared thermal imaging).[88] The authors suggest that this is evidence that KRG improves circulation (and, more specifically, microcirculation). In a pilot trial, KRG (3 g) improved FMD, an effect reproduced by the equivalent dose of isolated ginsenosides.[89]

5.12.10 Some dietary insights

Insights from an Indian paradox also point to other herbs that might be beneficial for microcirculatory and endothelial health. Briefly put, the prevalence of T2D in India is relatively high and with poor glycaemic control (average

HbA$_{1C}$ 9.2%). Yet microvascular complications, such as retinopathy, are only 16.6%,[90] compared with Europe, Japan, the United States, and Australia at around 30%.[91] Could it be that the many spices in the Indian diet, especially turmeric (*Curcuma longa*), cayenne (*Capsicum annuum*), and ginger (*Zingiber officinale*), support microcirculatory health? The physiomedicalists described ginger as a "diffusive stimulant", directly pointing to its effect on the microcirculation.

Consumption of spicy foods was inversely associated with total mortality and deaths from cancer, heart disease, and respiratory disease in a large population-based cohort study conducted in China.[92] Higher fresh fruit consumption was found to reduce T2D incidence as well as macrovascular and microvascular complications in a 7-year prospective study of 0.5 million Chinese adults, which is contrary to the traditional belief held within the Chinese population that excess fresh fruit consumption leads to T2D.[93]

5.13 The 5-point microvascular phytonutrient diet

Based on the above evidence, a 5-point phytonutrient dietary plan (in conjunction with herbs such as gotu kola, grape seed extract, Korean ginseng, and Ginkgo as additional treatments) is recommended for patients with poor microvascular/endothelial health.

The plan is as follows:

- Boost dietary nitrate: green leafy vegetables, but especially beetroot as juice (at least 200 mL/day) or a supplement.
- Increase cocoa intake: for example, 85% chocolate, 20 g/day.
- Increase berry anthocyanin intake: 50–100 g/day of blueberries, strawberries, raspberries, and blackberries.
- Use fresh-crushed raw garlic: ½–1 clove/day.
- Increase herbs and spices, especially green tea (3–4 cups/day), turmeric, and ginger.

5.14 Improving microcirculatory flow with herbs

Key herbal strategies to improve microcirculatory flow, based largely on the above review, are the following:

- to boost endothelial function: green tea, garlic, Korean ginseng, turmeric (curcumin), grape seed
- to enhance microvascular integrity: grape seed, bilberry, gotu kola
- to boost microvascular flow: Ginkgo, turmeric (curcumin), ginger, garlic, dan shen (*Salvia miltiorrhiza*), Coleus (*Coleus forskolii*)

5.15 A case history

Regardless of the aetiology (hypertension, diabetes mellitus, atherosclerosis, obesity, and so on), chronic kidney disease (CKD) universally associates with microvascular rarefaction. A progressive damage of the microcirculation deteriorates renal haemodynamics and perfusion, leading to a progressive loss of filtration, tubular function, and development of fibrosis, which, in turn, serves as a feedback mechanism that may further accelerate progression of CKD towards irreversible renal injury.[94]

A 61-year-old man presented with the main problem of declining kidney function. As well as having high blood pressure (controlled by multiple drugs), he also had T2D, although this was controlled well with just diet. His poor kidney function could have been caused by the diabetes, but a medical specialist advised that some type of autoimmune damage to the glomeruli might be at play as well. In addition, tests showed that the tissue around his glomeruli exhibited a high degree of fibrosis, leading to a main diagnosis of arterionephrosclerosis. His glomerular filtration rate (eGFR) was quite abnormal at 35, and his plasma creatinine was elevated. His renal specialist had advised that, based on his current rate of deterioration, he will probably be needing dialysis in 18–24 months.

The patient was recommended to follow the 5-point phytonutrient dietary plan above. In addition, he was prescribed tablets containing high doses of Echinacea root (for the autoimmune aspects), turmeric (Nrf2, anti-inflammatory and protective of the kidneys), and grape seed, gotu kola, and Ginkgo for his microcirculation. He was also advised to take a high-dose fish oil supplement for its anti-inflammatory omega-3 fatty acids.

He had another blood test conducted by his medical specialist 5 months later. To both their surprise, his creatinine level had fallen by 33%, and his eGFR had risen to 51. His specialist commented that it was very rare for the eGFR to come back in this way, especially with his damaged kidneys. Normally it is a one-way decline. Eighteen months after the patient's initial presentation for herbal treatment, his eGFR had returned to normal at 74. Six years later it is maintained at around these normal levels.

References

1. Aird WC. Spatial and temporal dynamics of the endothelium. *J Thromb Haemost.* 2005; **3**: 1392–1406.
2. Wiernsperger N, Rapin JR. Microvascular diseases: is a new era coming? *Cardiovasc Hematol Agents Med Chem.* 2012; **10**(2): 167–183. [p 167]
3. Ibid.
4. Ibid. [p 172]
5. Henriksson P, Lu Q, Diczfalusy U, et al. Immediate effect of passive smoking on microcirculatory flow. *Microcirculation.* 2014; **21**(7): 587–592.
6. Balaji SM. Tobacco smoking and surgical healing of oral tissues: a review. *Indian J Dent Res.* 2008; **19**(4): 344–348.
7. Tyagi SC, Lominadze D, Roberts AM. Homocysteine in microvascular endothelial cell barrier permeability. *Cell Biochem Biophys.* 2005; **43**(1): 37–44.
8. Chantler PD, Frisbee JC. Arterial function in cardio-metabolic diseases: from the microcirculation to the large conduits. *Prog Cardiovasc Dis.* 2015; **57**(5): 489–496.
9. Boillot A, Zoungas S, Mitchell P, et al. Obesity and the microvasculature: a systematic review and meta-analysis. *PloS One.* 2013; **8**(2): e52708. doi:10.1371/journal.pone.0052708.
10. Bentov I, Reed MJ. Anesthesia, microcirculation, and wound repair in aging. *Anesthesiology.* 2014; **120**(3): 760–772.
11. Findlay DM. Vascular pathology and osteoarthritis. *Rheumatology.* 2007; **46**(12): 1763–1768.
12. Conaghan PG, Vanharanta H, Dieppe PA. Is progressive osteoarthritis an atheromatous vascular disease? *Ann Rheum Dis.* 2005; **64**(11): 1539–1541.
13. Lee DH, Youn HJ, Choi YS et al. Coronary flow reserve is a comprehensive indicator of cardiovascular risk factors in subjects with chest pain and normal coronary angiogram. *Circ J.* 2010; **74**(7): 1405–1414.
14. Prescott E, Abildstrøm SZ, Aziz A, et al. Improving diagnosis and treatment of women with angina pectoris and microvascular disease: the iPOWER study design and rationale. *Am Heart J.* 2014; **167**(4): 452–458.
15. Wang X, Nie SP. The coronary slow flow phenomenon: characteristics, mechanisms

and implications. *Cardiovasc Diagn Ther.* 2011; **1**(1): 37–43. doi:10.3978/j.issn.2223-3652.2011.10.01.
16. Li N, Tian L, Ren J, Li Y, Liu Y. Evaluation of homocysteine in the diagnosis and prognosis of coronary slow flow syndrome. *Biomark Med.* 2019; **13**(17): 1439–1446. doi:10.2217/bmm-2018-0446.
17. Le Couteur DG, Fraser R, Hilmer S, et al. The hepatic sinusoid in aging and cirrhosis: effects on hepatic substrate disposition and drug clearance. *Clin Pharmacokinet.* 2005; **44**(2): 187–200.
18. Le Couteur DG, Warren A, Cogger VC, et al. Old age and the hepatic sinusoid. *Anat Rec (Hoboken).* 2008; **291**(6): 672–683.
19. Margo J. *The Australian.* 2006.
20. Wiernsperger N, Rapin JR. Microvascular diseases: is a new era coming? *Cardiovasc Hematol Agents Med Chem.* 2012; **10**(2): 167–183.
21. Boillot A, Zoungas S, Mitchell P, et al. Obesity and the microvasculature: a systematic review and meta-analysis. *PloS One.* 2013; **8**(2): e52708.
22. Castro AV, Kolka CM, Kim SP, et al. Obesity, insulin resistance and comorbidities? Mechanisms of association. *Arq Bras Endocrinol Metabol.* 2014; **58**(6): 600–609.
23. Muris DM, Houben AJ, Schram MT, et al. Microvascular dysfunction is associated with a higher incidence of type 2 diabetes mellitus: a systematic review and meta-analysis. *Arterioscler Thromb Vasc Biol.* 2012; **32**(12): 3082–3094. [p 3082]
24. Bone KM, Mills SY. *Principles and Practice of Phytotherapy: Modern Herbal Medicine*, 2nd ed. Elsevier, UK, 2013, pp 596–627.
25. Vasquez BP, Zakzanis KK. The neuropsychological profile of vascular cognitive impairment not demented: a meta-analysis. *J Neuropsychol.* 2015 Mar; **9**(1): 109–136.
26. Ibid.
27 www.sciencedaily.com/releases/2014/02/140224204806.htm
28. Stone J. What initiates the formation of senile plaques? The origin of Alzheimer-like dementias in capillary haemorrhages. *Med Hypotheses.* 2008 Sep; **71**(3): 347–359.
29. Ibid. [p 347]
30. www.abc.net.au/radionational/programs/ockhamsrazor/dementia3a-a-tale-of-two-organs/6051492#transcript
31. Stone J, Johnstone DM, Mitrofanis J, et al. The mechanical cause of age-related dementia (Alzheimer's disease): the brain is destroyed by the pulse. *J Alzheimers Dis* .2015; **44**(2): 355–373.
32. Rabkin SW. Arterial stiffness: detection and consequences in cognitive impairment and dementia of the elderly. *J Alzheimers Dis.* 2012; **32**: 541–549.
33. Laurent, S, Cockcroft, J, Van Bortel, L, et al. European Network for Non-Invasive, Investigation of Large Arteries. Expert consensus document on arterial stiffness: methodological issues and clinical applications. *Eur Heart J.* 2006; **27**: 2588–2605.
34. Mitchell GF. Effects of central arterial aging on the structure and function of the peripheral vasculature: implications for end-organ damage. *J Appl Physiol.* 2008; **105**(5): 1652–1660.
35. Hughes TM, Craft S, Lopez OL. Review of "The potential role of arterial stiffness in the pathogenesis of Alzheimer's disease". *Neurodegener Dis Manag.* 2015; **5**(2): 121–135.
36. Çalık AN, Özcan KS, Yüksel G, et al. Altered diastolic function and aortic stiffness in Alzheimer's disease. *Clin Interv Aging.* 2014 Jul; **16**(9): 1115–1121.
37. Jochemsen HM, Muller M, Bots ML, et al., SMART Study Group. Arterial stiffness and progression of structural brain changes: the SMART-MR study. *Neurology.* 2015 Feb 3; **84**(5): 448–455.

38. Tsao CW, Seshadri S, Beiser AS, et al. Relations of arterial stiffness and endothelial function to brain aging in the community. *Neurology.* 2013 Sep 10; **81**(11): 984–991.
39. Zhong W, Cruickshanks KJ, Schubert CR, et al. Pulse wave velocity and cognitive function in older adults. *Alzheimer Dis Assoc Disord.* 2014 Jan–Mar; **28**(1): 44–49.
40. Scuteri A, Wang H. Pulse wave velocity as a marker of cognitive impairment in the elderly. *J Alzheimers Dis.* 2014; **42**(Suppl 4): S401–410.
41. Pantoni L. Cerebral small vessel disease: from pathogenesis and clinical characteristics to therapeutic challenges. *Lancet Neurol.* 2010 Jul; **9**(7): 689–701.
42. Girouard H, Iadecola C. Neurovascular coupling in the normal brain and in hypertension, stroke, and Alzheimer disease. *J Appl Physiol(1985).* 2006 Jan; **100**(1): 328–335.
43. Meyer JS, Xu G, Thornby J, et al. Is mild cognitive impairment prodromal for vascular dementia like Alzheimer's disease? *Stroke.* 2002 Aug; **33**(8): 1981–1985.
44. Charidimou, A, Pantoni, L, Love, S. The concept of sporadic cerebral small vessel disease: a road map on key definitions and current concepts. *Int J Stroke.* 2016; **11**: 6–18.
45. Bell RD, Winkler EA, Sagare AP, et al. Pericytes control key neurovascular functions and neuronal phenotype in the adult brain and during brain aging. *Neuron.* 2010 Nov 4; **68**(3): 409–427.
46. Thomas, T., Miners, S, Love, S. Post-mortem assessment of hypoperfusion of cerebral cortex in Alzheimer's disease and vascular dementia. *Brain.* 2015; **138**: 1059–1069.
47. Barker, R, Ashby, EL, Wellington, D, et al. Pathophysiology of white matter perfusion in Alzheimer's disease and vascular dementia. *Brain.* 2014; **137**, 1524–1532.
48. Reriani MK, Lerman LO, Lerman A. Endothelial function as a functional expression of cardiovascular risk factors. *Biomark Med.* 2010; **4**(3): 351–360.
49. Mitidieri E, Cirino G, d'Emmanuele di Villa Bianca R, et al. Pharmacology and perspectives in erectile dysfunction in man. *Pharmacol Ther.* 2020 Apr; **208**: 107493. doi:10.1016/j.pharmthera.2020.107493.
50. Piovella C, Curri BS, Piovella M, et al. *Terapia Angiol.* 1979; **35**: 119.
51. Carmignani G. Lotta Contro La Tuberce Malattie. *Polm Soc.* 1983; **53**: 732.
52. Orsucci PL, Rossi M, Sabbatini G, et al. Trattamento della retonpatia diabetic con antocianosidil Indagine preliminare. *Clin Ocul.* 1983; **4**: 377.
53. Mattioli L, Dallari S, Galetti R. Vaccinium myrtillus L. *Fitoterapia.* 1988; **59**(Suppl 1): 41.
54. Repossi P, Malagola R, de Cadihac C. The role of anthocyanosides on vascular permeability in diabetic retinopathy. *Ann Ottal Clin Ocul.* 1987; **113**(4): 357–361.
55. Rodriguez-Mateos A, Rendeiro C, Bergillos-Meca T, et al. Intake and time dependence of blueberry flavonoid- induced improvements in vascular function: a randomized, controlled, double-blind, crossover intervention study with mechanistic insights into biological activity. *Am J Clin Nutr.* 2013; **98**(5): 1179–1191.
56. Johnson SA, Figueroa A, Navaei N, et al. Daily blueberry consumption improves blood pressure and arterial stiffness in postmenopausal women with pre- and stage 1-hypertension: a randomized, double-blind, placebo-controlled clinical trial. *J Acad Nutr Diet.* 2015; **115**(3): 369–377.
57. Jeong HS, Kim S, Hong SJ, et al. Black raspberry extract increased circulating endothelial progenitor cells and improved arterial stiffness in patients with metabolic syndrome: a randomized controlled trial. *Journal of Medicinal Food.* 2016; **19**(4): 346–352.
58. Jung EM, Jung F, Mrowietz C, et al. Influence of garlic powder on cutaneous microcirculation: a randomized placebo-controlled double-blind crossover study in apparently healthy subjects. *Arzneimittelforschung.* 1991; **41**(6): 626–630.
59. Anim-Nyame N, Sooranna SR, Johnson MR, et al. Garlic supplementation increases peripheral blood flow: a role for interleukin–6? *J Nutr Biochem.* 2004; **15**(1): 30–36.

60. Benavides GA, Squadrito GL, Mills RW, et al. Hydrogen sulfide mediates the vasoactivity of garlic. *Proc Natl Acad Sci USA*. 2007; **104**(46): 17977–17982. doi:10.1073/pnas.0705710104.
61. Incandela L, Belcaro G, Cesarone MR, et al. Treatment of diabetic microangiopathy and edema with total triterpenic fraction of *Centella asiatica*: a prospective, placebo-controlled randomized study. *Angiology*. 2001; **52**(Suppl 2): S27–S31.
62. Cesarone MR, Incandela L, De Sanctis MT, et al. Evaluation of treatment of diabetic microangiopathy with total triterpenic fraction of *Centella asiatica*: a clinical prospective randomized trial with a microcirculatory model. *Angiology*. 2001; **52**(Suppl 1–2): S49–S54.
63. Chung HS, Harris A, Kristinsson JK, et al. Ginkgo biloba extract increases ocular blood flow velocity. *J Ocul Pharmacol Ther*. 1999; **15**(3): 233–240.
64. Huang SY, Jeng C, Kao SC, et al. Improved haemorheological properties by Ginkgo biloba extract (Egb 761) in type 2 diabetes mellitus complicated with retinopathy. *Clin Nutr*. 2004; **23**(4): 615–621.
65. Quaranta L, Bettelli S, Uva MG, et al. Effect of Ginkgo biloba extract on preexisting visual field damage in normal tension glaucoma. *Ophthalmology*. 2003; **110**(2): 359–362.
66. Jung F, Mrowietz C, Kiesewetter H, et al. Effect of Ginkgo biloba on fluidity of blood and peripheral microcirculation in volunteers. *Arzneimittelforschung*. 1990 May; **40**(5): 589–593.
67. Mehlsen J, Drabaek H, Wiinberg N, et al. Effects of a Ginkgo biloba extract on forearm haemodynamics in healthy volunteers. *Clin Physiol Funct Imaging*. 2002 Nov; **22**(6): 375–378.
68. Jung F, Mrowietz C, Kiesewetter H, Wenzel E. Effect of Ginkgo biloba on fluidity of blood and peripheral microcirculation in volunteers. *Arzneimittelforschung*. 1990; **40**(5): 589–593. PMID 2383302.
69. Morgan M, Andrews C. *Nutritional Perspective*. 2007; **26**: 1–3.
70. Sano A, Tokutake S, Seo A. Proanthocyanidin-rich grape seed extract reduces leg swelling in healthy women during prolonged sitting. *J Sci Food Agric*. 2013; **93**(3): 457–462.
71. Lee DS, Kim J. Effects of grape seed extract supplementation on hemodynamic response and vascular endothelial function in postmenopausal women. *Iran J Public Health*. 2019; **48**(9): 1735–1737.
72. Moon SW, Shin YU, Cho H, Bae SH, Kim HK; and for the Mogen Study Group. Effect of grape seed proanthocyanidin extract on hard exudates in patients with non-proliferative diabetic retinopathy. *Medicine (Baltimore)*. 2019; **98**(21): e15515. doi:10.1097/MD.0000000000015515.
73. Grassi D, Desideri G, Necozione S, et al. Protective effects of flavanol-rich dark chocolate on endothelial function and wave reflection during acute hyperglycemia. *Hypertension*. 2012; **60**(3): 827–832.
74. Theunissen S, Schumacker J, Guerrero F, et al. Dark chocolate reduces endothelial dysfunction after successive breath-hold dives in cool water. *Eur J Appl Physiol*. 2013; **113**(12): 2967–2975.
75. Lamport DJ, Pal D, Moutsiana C, et al. The effect of flavanol-rich cocoa on cerebral perfusion in healthy older adults during conscious resting state: a placebo controlled, crossover, acute trial. *Psychopharmacology (Berl)*. 2015; **232**(17): 3227–3234.
76. Pereira T, Maldonado J, Laranjeiro M, et al. Central arterial hemodynamic effects of dark chocolate ingestion in young healthy people: a randomized and controlled trial. *Cardiol Res Pract*. 2014; **2014**: 945–951. doi:10.1155/2014/945951.
77. Taub PR, Ramirez-Sanchez I, Patel M, et al. Beneficial effects of dark chocolate on exercise capacity in sedentary subjects: underlying mechanisms. A double blind, randomized, placebo controlled trial. *Food Funct*. 2016 Sep 14; **7**(9): 3686–3693.

78. Okamoto T, Kobayashi R, Natsume M, et al. Habitual cocoa intake reduces arterial stiffness in postmenopausal women regardless of intake frequency: a randomized parallel-group study. *Clin Interv Aging*. 2016 Nov; **14**(11): 1645–1652.
79. Heiss C, Dejam A, Kleinbongard P, et al. Vascular effects of cocoa rich in flavan–3-ols. *JAMA*. 2003; **290**(8): 1030–1031.
80. Morgan M. Beet, greens & herbs for health & vitality. *Nutritional Perspective*. 2013; **38**: 1–7.
81. Nyakayiru J, Jonvik KL, Trommelen J, et al. Beetroot juice supplementation improves high-intensity intermittent type exercise performance in trained soccer players. *Nutrients*. 2017 Mar 22; **9**(3): E314. doi:10.3390/nu9030314.
82. Shannon OM, Barlow MJ, Duckworth L, et al. Dietary nitrate supplementation enhances short but not longer duration running time trial performance. *Eur J Appl Physiol*. April 2017; **117**(4): 775–785.
83. Alferink LJM, Fittipaldi J, Kiefte-de Jong JC, et al. Coffee and herbal tea consumption is associated with lower liver stiffness in the general population: the Rotterdam study. *J Hepatol*. 2017 Aug; **67**(2): 339–348.
84. Oyama J, Maeda T, Kouzuma K, et al. Green tea catechins improve human forearm endothelial dysfunction and have antiatherosclerotic effects in smokers. *Circ J*. 2010; **74**(3): 578–588.
85. Park CS, Kim W, Woo JS, et al. Green tea consumption improves endothelial function but not circulating endothelial progenitor cells in patients with chronic renal failure. *Int J Cardiol*. 2010; **145**(2): 261–262.
86. Lorenz M, Rauhut F, Hofer C, et al. Tea-induced improvement of endothelial function in humans: no role for epigallocatechin gallate (EGCG). *Sci Rep*. 2017; **7**(1): 2279. doi:10.1038/s41598-017-02384-x.
87. Park KS, Park KI, Kim JW, et al. Efficacy and safety of Korean red ginseng for cold hypersensitivity in the hands and feet: a randomized, double-blind, placebo-controlled trial. *J Ethnopharmacol*. 2014; **158** Pt A: 25–32.
88. Kang J, Lee N, Ahn Y, et al. Study on improving blood flow with Korean red ginseng substances using digital infrared thermal imaging and Doppler sonography: randomized, double blind, placebo-controlled clinical trial with parallel design. *J Tradit Chin Med*. 2013; **33**(1): 39–45.
89. Jovanovski E, Peeva V, Sievenpiper JL, et al. Modulation of endothelial function by Korean red ginseng (Panax ginseng C.A. Meyer) and its components in healthy individuals: a randomized controlled trial. *Cardiovasc Ther*. 2014; **32**(4): 163–169.
90. Mohan V, Shah S, Saboo B. Current glycemic status and diabetes related complications among type 2 diabetes patients in India: data from the A1chieve study. *J Assoc Physicians India*. 2013; **61**(1 Suppl): 12–15.
91. Raman R, Rani PK, Reddi Rachepalle S, et al. Prevalence of diabetic retinopathy in India: Sankara Nethralaya Diabetic Retinopathy Epidemiology and Molecular Genetics Study report 2. *Ophthalmology*. 2009; **116**(2): 311–318.
92. Lv J, Qi L, Yu C, et al. Consumption of spicy foods and total and cause specific mortality: population based cohort study. *BMJ*. 2015 Aug 4; **351**: h3942. doi:10.1136/bmj.h3942.
93. Du H, Li L, Bennett D, et al. Fresh fruit consumption in relation to incident diabetes and diabetic vascular complications: A 7-y prospective study of 0.5 million Chinese adults. *Plos MED*. 2017 Apr 11; **14**(4): e1002279. doi:10.1371/journal.pmed.1002279.
94. Chade AR. Small vessels, big role: renal microcirculation and progression of renal injury. *Hypertension*. 2017; **69**(4): 551–563. doi:10.1161/HYPERTENSIONAHA.116.08319.

6

Cellular protection and the Nrf2 pathway: a core FHT strategy

This chapter scopes the supporting evidence for and clinical ramifications of the core FHT strategy of supporting and enhancing cellular health and protection (cytoprotection). The central significance of priming the Nrf2 pathway forms much of the discussion. Ensuring good cytoprotection will minimise the damage caused by the constant exposure to both external and internal toxic factors that threaten cellular integrity.

6.1   Basic redox chemistry and definitions

Redox (short for reduction-oxidation) describes chemical reactions where the oxidative state of the component atoms in a molecule changes. With oxidation (one half of the redox reaction), there is a loss of electrons or an addition of oxygen. With reduction (the other half of the redox reaction), there is a gain of electrons or an addition of hydrogen. The two reactions occur simultaneously, hence the combined term redox.

In a redox reaction the oxidant (oxidising agent) is reduced and the reducing agent is oxidised. Hence there is potentially a flow of electrons from the reducing agent to the oxidant. A chemical that is good at giving away electrons is a powerful reducing agent.

Similarly, a chemical that actively seeks electrons (an electrophile) is a powerful oxidising agent. Because electron flow is often involved, chemicals involved in redox reactions can be placed in an electrochemical series, depending on their redox potentials (measured in volts).

The more negative the redox potential, the more powerful the reducing agent. The more positive the potential, the more powerful the oxidant. When a chemical is placed in this series, anything with a more negative redox potential can reduce it, anything with a more positive potential can oxidise it. Hence, depending on the environment and what it reacts with, an antioxidant (reducing) chemical can become a pro-oxidant (oxidising agent). Moreover, *any* chemical entity involved in a redox reaction has both an oxidised form (that can act as pro-oxidant) and a reduced form (that can act as an antioxidant).

In the human body, many key oxidising agents are based on oxygen and are called reactive oxygen species (ROS). ROS are produced as a normal product of cellular metabolism. Many ROS have unpaired electrons that need to find a pair: such chemicals are known as free radicals. Free radicals can damage tissue by causing cross-linking of molecules and chain reactions.

6.2 The herbal antioxidant cliché

We all hear about antioxidants! They are the good things in our diet that protect us against the evils of damage caused by free radicals. However, in both scientific circles and to a lesser extent consumer opinion, there has been a rethink of the value of antioxidants, largely led by the negative publicity from certain clinical trials (such as the one on beta-carotene).[1] Unfortunately, this more informed perspective has not yet reached the mainstream media or even some marketers of natural remedies.

The rethink was highlighted in a 2012 article in the industry newsletter *newhope360*:

> Antioxidants as an ingredient category have suffered from the "magic pill" syndrome. In the past 15 years these ingredients have soared on promises that remain mostly unfulfilled and crashed on doubts that were overstated.[2]

The author, Hank Schultz, went on to write:[3]

> More than a decade ago information about the damage that free oxygen radicals can do in cells was becoming fixed in consumers' consciousness. In a society focused on the attainment of eternal youth, free radicals, which had

been linked to premature aging, had become the new bogeymen. And new miracle molecules – antioxidants – were coming to the rescue, armed with the powerful weapon of high ORAC values. ORAC numbers (oxygen radical absorption capacity) began to be quoted on package labels. . . . This quick climb to the top began to be clouded by wavering doubts.

First, there was the question of the ORAC test itself. . . . Then there is the *in vitro* versus *in vivo* question. It doesn't matter how good the sponge might be if you can't use it to clean your kitchen.

The "*in vitro* versus *in vivo* question" means that not all results produced in test tubes, such as ORAC values, translate into meaningful effects in living bodies.

6.3 Concerns over "antioxidants"

In scientific circles, concerns over the value of antioxidants go much further than this. The key free radicals produced in the body, the reactive oxygen species (ROS, which may be described as energised forms of oxygen), might sometimes be beneficial. ROS are a byproduct of cellular metabolism, for instance, in our mitochondria. As noted above, many ROS contain unpaired electrons that, desirous of finding a pair, strip electrons from covalent bonds, disrupting them and creating further free radicals. As a result, these free radicals cause damage to tissues via molecular cross linkages and chain reactions.

The discovery of ROS signalling (where free radicals trigger essential healthy responses) has been verified as important pathway in a variety of physiological functions, including glucose-stimulated insulin secretion and the arming of defences against invading micro-organisms.[4] ROS can also promote anti-tumour signalling, initiating oxidative stress-induced tumour cell death (part of the basis of concern over taking "antioxidants" during chemotherapy).

To add fuel to the fire, there are even new doubts over the oxidative stress theory of ageing. This theory was first proposed in 1956 by Harman, as follows: ROS inflict indiscriminate oxidative damage to cells that is not completely neutralised by antioxidants and/or repaired. Damage then accumulates with time, causing the changes we know as ageing. "Despite the intuitive logic and vast support for this theory, a causal link between oxidative stress and the rate of ageing has not been clearly established."[5]

Also, as noted above, antioxidants might become pro-oxidants in the right environment: examples include the tumour-killing ability of intravenous ascorbic acid and the negative clinical results for isolated beta-carotene in smokers.

Ironically, at the same time there has been an intriguing new insight into how plant-based chemicals (phytochemicals) might exert antioxidant activity in the body. This new understanding completely dismisses most negative concerns about using herbs for antioxidant protection and, furthermore, provides intriguing insights into the primordial relationship between plant intake and cellular health in the human body. It will also hopefully change the way you think about phytochemical antioxidants forever.

6.4 Biological versus chemical antioxidation

Any given antioxidant molecule can certainly prevent the damage induced by ROS, namely to DNA, protein, and other important biomolecules. However, the use of antioxidant nutrient supplements in isolation (e.g., vitamins C and E) is not an ideal approach, nor is it targeted. An unstated aspect of the antioxidant theory is that they act as passive sponges of free radicals, usually operating outside the cell. Hence, to gain a significant protection against damaging free radicals, we need to take large (possibly unrealistic) amounts to flood the body tissues with enough activity. Moreover, once they are inside our body, we cannot control any potentially negative radical-scavenging effects, because they are just acting passively. Hence, this blanket approach to antioxidation might interfere with the important positive functions of ROS noted above.

In essence, antioxidants are a very useful clinical tool, but the manner in which they are administered and utilised must be targeted and controlled. We can call this targeted approach "biological" antioxidation. The important differences between biological and chemical antioxidation are outlined in **Table 6.1**.

Expanding on the above, a chemical antioxidant (such as ascorbic acid) has uncertain access to the cell in a living organism, because it must potentially cross three barriers: the gut, the cell membrane, and the blood–brain

Table 6.1 Contrasting biological and chemical antioxidation

Biological antioxidation	Chemical antioxidation
▷ occurs inside the cell	▷ uncertain access to the cell (via traversing the gut wall, cell membrane, and possibly the blood–brain barrier)
▷ compatible with cellular physiology	▷ may interfere with cellular physiology
▷ activated only when needed	▷ passive blanket effect
▷ enzymatic – hence constantly renewed	▷ chemical – hence readily depleted and limited

barrier, in the case of the central nervous system (the three barrier criteria). Biological antioxidants are already present where they are needed most, inside all the cells of the body.

Fundamentally, our biological antioxidants (such as catalase, superoxide dismutase, thioredoxin, and so on) are generally enzymatic (with the important exception of glutathione), which means they are constantly renewed. In contrast, a chemical antioxidant needs to be regenerated once it is depleted. This might happen, depending on the environment in the cell. But in some cases it might not be regenerated and is thereby rendered useless or possibly harmful in its oxidised form. One molecule of ascorbic acid can quench one free radical. In contrast, one molecule of superoxide dismutase quenches an estimated one billion free radicals per second.

We can only wonder why so much attention is devoted to the stale and limited concepts backing chemical antioxidation when, instead, we can now understand and harness biological antioxidation to deliver more effective clinical outcomes. But how is this achieved?

6.5 The Nrf2/ARE pathway

Can biological antioxidant protection be optimised in a safe and effective manner? Recent discoveries endorse that this goal can indeed be readily achieved, via priming the Keap1/Nrf2/ARE pathway. The discovery of this pathway is revolutionary and is a game-changing concept for natural therapies, especially for herbal (phytochemical) cytoprotection and detoxification. It might be considered as significant a development for herbal therapy as the discovery of vitamins was for the nutritional world. Others share this view, as per the following quotation concerning the discovery of this pathway:[6] ". . . may well become the most extraordinary therapeutic and most extraordinary preventative breakthrough in the history of medicine." The authors go on to note that Nrf2 regulates around 500 genes, roughly 2% of our genome.

The Nrf2/ARE pathway describes a targeted approach to antioxidant protection *within* each living cell in our bodies (except for cells that contain no nucleus, such as mature red blood cells and cornified cells in the skin, hair, and nails). This pathway, fundamental to all animal cells, is a dynamic response induced by oxidative or chemical stress on the cell. It is a switch-on, switch-off mechanism, and most of the known priming agents that facilitate its action are natural plant chemicals.

A transcription factor is a cellular chemical that activates the DNA of the cell leading to the manufacture of specific proteins via the transcription process. The proteins that are manufactured depend on the transcription factor. Nrf2 (nuclear factor erythroid 2-related factor 2) is such a factor, normally anchored in the cell cytoplasm (outside the nucleus) by a molecule known as Keap1 (Kelch-like ECH-associated protein 1). Chemical stress on the cell disrupts the tethering of Keap1 to Nrf2, releasing it. The free Nrf2 moves (translocates) to the nucleus, being activated on the way, and there binds to the antioxidant response element (ARE) of our DNA. This induces the new synthesis of a range of antioxidant, detoxifying, protective, and anti-inflammatory enzymes. Hence, it is not just antioxidant activity that is induced by the Nrf2/ARE pathway, but also the activity of a series of beneficial genes. This cellular mechanism is thereby the key cytoprotective pathway and the master regulator of cellular redox homeostasis.[7]

Put another way, the Keap1/Nrf2/ARE transcriptional pathway provides an effective "backup system" for cysteine-based redox regulation (provided predominantly by glutathione, GSH) via activation of endogenous gene networks involved in antioxidant defence. It is at the centre of our daily biological responses to oxidative stress in the body and not only mediates the transcription of many antioxidant genes that maintain cellular homeostasis, it also activates detoxification genes that eliminate potentially damaging carcinogens, and toxins.[8]

Additional experimental evidence suggests that Nrf2 is an important component for the maintenance of mitochondrial homeostasis and structural integrity. This becomes particularly important under conditions of oxidative, electrophilic, and inflammatory stress.

6.5.1 The key outcomes of Nrf2 activation

The key activities resulting from Nrf2 activation include:

- antioxidant
- anti-inflammatory
- detoxifying
- cytoprotection/repair
- metabolic correction

In more detail, the following outcomes are initiated:[9]

1. synthesis of enzymatic antioxidants targeted at ROS excess: catalase, SOD (superoxide-dismutase), GSH-peroxidases, GSH-reductase, GSH-transferase, NQO1 (NADPH-quinone oxidoreductase), the cytochrome P450 monooxygenase system, thioredoxin and thioredoxin reductase, and HSP70 (heat shock protein 70)
2. activation of glutathione synthase with a consequent increase of intracellular GSH
3. enhancement of key phase II detoxifying enzymes such as UDP-glucuronosyltransferase, N-acetyltransferases, and sulfotransferases
4. upregulation of HO-1 (haem oxygenase–1), which is highly cytoprotective (especially for neuronal tissue) and, with NO, allows vasodilation in ischaemic tissues
5. reduction of iron overload via elevated ferritin and bilirubin as a lipophilic antioxidant
6. upregulation of phase III transporter proteins (that remove toxins and damaged cellular components)
7. under homeostatic conditions: support of mitochondrial function by increasing mitochondrial membrane potential, fatty acid oxidation, and ATP (adenosine triphosphate) synthesis

8 under cellular stress: reduction of increased ROS in mitochondria and an increase in mitochondrial biogenesis (e.g., by increasing PGC-1α)

In summary, as well as inducing biological antioxidant protection for the cell, Nrf2 activation enhances DNA repair, haem metabolism, GSH synthesis, and removal and breakdown of toxins. It activates detoxification, stabilises proteins, strengthens cellular integrity, reduces inflammatory responses (see Section 13.2.2), and optimises mitochondrial function.[10] Phase II detoxifying enzymes were thought to only occur in our liver, gut, and kidney and nowhere else; so that was where any detoxification took place. But now, with the discovery of this pathway, we know that every cell in the body can produce these phase II detoxifying enzymes.

Figure 6.1 illustrates the basics of the Nrf2/ARE pathway and how calorie restriction, moderate physical exercise and polyphenol (herbal) supplementation have the potential to activate it. The Keap1 protein contains sulfur groups that are sensitive to the environment – specifically to electrophiles (oxidant molecules). If these are present in sufficient amounts, this stimulates the release of Nrf2 from Keap1. Nrf2 becomes free and moves into the nucleus where it dimerises with members of the small Maf (masculoaponeurotic fibrosarcoma) protein family and then binds to the ARE (electrophile response elements) located in the regulatory regions of the cellular defence enzyme genes. It is thought that individual variations in expression of Maf proteins exist, so not everyone switches on this pathway as well as might be needed.

6.5.2 Nrf2, oxidative stress, and inflammation

There are three stages of response that occur when a cell is stressed, especially by oxidative and toxic stress. The first invokes the Nrf2 response. If that is insufficient to deal with the threat, nuclear factor kappa-light-chain-enhancer of activated B cells (NFκB) is invoked, which is another transcription factor that specifically up-regulates an inflammatory response. If that fails to maintain cellular integrity, activator protein 1 is induced, which then initiates apoptosis to kill the cell. If Nrf2 is functioning properly, it blocks the impact of chemical stress on the cell. This then reduces the need for the up-regulation of inflammation via NFκB activation (see **Figure 6.2**).

The specifics of this anti-inflammatory mechanism for Nrf2 are as follows. When oxidative stress triggers the release of Nrf2 from Keap1, the resultant increase in the intracellular pool of unbound Keap1 is available to capture more intracellular IKKβ (I-kappa-B-kinase beta), thereby inhibiting NFκB target gene expression. (IKKβ is involved in NFκB activation under conditions of mild to moderate oxidative stress.) This creates a cross-talk between cellular inflammation and cytoprotection, between NFκB nuclear transcription and Nrf2 nuclear transcription.

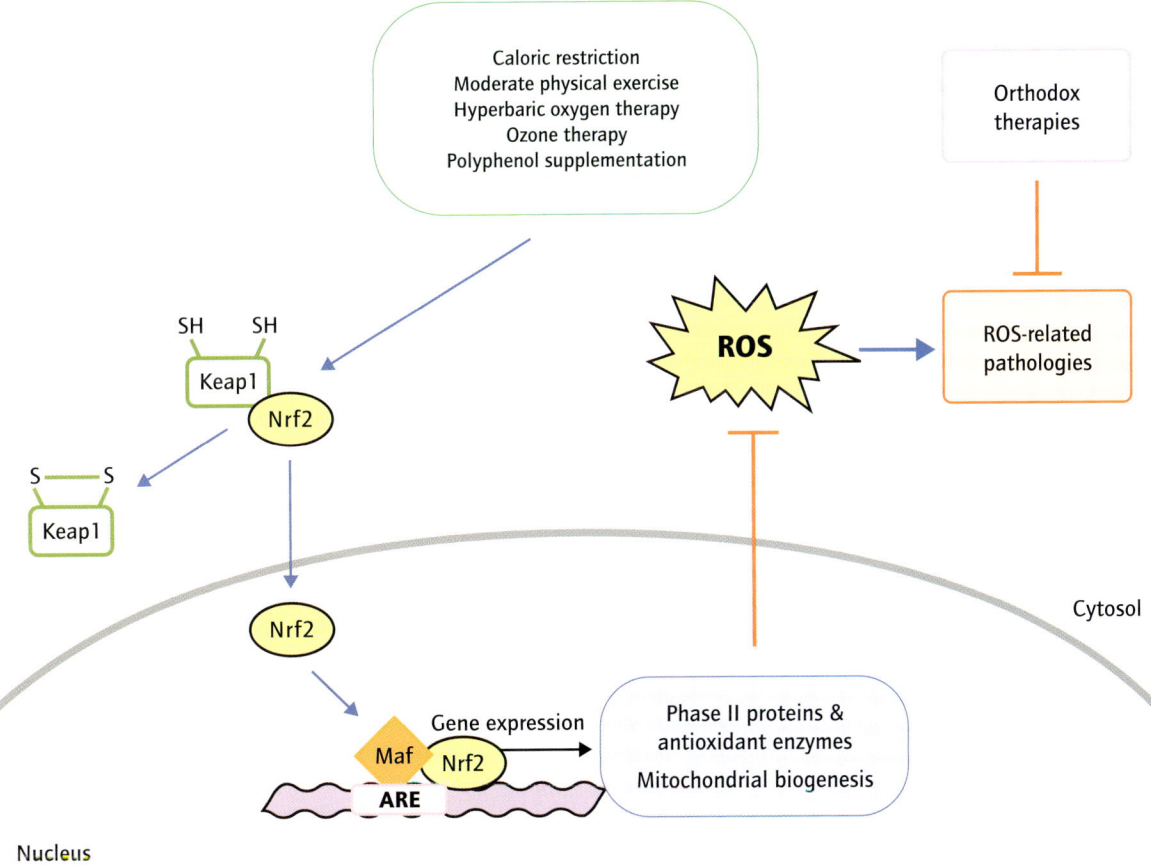

Figure 6.1 The Keap1/Nrf2/ARE pathway.[11] [ROS = reactive oxygen species; ARE = antioxidant response element.]

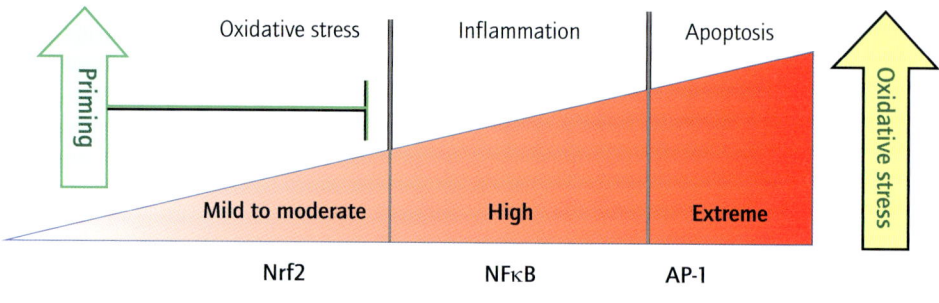

Figure 6.2 Differential cellular responses to rising oxidative stress.[12]

6.5.3 Diet and the Nrf2/ARE pathway

The Nrf2/ARE pathway is mainly primed by plant chemicals. In fact, with the discovery of this pathway there are some highly credible researchers who are suggesting that a recommended daily allowance for phytonutrients may now be necessary. This is because of the idea that this pathway only works well if we have a baseline intake of phytonutrients.[13] Considering our modern phytonutrient deficient diet, this might well result in an Nrf2/ARE pathway that is sub-par.

6.5.4 NQO1 and coenzyme Q10

Coenzyme Q10 exists in two forms in the body: ubiquinone is the inactive form and ubiquinol the active form. Ubiquinol is generated by the enzymes thioredoxin reductase and NQO1. NQO1 is a phase II enzyme induced by the Nrf2/ARE pathway. Its genetic variations (polymorphisms) have been studied extensively : there are inactive single nucleotide polymorphisms (SNPs) of this enzyme, especially NQO1*2. The frequency of the inactive homozygous polymorphism NQO1*2/*2 is 4% in Caucasians, 5% in African–Americans, and 22% in Chinese populations.[14] A pilot study found that NQO1 polymorphism influences CoQ10 status in humans.[15] By harnessing the Nrf2/ARE pathway, there is the potential to improve a person's ubiquinol status, especially if they are heterozygous for NQO1*2.

6.6 Therapeutic impact of Nrf2/ARE pathway priming

Obviously, harnessing a mechanism as powerful as the Nrf2/ARE pathway can have profound effects on health maintenance and disease management. Current research has identified several important benefits to priming the pathway in the quest to maintain health and prevent disease:[16]

- providing clinically relevant, safe, targeted antioxidant cover
- supporting antiageing/healthy longevity protocols
- supporting the detoxification of any toxin: drugs, alcohol, smoking, heavy metals
- facilitating protection against any physical or biological stressor: especially radiation and heat stress
- reducing cancer incidence – the cancer preventative effect of activating this pathway is well demonstrated in animal models
- reducing cancer recurrence – but they are not to be used during chemotherapy or radiotherapy (see Section 6.9)
- reducing neurodegeneration, as in macular degeneration (AMD), Alzheimer's disease (AD), and Parkinson's diseases (PD), stroke recovery, and diabetic neuropathy
- acting as key moderators in any chronic inflammatory disease, such as osteoarthritis and autoimmune diseases
- acting as key preventative and palliative agents in cardiovascular disease, especially for arterial and endothelial damage/dysfunction
- helping to counter the negative metabolic effects of a high-fat and/or high fried-food diet
- providing protective cover during weight loss
- improving metabolism in diabetes and metabolic syndrome
- supporting the lungs in any chronic lung disease
- benefits in diseases involving oxidative damage and inflammation
- potential benefit in diseases resulting from accumulated toxins, even heavy metals
- the pathway also upregulates GSH levels, in itself an important cellular antioxidant and protective agent (GSH also binds to the products of phase II detoxification)

Examining some of these applications in more detail, let us first revisit the oxidative stress theory of ageing. Comparing different animals, short-lived species have lower levels of Nrf2, together with reduced nuclear binding activity, higher levels of Keap1, and lower production of ARE enzymes following Nrf2 activation. In other words, healthy longevity may not be so much about the degree of exposure to free radicals; it might instead be about how well protected the organism's cells are by this pathway from such ROS damage.[17]

Improving Nrf2/ARE responses can protect against cancer, as suggested by many experimental models. Many of the key phytochemicals known to prevent cancer in animal models of carcinogenesis are thought to prime the Nrf2/ARE pathway. The combination of anti-inflammatory and antioxidant activity with detoxification represents a very powerful mechanism to resist the cancer-causing potential of carcinogenic agents.[18,19]

A growing body of experimental evidence suggests that the pharmacological activation of Nrf2 can effectively counteract several pathological processes occurring in neurodegenerative diseases. Targeting Nrf2 signalling could lead to therapeutic options that delay onset, slow progression, and decrease symptoms of a wide range of neurodegenerative conditions.[20] Nervous tissue is richly endowed with fat and highly prone to free radical damage. Beneficial effects of Nrf2/ARE priming/activation have been suggested for diabetic neuropathy,[21] AD,[22] PD,[23] and AMD.[24] HO-1 is a known neuroprotective heat-shock enzyme (induced by Nrf2) that protects against brain injury: for example, in stroke.[25] In one study, cells from a biopsy of the olfactory mucosa expressed lower GSH levels and detoxifying capacity in PD patients compared to those from healthy control donors. These cells from the PD patients were also in a state of oxidative stress due to higher levels of hydrogen peroxide (a key ROS). Significantly, activation of the Nrf2/ARE pathway restored those defective cells to normal.[26]

Positive effects of Nrf2/ARE priming have been suggested for lung disease, including in cigarette smokers, and for asthma, pulmonary fibrosis, and emphysema. The lungs are highly exposed to oxygen because of both their function and very high surface area, and often suffer greatly from damage by ROS.

Cardiovascular and autoimmune diseases are also in the list of diseases that might benefit.[27] **Figure 6.3** illustrates an extensive list of diseases that may be linked to Nrf2 dysregulation (the Nrf2 diseasome).

CELLULAR PROTECTION AND THE Nrf2 PATHWAY

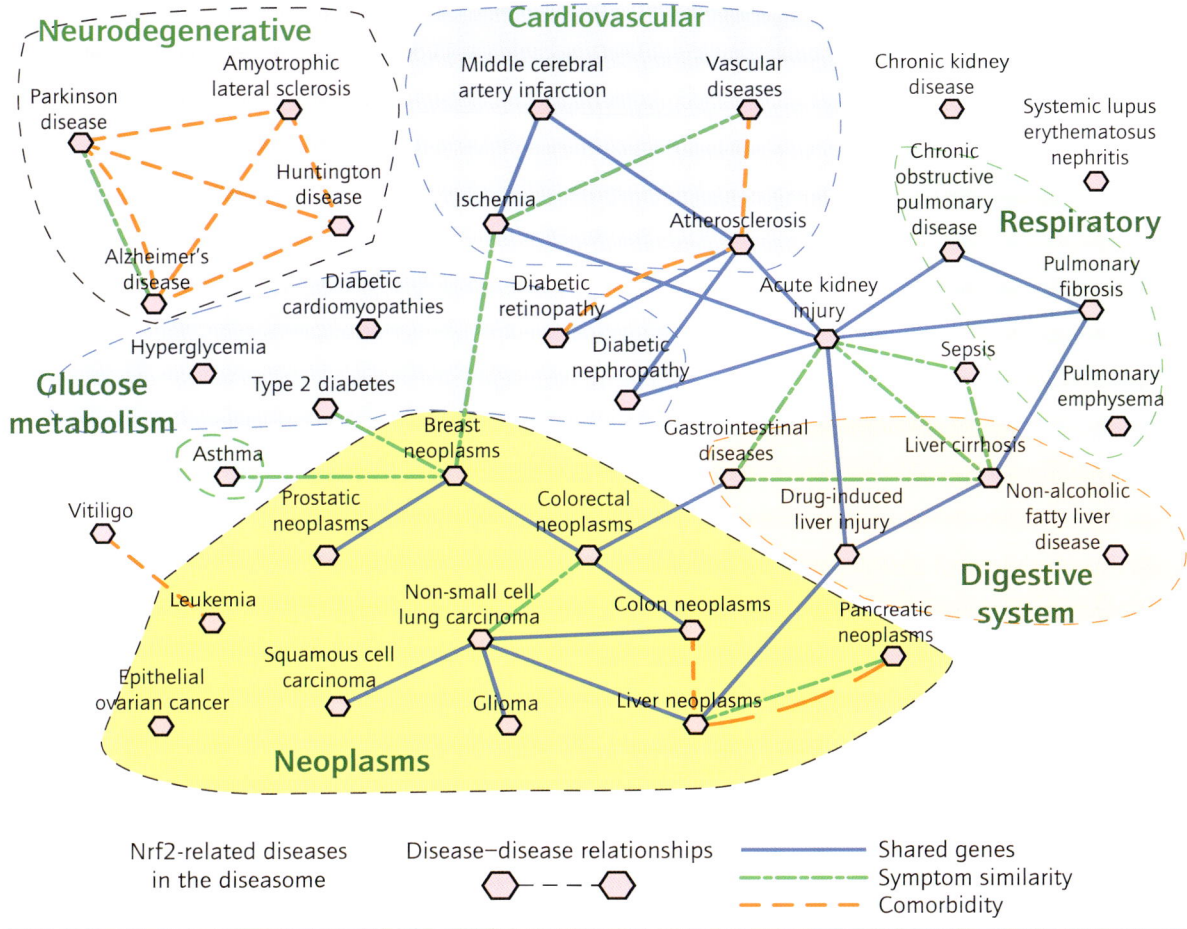

Figure 6.3 Diseases linked to Nrf2 dysregulation.[28]

6.6.1 Nrf2 and diabetes

Recently, the role of Nrf2 has been acknowledged as a factor in delaying the progression of type 2 diabetes mellitus (T2D) and associated co-morbidities, due to its antioxidant and anti-inflammatory impact.[29] Nrf2 activators that might assist in diabetes management include curcumin, sulforaphane, resveratrol, and micronutrients (zinc, chromium, and vitamin D). These can activate nuclear Nrf2 translocation to augment β-cell function (in pre-diabetes) and avert the complications of diabetes when the antioxidant

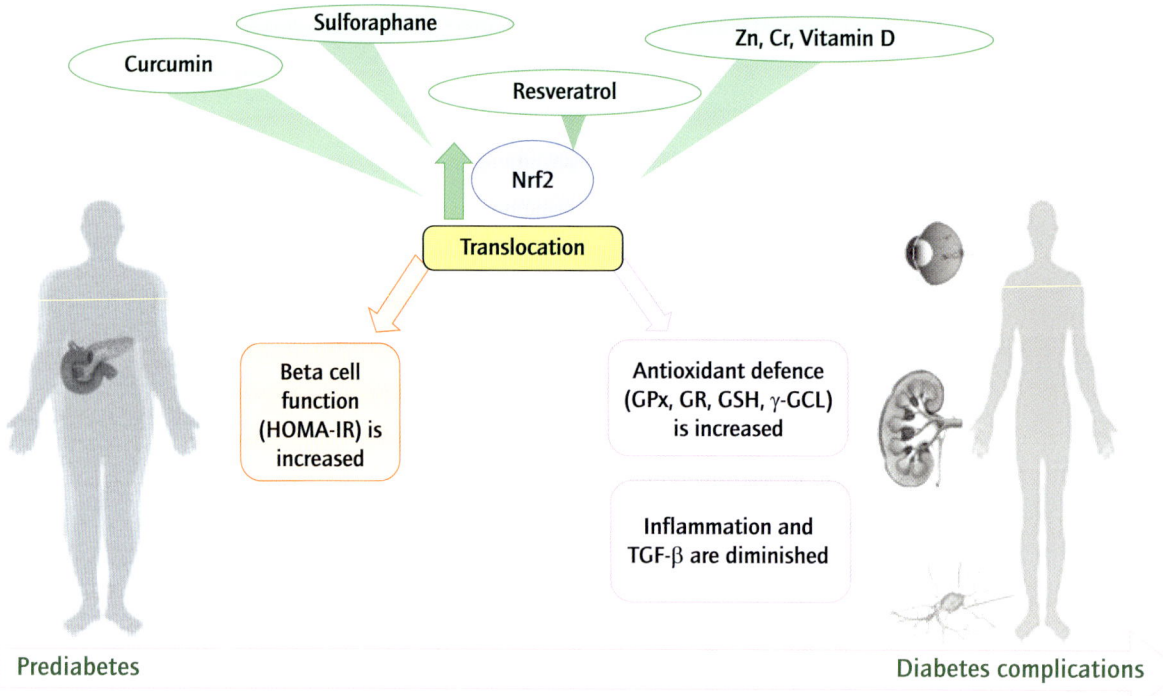

Figure 6.4 The role of natural activators of Nrf2 from prediabetes to diabetes complications. [HOMA-IR = homeostasis model assessment for insulin resistance; GPx = glutathione peroxidase; GR = glutathione reductase; GSH = glutathione; γGCL = gamma-glutamate cysteine ligase; TGFβ = transforming growth factor-beta.]

defences are triggered and inflammation is counteracted (see **Figure 6.4**). Under hyperglycaemic conditions, inflammation, ROS production, protein kinase C, and the hexosamine pathways were all inhibited by Nrf2 activation.

6.7 Herbs that prime the Nrf2/ARE response

What are the key herbs and phytochemicals with Nrf2/ARE priming activity? The research has focused on a few key ones: sulforaphane from broccoli (especially the sprouts), curcumin from turmeric, resveratrol, carnosol from rosemary, Ginkgo extract, the polyphenols from green tea, and the sulfur compounds in garlic.

6.7.1 Broccoli sprouts

The consumption of cruciferous vegetables has long been associated with a reduced risk of cancer at various sites in the body. The key chemopreventive phytochemical sulforaphane is found in certain cruciferous vegetables and is especially high in broccoli sprouts (BS).[30] It is believed to interact with the cysteine amino acid residues in Keap1, thereby enhancing its release. In addition to the Nrf2-mediated induction of cellular defences, many other mechanisms have also been proposed for cancer chemoprevention by sulforaphane, and these appear to act synergistically.[31]

Efficacy of sulforaphane in chemoprevention was evident following sulforaphane administration during either the initiation or the post-initiation stages of carcinogenesis.[32] In a mouse skin carcinogenesis model, sulforaphane inhibited both the incidence and multiplicity of tumours.[33] However, no chemoprotective effect was observed with sulforaphane pre-treatment when Nrf2-knockout mice were used, supporting the notion that the Keap1–Nrf2 pathway plays an essential role in the mechanism of action of sulforaphane against cancer.

BS have reduced measures of oxidative stress in type 2 diabetes patients in a clinical trial.[34] In an open-label trial, 440 mg/day of broccoli sprout extract administered to moderately asthmatic patients for 14 days led to improved lung function and increased NQO-1 gene expression.[35] In a randomised controlled trial (RCT) over 12 weeks in 291 people, a broccoli sprout drink increased the detoxification of inhaled airborne pollutants (especially as GSH phase II products); increased Nrf2 activity can be inferred by this result.[36] Sulforaphane increased blood GSH levels in healthy human participants following 7 days of daily oral administration. A significant positive correlation between blood and thalamic GSH ratios post- and pre-sulforaphane treatment was also observed, in addition to a consistent increase in brain GSH levels in response to treatment.[37]

Since there has been a growing appreciation of the role of oxidative stress in asthma and allergy, a team of US scientists investigated the impact of BS on phase II enzymes in upper airway cells sampled by nasal lavage.[38] A placebo-controlled dose escalation trial was conducted in 65 healthy volunteers to investigate the clinical impact of sulforaphane on expression of the phase II enzymes GSTM1 (glutathione-S-transferase M1), GSTP1 (glutathione-S-transferase P1), NQO1, and HO-1. Prior to starting the single-blind study, volunteers were provided with a list of sulforaphane-containing foods and were instructed to avoid these foods during the study period. Baseline nasal lavage and blood samples were collected from each enrolled volunteer on Day 1 to assess baseline phase II enzyme expression. Volunteers subsequently ingested a measured amount of broccoli sprout homogenate (BSH) once daily on Days 1, 2, and 3. Once safety and tolerability were established, volunteers were enrolled at doses of 125, 150, 175, and 200 g to examine a dose–response effect. Five volunteers took an alfalfa sprout homogenate at 200 g as a control group. No serious adverse events were reported, and the BSH was well tolerated by the volunteers, even at relatively high doses. BS were found to significantly increase phase II enzymes in a dose-dependent manner. The effect was highest for BSH doses higher than 100 g, corresponding to about 55 g of original fresh sprouts. The effects observed were quite marked, with the increase in mean expression of phase II enzymes ranging from 101% for GSTP1 to 199% for NQO1 at the highest dose of BSH administration. This represents a doubling to tripling of baseline enzyme expression rates. Also significant was the observation that all the phase II enzymes tested were increased. This is consistent with the current understanding that sulforaphane acts by a single mechanism, namely by activating the Nrf2 transcription factor.

This study yielded two important pieces of new information. It was the first study to show that BS can induce phase II enzymes in the human respiratory tract, suggesting a role for this herb in asthma and allergic rhinitis, and perhaps even severe respiratory infections. The study also clearly demonstrated that BS are a potent and clinically relevant inducer of phase II enzymes, and they do so in a dose-dependent manner. This has clear implications for the use of BS in the enhancement of xenobiotic detoxification by the liver and other organs and provides strong evidence for such an application.

6.7.2 Turmeric and curcumin

Multiple animal laboratory studies have demonstrated chemopreventive activity for curcumin and turmeric.[39] The Nrf2/ARE pathway is thought to be an important platform for these effects. For example, the epigenetic silencing of Nrf2 during the progression of prostate tumours in a mouse model was reversed by curcumin.[40]

Brain and liver injury were reduced by curcumin through Nrf2-mediated induction of HO-1.[41,42] Dietary curcumin led to increased Nrf2 protein levels and enhanced ARE binding in the liver and lungs of mice.[43]

The therapeutic value of curcumin in treating diabetic kidney disease was investigated in an open-label trial, where 500 mg was administered per day. It led to decreased urinary microalbumin excretion, increased NQO1 and other anti-oxidative enzymes (indicating Nrf2 activity), and increased IκB (an inhibitory protein on inflammatory signalling within lymphocytes).[44] Curcumin also demonstrated the capacity to decrease the Nrf2-signalling defects imposed by a high-fat diet *in vivo*.[45]

In a highly relevant RCT, 60 people experiencing occupational stress-related anxiety and fatigue were randomised to receive CGM (containing 400 mg/day curcuminoids), standard curcumin, or placebo for 30 days. CGM is curcumagalactomannoside, a formulation of natural curcumin with fenugreek dietary fibre that has been shown to possess improved bioavailability.[46] A significant improvement in quality of life ($p < 0.05$), with considerable reductions in stress ($p < 0.001$), anxiety ($p < 0.001$), and fatigue ($p < 0.001$), was observed among the CGM-treated group, as compared with the standard curcumin group. These improvements in quality of life were further correlated with a significant enhancement in endogenous antioxidant markers ($p < 0.01$) and a reduction in lipid peroxidation ($p < 0.001$). Further comparison revealed enhanced absorption and improved pharmacokinetics of CGM compared to standard curcumin upon both single- (30.7-fold) and repeated-dose (39.1-fold) administrations. Most importantly, levels of the antioxidant targets of the Nrf2 pathway were significantly elevated for both forms of curcumin, but with the enhanced product showing a substantially higher response (see **Figure 6.5**).

6.7.3 Green tea

A significant proportion of green tea's health-promoting activity is linked to its key component, epigallocatechin gallate (EGCG), activating the Nrf2/ARE pathway.[47] These activities include chemopreventive, neuroprotective,

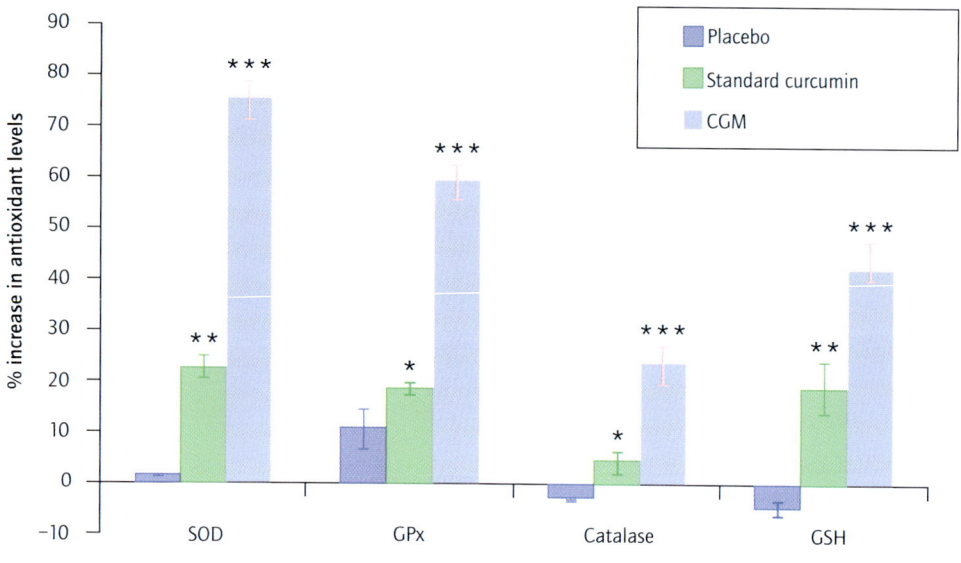

Figure 6.5 Clinical influence of standard and enhanced curcumin (CGM) on Nrf2 antioxidant targets. [SOD = superoxide-dismutase; GPx = glutathione peroxidase; GSH = glutathione.]

detoxifying, and antioxidant outcomes. These beneficial effects for green tea are not seen in Nrf2-deficient animal models. One *in vivo* study evaluated the effects of EGCG on arsenic-induced hepatotoxicity. It found that EGCG inhibited hepatic pathological damage, the level of reactive oxygen species in the liver, and the level of oxidative stress biomarker malondialdehyde (MDA) by enhancing expressions of Nrf2-signalling related genes (Nrf2, NQO1, and HO-1).[48] Green tea supplementation increased whole blood GSH and plasma antioxidant capacity in adults with metabolic syndrome, presumably via the Nrf2 mechanism.[49]

6.7.4 Resveratrol

Resveratrol is a very active primer of the Nrf2/ARE pathway. Favourable Nrf2-mediated protection has been demonstrated in many body systems, including the endocrine, cardiovascular, and nervous systems. For example, the endothelial (circulatory) protective effects of resveratrol against a high-fat diet were largely diminished in Nrf2 knockout mice.[50]

In a double-blind, randomised, crossover study, 10 normal healthy men and women were given a high-fat, high-carbohydrate (HFHC) meal (930 kcal), either with a placebo or with a product containing 100 mg of resveratrol from *Polygonum cuspidatum* plus 75 mg of total polyphenols from a grape extract.[51] DNA binding activity of Nrf2 in white cells was increased significantly by 150 ± 39% over baseline at 3 hours after the meal and supplement intake, whereas meal consumption in the placebo group resulted in a significant reduction in Nrf2 binding activity at 5 hours. These effects were associated with a significant reduction of Keap1 by 48% in the supplement group and a significant increase by 66% in the placebo group.

6.7.5 Ginkgo

Ginkgo is well known as a powerful clinical antioxidant. Its antioxidant properties play an important role in protection against radiation damage and are mediated by Nrf2. In an uncontrolled trial conducted in 1995, Ginkgo extract protected against radiation-induced DNA damage in Chernobyl workers.[52] More recently, the same dose of extract (120 mg/day) protected against the DNA damage caused by radioactive iodine treatment in patients with thyroid disease.[53] There have been many trials of Ginkgo for stroke recovery in China, and the Cochrane Collaboration published a systematic review and meta-analysis on this topic.[54] While the review expressed concerns about the quality of most trials, it did find that Ginkgo was associated with a significant increase in the number of improved patients, based on neurological symptoms. Induction of HO-1 via Nrf2/ARE activation by Ginkgo was suggested as a significant mechanism for neuroprotection and recovery following cerebral ischemia.[55,56]

6.7.6 Garlic

Garlic primes the NRF2/ARE pathway *in vivo*, as shown, for example, in a veterinary study,[57] and numerous laboratory studies also support its activity against heavy metal toxicity. For example, diallyl trisulfide, a garlic polysulfide, protected against arsenic-induced renal oxidative nephrotoxicity, apoptosis, and inflammation *in vivo* by activating the Nrf2/ARE signalling pathway.[58]

6.7.7 Grape seed

Several animal models have shown that grape seed extract (GSE) mediates favourable health effects via the Nrf2 pathway.[59,60] A double-blind RCT found that GSE significantly improved markers of inflammation and glycaemia and a sole marker of oxidative stress (whole blood GSH) in obese type 2 diabetic patients at high risk of cardiovascular events over a 4-week period. The findings suggest GSE may have a significant therapeutic role in decreasing cardiovascular risk.[61] The increase in GSH was probably mediated by activation of the Nrf2 pathway.

6.7.8 Nrf2 primers everywhere?

Nrf2 is a sensitive cellular mechanism and, as such, is readily triggered under *in vitro* conditions. This can lead to assertions that certain herbs or phytochemicals might have clinically relevant Nrf2 activity, when in fact they do not. For *in vivo* translation of *in vitro* activity, we need to consider factors such as metabolism, traversing body barriers, and concentration/dosage issues (see also Section 9.5.3). The best candidates will be herbs or phytochemicals with known chemopreventive and detoxifying activities (from oral doses). Furthermore, preference should be given to those herbs with proven activity via Nrf2 pathways in clinical trials and to those exhibiting good human bioavailability (as per the examples above).

So, the warning is to not over-interpret the literature. We are probably now seeing false positives from test-tube studies, as the number of experiments continues to grow. The recommended clinically relevant herbs/phytochemicals for priming the Nrf2 response are the following:

- broccoli sprouts/sulforaphane
- turmeric/curcumin
- rosemary/carnosol and carnosic acid (see Section 6.8)
- green tea/EGCG
- Polygonum (fallopia)/resveratrol
- garlic
- Ginkgo
- grape seed
- Korean ginseng

6.8 Why do phytochemicals beneficially influence the Nrf2/ARE pathway?

A toxic chemical and a beneficial chemical (such as a phytochemical) can both activate the same Nrf2/ARE pathway. How can it, then, be good if sulforaphane activates that pathway and bad when a toxin activates the same pathway? The answer appears to be all about dose-response, as illustrated in **Figure 6.6**.

As represented in Figure 6.6, EPs are electrophiles (positively polarised compounds that are attracted to and react with an electron-rich centre). They also exert pro-oxidant activity.[62] EPs activate potent cellular defence systems, such as the Keap1/Nrf2/ARE pathway against oxidative stress. In the figure, EP1 is a toxic chemical (doxorubicin); EP3 is the beneficial carnosic acid (CA) from the herb rosemary; and EP2 is an investigational drug for the Nrf2 pathway (NEPP11), which is somewhere between beneficial and toxic. (Note that carnosic acid and carnosol from rosemary are not ordinarily electrophilic, but become so due to oxidation. These oxidation products then activate Nrf2, see Section 6.9.)

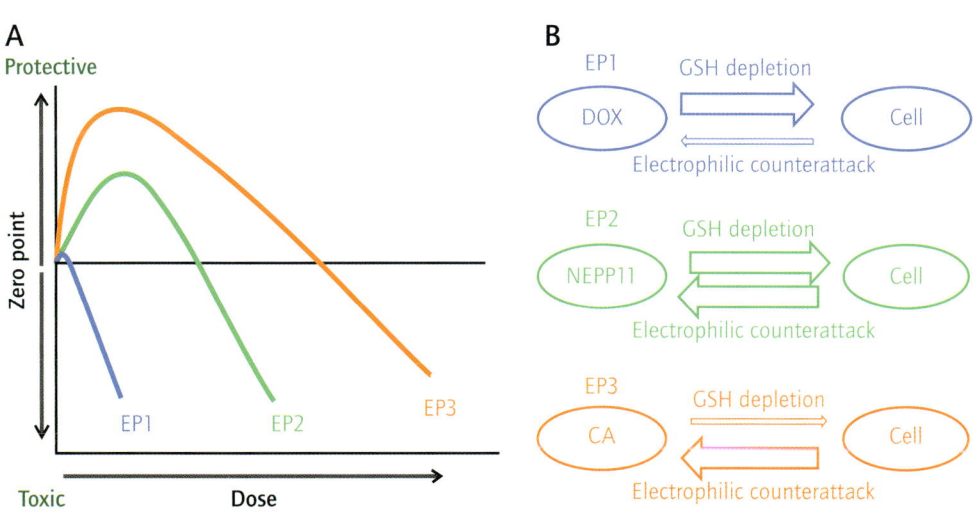

Figure 6.6 Benign and harmful Nrf2 activators. [GSH = glutathione DOX = doxorubicin; CA = carnosic acid.]

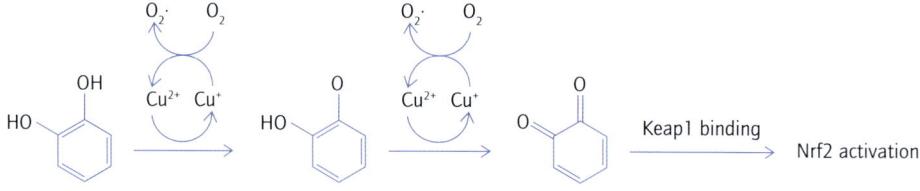

Figure 6.7 Carnosol and carnosic acid are activated by oxidation.

The most basic distinction after cellular exposure to an electrophile involves two opposing actions. The first involves GSH depletion, which contributes to the toxic effect on the cell, and the second is "electrophilic counterattack" via Nrf2, affording cellular protection from the oxidative insult. With EP1, damage and GSH depletion happen at a very early stage in the process (low exposure), so there is very little Nrf2 protection induced by that chemical before toxic effects predominate. In other words, EP1 predominantly causes cell death by depletion of GSH, while barely activating the electrophilic counterattack that affords protection. In contrast, before carnosic acid's influence on the cell is liable to cause any damage via GSH depletion, it initiates a marked up-regulation of the protective Nrf2 pathway.

As alluded to above, there is something unique about the Nrf2 priming activity of rosemary: carnosic acid and carnosol from rosemary are not ordinarily strongly electrophilic, but they become so after oxidation. In **Figure 6.7**, carnosic acid and carnosol are represented by the general structure of two adjacent hydroxyl groups on their benzene ring (the catechol structure).[63] Under conditions of oxidative stress, the ortho-quinone version of the catechol molecule is created by oxidation, and it is only this quinone version that can then activate the Nrf2/ARE pathway.

So, when a person ingests rosemary, carnosol and carnosic acid circulate in the body's tissues. When these phytochemicals reach a tissue environment that is under electrophilic or toxic attack, they are converted to their quinone forms that subsequently activate the Nrf2 pathway. This is an ideal situation, because carnosol and carnosic acid will only act in those tissues that need it. It is the safest and most targeted way of activating the Nrf2/ARE pathway possible, and as a result probably makes rosemary **the** most important herb for priming this pathway.

Both carnosol and carnosic acid have a high bioavailability and, as per above, are now understood to be potent indirect primers of the Nrf2/ARE pathway. They have demonstrated neuroprotective activity by this pathway, which may reflect on rosemary's traditional use for memory.[64,65] Supporting this, a single 750 mg dose of rosemary improved the speed of memory and alertness of healthy older adults.[66] The results of another study investigating the cytoprotective and chemopreventive potential of rosemary established that the expression of Sestrin2 and MRP2 was increased after treatment with rosemary extracts. These are two functional proteins regulated by Nrf2.[67] Carnosol from rosemary also exhibited potent lung protective action *in vivo*, via Nrf2 activation.[68] This is just a small selection of the many studies.

6.9   Nrf2 and cancer

There is one important cautionary note: Nrf2 and its downstream genes are over-expressed in many experimental cancer cell lines and human cancers, giving cancer cells a survival and growth advantage (see **Figure 6.8**). Nrf2 is particularly upregulated in cancer cells resistant to chemotherapy and is thought to be largely responsible for acquired chemoresistance. It might

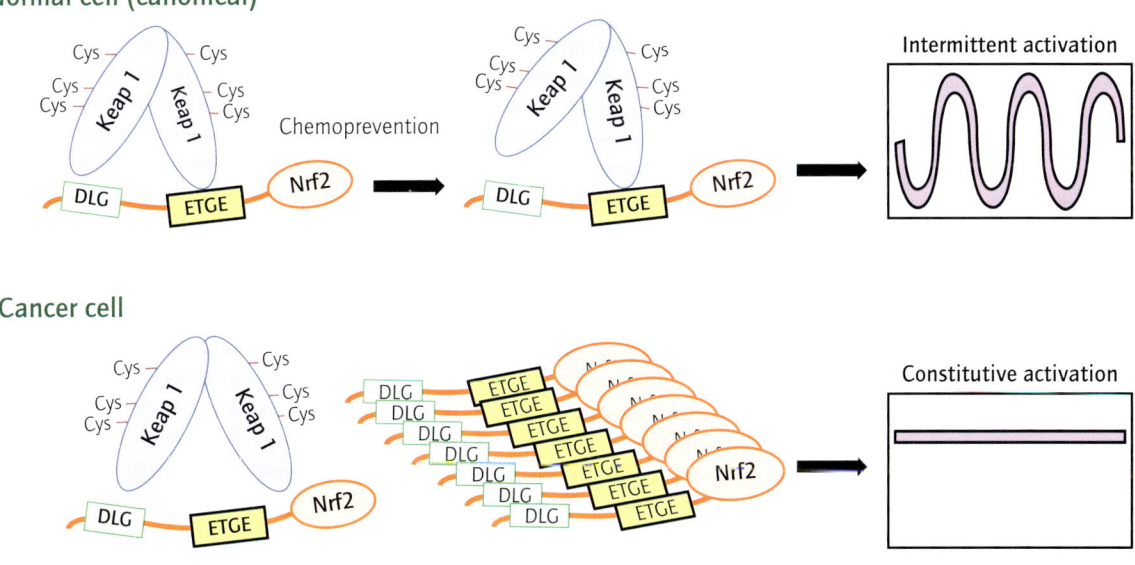

Figure 6.8   Nrf2 activation in normal and cancer cells.

therefore even be advantageous to inhibit the Nrf2/ARE pathway during chemotherapy.[69] There are still many questions to be answered. However, caution dictates that any known Nrf2/ARE upregulating herbs should not be taken at least 24 hours either side of each chemotherapy or radiotherapy treatment, so there is no potential interference with the cancer killing effects of these treatments.

References

1. Albanes D, Heinonen OP, Huttunen JK, Taylor PR, Virtamo J, Edwards BK, Haapakoski J, Rautalahti M, Hartman AM, Palmgren J. Effects of alpha-tocopherol and beta-carotene supplements on cancer incidence in the Alpha-Tocopherol Beta-Carotene Cancer Prevention Study. *Am J Clin Nutr*. 1995 Dec; **62**(6 Suppl): 1427S–1430S. doi:10.1093/ajcn/62.6.1427S. PMID: 7495243.
2. Schultz H. Is the future of antioxidants in fighting inflammation? 2012 March 1. https://www.newhope.com/supplements/future-antioxidants-fighting-inflammation
3. *Ibid.*
4. Zhang Q, Pi J, Woods CG, et al. A systems biology perspective on Nrf2-mediated antioxidant response. *Toxicol Appl Pharmacol*. 2010; **244**(1): 84–97.
5. Lewis KN, Mele J, Hayes JD, et al. Nrf2, a guardian of healthspan and gatekeeper of species longevity. *Integr Comp Biol*. 2010; **50**(5): 829–843.
6. Pall ML, Levine S. Nrf2, a master regulator of detoxification and also antioxidant, anti-inflammatory and other cytoprotective mechanisms, is raised by health promoting factors. *Sheng Li Xue Bao*. 2015; **67**(1): 1–18.
7. Dinkova-Kostova AT, Abramov AY. The emerging role of Nrf2 in mitochondrial function. *Free Radic Biol Med*. 2015 Nov; **88**(Pt B): 179–188.
8. Stefanson AL, Bakovic M. Dietary regulation of Keap1/Nrf2/ARE pathway: focus on plant-derived compounds and trace minerals. *Nutrients*. 2014 Sep 19; **6**(9): 3777–3801.
9. Dinkova-Kostova AT, Abramov AY. The emerging role of Nrf2 in mitochondrial function. *Free Radic Biol Med*. 2015 Nov; **88**(Pt B): 179–188.
10. Harder B, Jiang T, Wu T, et al. Molecular mechanisms of Nrf2 regulation and how these influence chemical modulation for disease intervention. *Biochem Soc Trans*. 2015 Aug; **43**(4): 680–686.
11. Bocci V, Valacchi G. Nrf2 activation as target to implement therapeutic treatments. *Front Chem*. 2015 Feb 2; **3**:4. doi:10.3389/fchem.2015.00004.eCollection 2015.
12. Stefanson AL, Bakovic M. Dietary regulation of Keap1/Nrf2/ARE pathway: focus on plant-derived compounds and trace minerals. *Nutrients*. 2014 Sep 19; **6**(9): 3777–3801.
13. Senger DR, Li D, Jaminet SC, Cao S. Activation of the Nrf2 cell defense pathway by ancient foods: disease prevention by important molecules and microbes lost from the modern western diet. *PloS One*. 2016; **11**(2): e0148042. doi:10.1371/journal.pone.0148042.
14. Ross D, Kepa JK, Winski SL, et al. NAD(P)H:quinone oxidoreductase 1 (NQO1): chemoprotection, bioactivation, gene regulation and genetic polymorphisms. *Chem Biol Interact*. 2000 Dec 1; **129**(1–2): 77–97.
15. Fischer A, Schmelzer C, Rimbach G, Niklowitz P, Menke T, Döring F. Association between

genetic variants in the Coenzyme Q10 metabolism and Coenzyme Q10 status in humans. *BMC Res Notes.* 2011 Jul 21; **4**: 245. doi:10.1186/1756-0500-4-245.
16. Tu W, Wang H, Li S, Liu Q, Sha H. The anti-inflammatory and anti-oxidant mechanisms of the Keap1/Nrf2/ARE signaling pathway in chronic diseases. *Aging Dis.* 2019; **10**(3): 637–651. doi:10.14336/AD.2018.0513.
17. Lewis KN, Mele J, Hayes JD, et al. Nrf2, a guardian of healthspan and gatekeeper of species longevity. *Integr Comp Biol.* 2010; **50**(5): 829–843.
18. Kwak MK, Kensler TW. Targeting NRF2 signaling for cancer chemoprevention. *Toxicol Appl Pharmacol* 2010; **244**(1): 66–76.
19. Khor TO, Yu S, Kong AN. Dietary cancer chemopreventive agents: targeting inflammation and Nrf2 signaling pathway. *Planta Med* 2008; **74**(13): 1540–1547.
20. Dinkova-Kostova AT, Kostov RV, Kazantsev AG. The role of Nrf2 signaling in counteracting neurodegenerative diseases. *FEBS J.* 2018 Jan 11. doi:10.1111/febs.14379.
21. Negi G, Kumar A, Joshi RP, et al. Oxidative stress and Nrf2 in the pathophysiology of diabetic neuropathy: old perspective with a new angle. *Biochem Biophys Res Commun.* 2011; **408**(1): 1–5.
22. Calkins MJ, Johnson DA, Townsend JA, et al. The Nrf2/ARE pathway as a potential therapeutic target in neurodegenerative disease. *Antioxid Redox Signal.* 2009; **11**(3): 497–508.
23. Cuadrado A, Moreno-Murciano P, Pedraza-Chaverri J. The transcription factor Nrf2 as a new therapeutic target in Parkinson's disease. *Expert Opin Ther Targets.* 2009; **13**(3): 319–329.
24. Plafker SM. Oxidative stress and the ubiquitin proteolytic system in age-related macular degeneration. *Adv Exp Med Biol.* 2010; **664**: 447–456.
25. Jazwa A, Cuadrado A. Targeting heme oxygenase-1 for neuroprotection and neuroinflammation in neurodegenerative diseases. *Curr Drug Targets.* 2010; **11**(12): 1517–1531.
26. Cook AL, Vitale AM, Ravishankar S, et al. NRF2 activation restores disease related metabolic deficiencies in olfactory neurosphere-derived cells from patients with sporadic Parkinson's disease. *PloS One.* 2011; **6**(7): e21907.
27. Singh S, Vrishni S, Singh BK, et al. Nrf2-ARE stress response mechanism: a control point in oxidative stress-mediated dysfunctions and chronic inflammatory diseases. *Free Radic Res.* 2010; **44**(11): 1267–1288.
28. Cuadrado A, Manda G, Hassan A, et al. Transcription factor NRF2 as a therapeutic target for chronic diseases: a systems medicine approach. *Pharmacol Rev.* 2018 Apr; **70**(2): 348–383.
29. Jiménez-Osorio AS, González-Reyes S, Pedraza-Chaverri J. Natural Nrf2 activators in diabetes. *Clin Chim Acta.* 2015; **448**: 182–192. doi:10.1016/j.cca.2015.07.009.
30. Keum YS. Regulation of the Keap1/Nrf2 system by chemopreventive sulforaphane: implications of posttranslational modifications. *Ann NY Acad Sci.* 2011; **1229**: 184–189.
31. Juge N, Mithen RF, Traka M. Molecular basis for chemoprevention by sulforaphane: a comprehensive review. *Cell Mol Life Sci.* 2007; **64**(9): 1105–1127.
32. Dinkova-Kostova AT, Fahey JW, Kostov RV, Kensler TW. KEAP1 and done? Targeting the NRF2 pathway with sulforaphane. *Trends Food Sci Technol.* 2017 Nov; **69**(Pt B): 257–269.
33. Gills JJ, Jeffery EH, Matusheski NV, et al. Sulforaphane prevents mouse skin tumorigenesis during the stage of promotion. *Cancer Lett.* 2006 May 8; **236**(1): 72–79.
34. Lyu JH, Kim KH, Kim HW, et al. Dangkwisoo-san, an herbal medicinal formula, ameliorates acute lung inflammation via activation of Nrf2 and suppression of NF-κB. *J Ethnopharmacol.* 2012; **140**(1): 107–116.
35. Brown RH, Reynolds C, Brooker A, et al. Sulforaphane improves the bronchoprotective response in asthmatics through Nrf2-mediated gene pathways. *Respir Res.* 2015 Sep 15; **16**: 106. doi:10.1186/s12931-015-0253-z.

36. Yang L, Palliyaguru DL, Kensler TW. Frugal chemoprevention: targeting Nrf2 with foods rich in sulforaphane. *Semin Oncol.* 2016 Feb; **43**(1): 146–153.
37. Sedlak TW, Nucifora LG, Koga M, et al. Sulforaphane Augments Glutathione and Influences Brain Metabolites in Human Subjects: A Clinical Pilot Study. *Mol Neuropsychiatry.* 2018; **3**(4): 214 222. doi:10.1159/000487639.
38. Riedl MA, Saxon A, Diaz-Sanchez D. Oral sulforaphane increases Phase II antioxidant enzymes in the human upper airway. *Clin Immunol.* 2009; **130**(3): 244–251. doi:10.1016/j.clim.2008.10.007.
39. Aggarwal BB, Surh YJ, Shisodia S (Eds). The molecular targets and therapeutic uses of curcumin in health and disease. *Adv Exptl Med Biol.* 2007; **595**; 1–489.
40. Khor TO, Huang Y, Wu TY, et al. Pharmacodynamics of curcumin as DNA hypomethylation agent in restoring the expression of Nrf2 via promoter CpGs demethylation. *Biochem Pharmacol.* 2011; **82**(9): 1073–1078.
41. Yang C, Zhang X, Fan H, et al. Curcumin upregulates transcription factor Nrf2, HO–1 expression and protects rat brains against focal ischemia. *Brain Res,* 2009; **1282**: 133–141.
42. Farombi EO, Shrotriya S, Na HK, et al. Curcumin attenuates dimethylnitrosamine-induced liver injury in rats through Nrf2-mediated induction of heme oxygenase–1. *Food Chem Toxicol.* 2008; **46**(4): 1279–1287.
43. Garg R, Gupta S, Maru GB. Dietary curcumin modulates transcriptional regulators of phase I and phase II enzymes in benzo[a]pyrene-treated mice: mechanism of its anti-initiating action. *Carcinogenesis.* 2008; **29**(5): 1022–1032.
44. Yang H, Xu W, Zhou Z, et al. Curcumin attenuates urinary excretion of albumin in type II diabetic patients with enhancing nuclear factor erythroid-derived 2-like 2 (Nrf2) system and repressing inflammatory signaling efficacies. *Exp Clin Endocrinol Diabetes.* 2015 Jun; **123**(6): 360–367.
45. He HJ, Wang GY, Gao Y, et al. Curcumin attenuates Nrf2 signalling defect, oxidative stress in muscle and glucose intolerance in high fat diet-fed mice. *World J Diabetes.* 2012 May 15; **3**(5): 94–104.
46. Pandaran Sudheeran S, Jacob D, Natinga Mulakal J, et al. Safety, tolerance, and enhanced efficacy of a bioavailable formulation of curcumin with fenugreek dietary fiber on occupational stress: a randomized, double-blind, placebo-controlled pilot study. *J Clin Psychopharmacol.* 2016; **36**(3): 236–243. doi:10.1097/JCP.0000000000000508.
47. Na HK, Surh YJ. Modulation of Nrf2-mediated antioxidant and detoxifying enzyme induction by the green tea polyphenol EGCG. *Food Chem Toxicol.* 2008; **46**(4): 1271–1278.
48. Han XD, Zhang YY, Wang KL, et al. The involvement of Nrf2 in the protective effects of (−)-Epigallocatechin–3-gallate (EGCG) on NaAsO(2)-induced hepatotoxicity. *Oncotarget.* 2017 Jun 21; **8**(39): 65302–65312.
49. Basu A, Betts NM, Mulugeta A, et al. Green tea supplementation increases glutathione and plasma antioxidant capacity in adults with the metabolic syndrome. *Nutr Res.* 2013; **33**(3): 180–187. doi:10.1016/j.nutres.2012.12.010.
50. Haskó G, Pacher P. Endothelial Nrf2 activation: a new target for resveratrol? *Am J Physiol Heart Circ Physiol.* 2010; **299**(1): H10–H12.
51. Ghanim H, Sia CL, Korzeniewski K, et al. A resveratrol and polyphenol preparation suppresses oxidative and inflammatory stress response to a high-fat, high-carbohydrate meal. *J Clin Endocrinol Metab.* 2011; **96**(5): 1409–1414.
52. Emerit I, Oganesian N, Sarkisian T, et al. Clastogenic factors in the plasma of Chernobyl accident recovery workers: anticlastogenic effect of Ginkgo biloba extract. *Radiat Res.* 1995; **144**(2): 198–205.
53. Dardano A, Ballardin M, Ferdeghini M, et al. Anticlastogenic effect of Ginkgo biloba

extract in Graves' disease patients receiving radioiodine therapy. *J Clin Endocrinol Metab.* 2007; **92**(11): 4286–4289.
54. Zeng X, Liu M, Yang Y, et al. Ginkgo biloba for acute ischaemic stroke. *Cochrane Database Syst Rev.* 2005; **4**: CD003691.
55. Saleem S, Zhuang H, Biswal S, et al. Ginkgo biloba extract neuroprotective action is dependent on heme oxygenase 1 in ischemic reperfusion brain injury. *Stroke.* 2008; **39**(12): 3389–3396.
56. Chen JS, Huang PH, Wang CH, et al. Nrf–2 mediated heme oxygenase–1 expression, an antioxidant-independent mechanism, contributes to anti-atherogenesis and vascular protective effects of Ginkgo biloba extract. *Atherosclerosis.* 2011; **214**(2): 301–309.
57. Yamato O, Tsuneyoshi T, Ushijima M, Jikihara H, Yabuki A. Safety and efficacy of aged garlic extract in dogs: upregulation of the nuclear factor erythroid 2-related factor 2 (Nrf2) signaling pathway and Nrf2-regulated phase II antioxidant enzymes. *BMC Vet Res.* 2018 Nov 29; **14**(1): 373. doi:10.1186/s12917-018-1699-2. PMID: 30497454.
58. Miltonprabu S, Sumedha NC, Senthilraja P. Diallyl trisulfide, a garlic polysulfide protects against As-induced renal oxidative nephrotoxicity, apoptosis and inflammation in rats by activating the Nrf2/ARE signaling pathway. *Int Immunopharmacol.* 2017; **50**: 107–120. doi:10.1016/j.intimp.2017.06.011.
59. Chen S, Zhu Y, Liu Z, et al. Grape seed proanthocyanidin extract ameliorates diabetic bladder dysfunction via the activation of the Nrf2 pathway. *PloS One.* 2015 May 14; **10**(5): e0126457. doi:10.1371/journal.pone.0126457.
60. Nazimabashir, Manoharan V, Miltonprabu S. Cadmium induced cardiac oxidative stress in rats and its attenuation by GSP through the activation of Nrf2 signaling pathway. *Chem Biol Interact.* 2015; **242**: 179–193. doi:10.1016/j.cbi.2015.10.005.
61. Kar P, Laight D, Rooprai HK, Shaw KM, Cummings M. Effects of grape seed extract in Type 2 diabetic subjects at high cardiovascular risk: a double blind randomized placebo controlled trial examining metabolic markers, vascular tone, inflammation, oxidative stress and insulin sensitivity. *Diabet Med.* 2009; **26**(5): 526–531. doi:10.1111/j.1464-5491.2009.02727.x.
62. Satoh T, McKercher SR, Lipton SA. Reprint of: Nrf2/ARE-mediated antioxidant actions of pro-electrophilic drugs. *Free Radic Biol Med.* 2014 Jan; **66**: 45–57.
63. Ibid.
64. Kosaka K, Mimura J, Itoh K, et al. Role of Nrf2 and p62/ZIP in the neurite outgrowth by carnosic acid in PC12h cells. *J Biochem.* 2010; **147**(1): 73–81.
65. Martin D, Rojo AI, Salinas M, et al. Regulation of heme oxygenase–1 expression through the phosphatidylinositol 3-kinase/Akt pathway and the Nrf2 transcription factor in response to the antioxidant phytochemical carnosol. *Biol Chem.* 2004; **279**(10): 8919–8929.
66. Pengelly A, Snow J, Mills SY, et al. Short-term study on the effects of rosemary on cognitive function in an elderly population. *J Med Food.* 2012; **15**(1): 10–17.
67. Tong XP, Ma YX, Quan DN, et al. Rosemary extracts upregulate Nrf2, sestrin2, and MRP2 protein level in human hepatoma HepG2 cells. *Evid Based Complement Alternat Med.* 2017; **2017**: 7359806. doi:10.1155/2017/7359806. Epub 2017 Feb 13.
68. Kawamura T, Momozane T, Sanosaka M, et al. Carnosol is a potent lung protective agent: experimental study on mice. *Transplant Proc.* 2015 Jul–Aug; **47**(6): 1657–1661.
69. Lau A, Villeneuve NF, Sun Z, et al. Dual roles of Nrf2 in cancer. *Pharmacol Res* 2008; **58**(5–6): 262–270.

7

FHT strategies to reduce the health impact of environmental toxin exposure

This chapter scopes the supporting evidence for and clinical ramifications of the core FHT strategy of protecting the body against toxic exposure and supporting detoxification processes in the body. It builds on the discussion in Chapter 6 of the important role of the Nrf2 pathway in cellular protection and detoxification and arrives at precise evidence-based protocols for enhancing the whole-body removal of specific toxins and/or up-regulating protection against their damaging effects, especially at the cellular level.

The chapter begins with an examination of the different types of environmental toxins and their negative impact on health. It then goes on to explore effective, practical measures to reduce toxin exposure and increase toxin clearance. Ensuring good cytoprotection will help to minimise the damage caused by constant exposure to both external and internal toxic factors that threaten cellular integrity, and this is further examined at the end of this chapter.

7.1 Overview: the controversial role of environmental toxins in chronic disease

The incidence of complex brain disorders in children seems to be rising, especially severe autism and attention deficit hyperactivity disorder (ADHD). It is estimated there are 80,000 new chemicals in our environment of human origin, of which only about 5% have been tested thoroughly for their toxicity.

Perhaps these, in combination with an environmentally vulnerable physiology, are triggering or aggravating these conditions? Is there a role that cytoprotection and detoxification can play in these disorders? Is there proof of any relationship between toxicity and autism or ADHD?

Studies from Mexico City have found that air pollution is neurotoxic, and when brain images of children in Mexico City were examined, brain changes similar to those visible in early stages of AD were found.[1]

Due to their archaic plumbing systems, US schools are grappling with lead in their children's water supply. This is just one example of an unexpected source of heavy metal exposure. As a result, children in 30–40 US schools are given bottled water to drink. But it is known that the bisphenol A (BPA) in the plastic bottles the children have for drinking water is also linked to health problems in children, for example asthma.[2] BPA is also an endocrine disruptor.[3]

The World Health Organization has declared glyphosate a possible carcinogen (see Section 7.2.8). There are some authors suggesting that glyphosate, which can be detected in the bloodstream, might be implicated in adding to the toxic burden in autistic children.[4]

Despite these examples and other mounting evidence, the concept of detoxification has become a controversial issue. The debate over its value and safety has made headlines around the world. In 2009, even Prince Charles was accused of quackery and exploitation over his company's promotion of a herbal "Detox Tincture".[5] Using herbal potions to detoxify the body was described as "implausible, unproven and dangerous".

The detractors maintain there is no convincing evidence that exposure to environmental toxins is linked to chronic health problems, and, furthermore, there is no clear indication that the removal of environmental toxins benefits health. They also suggest that there is no evidence that natural treatments can reduce either the level or the negative impact of environmental toxins in the body. Hence, any clinician promoting natural detoxification treatments is a fraud, a charlatan, and a quack: a snake-oil seller.

However, the fact that the value of detoxification does not have mainstream acceptance actually represents a major clinical opportunity for natural health practitioners. In fact, detoxification was probably always part of the herbalist's agenda, and now there is the science to support it. On the other hand, to avoid being labelled as "snake-oil sellers" we should confine ourselves to situations and treatments that have evidence behind them and avoid unproven fads and myths (such as using coriander leaf for heavy metal detoxification).

7.2   Our exposome in a potentially toxic modern world

An important review published in the prestigious journal *Science* proposed the following:[6]

> Despite extensive evidence showing that exposure to specific chemicals can lead to disease, current research approaches and regulatory policies fail to address the chemical complexity of our world. To safeguard current and future generations from the increasing number of chemicals polluting our environment, a systematic and agnostic approach is needed. The "exposome" concept strives to capture the diversity and range of exposures to synthetic chemicals, dietary constituents, psychosocial stressors, and physical factors, as well as their corresponding biological responses. Technological advances such as high-resolution mass spectrometry and network science have allowed us to take the first steps toward a comprehensive assessment of the exposome. Given the increased recognition of the dominant role that nongenetic factors play in disease, an effort to characterize the exposome at a scale comparable to that of the human genome is warranted.

The major chemical toxin exposures resulting from our modern industrialised world can broadly be divided into two categories: inorganic (mineral) and organic (molecules containing carbon). The main inorganic toxins of concern are the heavy metals (HMs), such as lead, cadmium, arsenic, and mercury, and certain indoor and outdoor air pollutants (oxides of nitrogen, fine mineral particles, and so on).

Organic toxins of major focus are many (as noted in **Figure 7.1**):

- persistent organic pollutants
- pseudo-POPs (see Section 7.2.4)
- biotoxins
- herbicides
- organic air pollutants (diesel particles)
- food additives (potentially)

- drugs in the environment (potentially)
- personal care chemicals (potentially)
- household chemicals (potentially)
- microplastics
- solvents

One organisation, the Environmental Working Group (EWG), is conducting interesting research in this area. A 2005 study by the EWG identified 287 environmental contaminants in umbilical cord blood.[8] Of these 287 chemicals detected, 180 cause cancer in humans or animals, 217 are toxic to the brain and nervous system, and 208 cause birth defects or abnormal development in animal tests. The dangers of pre- or post-natal exposure to this complex mixture of carcinogens, developmental toxins, and neurotoxins have never been studied.

In another study from the EWG, the urine of every one of 22 mothers and 26 children tested yielded evidence of exposure to TDCPP, a carcinogenic fire retardant.[9] In children, the average concentration of a chemical biomarker

Ecosystems
Food outlets, alcohol outlets
Built environment and
  urban land uses
Population density
Walkability
Green/blue space

Lifestyle
Physical activity
Sleep behaviour
Diet
Drug use
Smoking
Alcohol use

Social
Household income
Inequality
Social capital
Social networks
Cultural norms
Cultural capital
Psychological and mental stress

Physical–Chemical
Temperature/humidity
Electromagnetic fields
Ambient light
Odour and noise
Point, line sources,
  e.g. factories, ports
Outdoor and indoor air
  pollution
Agricultural activities,
  livestock
Pollen/mould/fungus
Pesticides
Fragrance products
Flame retardants (PBDEs)
Persistent organic pollutants
Plastic and plasticisers
Food contaminants
Soil contaminants
Drinking water contamination
Groundwater contamination
Surface water contamination
Occupational exposures

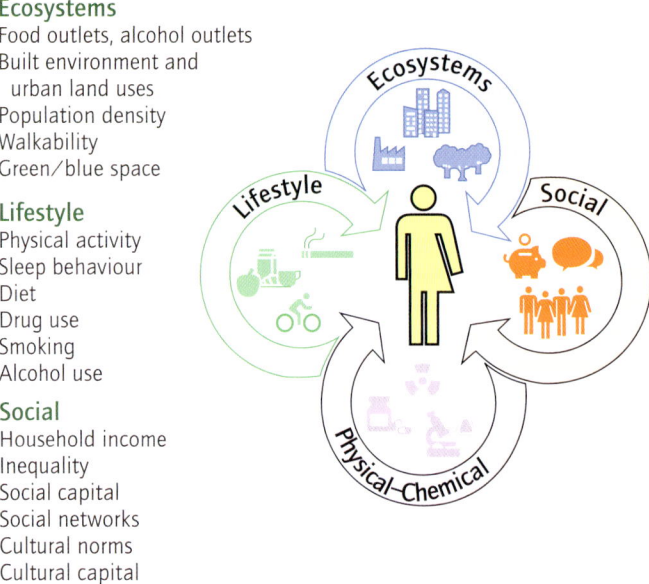

Figure 7.1 Our modern human exposome.[7] [PBDE = polybrominated diphenyl ether.]

left when TDCPP breaks down was nearly five times the average in the mothers. In the most extreme case, a child had 23 times the level measured in the mother. Modern treated furniture is a significant source of exposure to TDCPP.

In the past, research has focused on the impact of individual chemicals in terms of their detrimental effects on people and the environment. But, as intimated above, it has become apparent that this approach falls well short of the mark. This is because the real world is marked by multiple stressors. Among these stressors, and forming a significant part of our exposome, are cocktails of environmental chemicals. Some might claim that these exposures are at levels that do not cause concern for each individual chemical, but collectively they have increased potential to do harm. This realisation casts doubt on current regulations and testing, which only deal with the evaluation of individual chemicals before they are allowed to be used in circumstances that might result in human exposure. Such concerns are now mainstream, with another review article published in *Science* highlighting the urgent need to gain a better understanding of how the total chemical exposome impacts human health.[10]

7.2.1 Persistent organic pollutants

A significant class of organic toxins are the persistent organic pollutants (POPs). These are mainly organochlorine molecules, which largely comprise the PCBs, and DDT (dichlorodiphenyltrichloroethane) and its metabolites. PCBs are industrial polychlorinated biphenyls that were mainly used as transformer oil, since they had high dielectric strength and were not flammable. Other POPs include pesticides, the products of industrial activity, such as high-temperature incinerators and power stations, and chemicals like dioxins.

POPs were originally defined by the Stockholm Convention in 2001. The 12 initial POPs were:

- pesticides: aldrin, chlordane, DDT, dieldrin, endrin, heptachlor, hexachlorobenzene, mirex, toxaphene

- industrial chemicals: hexachlorobenzene, PCBs
- by-products: hexachlorobenzene; PCDDs (polychlorinated dibenzo-p-dioxins) and PCDFs (polychlorinated dibenzofurans); and PCBs

They have been banned from use in industrialised countries for several decades but are incredibly stable in the environment and accumulate in body fat. POPs can act as potent endocrine disruptors – especially for thyroid hormone, insulin, and sex hormones. They have also been implicated in cancer and autoimmunity. The body struggles to eliminate this persistent menace from its tissues, because of their pronounced chemical stability and high solubility in fat tissue. Because of these properties, they can accumulate and endlessly cycle in the biosphere. With the extremely sensitive analytical chemical techniques available today, they can be readily measured in most people.

Newer POPs added later under the Stockholm Convention included polycyclic aromatic hydrocarbons found in cigarette smoke and the brominated flame retardants (used in furniture fabrics, for example). More recently, the endosulfan pesticides and PFAS (see Section 7.2.2) were added to the POP classification.

7.2.2 PFAS and PFOS

Perfluoroalkyl and polyfluoroalkyl substances, or PFAS, are synthetic chemicals found in many products, including food packaging, household cleaners, fabrics, furniture, non-stick cookware, and in other grease- and water-resistant coatings. Notably, they are also used in firefighting foam. Certain types of PFAS, particularly perfluorooctanoic acid (PFOA) and perfluorooctane sulfonate (PFOS), do not break down in the environment or in the human body. They are "forever chemicals", and as such have been classified as new POPs under the Stockholm Convention.

PFAS have been linked to a variety of cancers and are known to interfere with immune function, endocrine function, and breast development. Women firefighters face high exposure to toxic PFAS chemicals, as verified in a study that was part of a larger investigation into the breast cancer risks experienced by women in the firefighting force.[11]

7.2.3   Organophosphate pesticides

Organophosphate (OP) compounds were originally developed as human nerve gas agents during the 1930s and 1940s, and some were later adapted as insecticides at lower doses. They are chemical substances produced by the process of esterification between phosphoric acid and alcohol. Hence, OPs can readily undergo hydrolysis on exposure to sunlight, air, and soil and, as a result, are not persistent in the environment.[12] However, they can occur at low levels in water and sprayed food.[13] In the United States, many OP pesticides, including malathion, dichlorvos, azinphos-methyl, and chlorpyrifos, were licensed for insecticidal use before the requirements to evaluate human toxicity or ecological effects were established.[14] Acute or chronic exposure to OPs can produce varying levels of toxicity in humans, animals, plants, and insects.[15]

Studies have shown that prolonged, repeated exposure to organophosphate pesticides (OPPs), as in the case of farm workers, can lead to significant health problems, including increased risks for cardiovascular and respiratory disease and cancer.[16] A high-level policy forum recently made the following recommendations:[17]

- Widespread use of OPPs to control insects has resulted in ubiquitous human exposures.
- High exposures to OPPs are responsible for poisonings and deaths, particularly in developing countries.
- Compelling evidence indicates that prenatal exposure at low levels is putting children at risk for cognitive and behavioural deficits and for neurodevelopmental disorders.

To protect children worldwide, their recommendations included the following:

- Governments should phase out chlorpyrifos and other OPPs, monitor watersheds and other sources of human exposures, promote the use of integrated pest management (IPM) through incentives and training in agroecology, and implement mandatory surveillance of pesticide-related illness.

Organophosphorus compounds cause four main neurotoxic effects in humans: cholinergic syndrome, intermediate syndrome (a spectrum disorder affecting the neuromuscular junction), organophosphate-induced delayed polyneuropathy, and chronic organophosphate-induced neuropsychiatric disorder.[18] There is also a possible link between chronic, low-level exposure to OPPs and neurodegenerative diseases, such as dementia, ADHD, and Parkinson's disease.

7.2.4 The pseudo-POPs

Pseudo-POPS can be so-called because, while they lack the environmental stability of POPs, they are consistently present in the environment. This is due either to their constant release from contaminating sources and/or our consistent exposure to them. Unlike POPs, they do not accumulate in fat tissue and are readily excreted. Our consistent exposure is not because they are biosphere accumulators, but because we are in contact with them every day. BPA is an example of a pseudo-POP in plastic bottles and canned food, but there are also other such toxins, including phthalates used as plasticisers, tributyltin, an industrial chemical, and perchlorate (a chemical used in solid rocket propellants, ordnance, fireworks, and airbag deployment systems that is ubiquitously detected in water and food).[19]

We are exposed to these pseudo-POPs every day from the containers we use for food and water, the personal care products we apply to our skin, the surfaces we touch, and the food and water we ingest. They are being investigated as significant endocrine disruptors, among other issues.[20]

7.2.5 Heavy metals

Heavy metals (HMs) are metallic elements that have a high atomic weight and a density much greater (at least 5 times) than water (aluminium is therefore not a heavy metal and exhibits different chemical behaviour). There are more than 20 heavy metals, but four are of particular concern to human health because they are highly toxic: lead (Pb), cadmium (Cd), mercury (Hg), and inorganic arsenic (As). HMs have been used by humans for thousands of years, and although their adverse health effects have been known for a long time, exposure to them continues. Being elements that cannot break down further, once they are released into the environment by industrial or agricultural activity, they will persist forever. HMs tend to accumulate in the food chain and in the body and can be stored in soft tissue (such as liver and kidney) and hard tissue (such as bone).[21]

These metals have been studied extensively and their effects on human health regularly reviewed by international bodies such as the WHO. There is a consensus that high-level exposure to HMs can cause several well-described acute symptoms and toxicities. What is more controversial is whether these same or similar toxic effects and symptoms might result from chronic, low-level exposure in sensitive individuals. In addition, other subtler effects might also result from low-level exposure, including subtle endocrine, neurological, and immunological dysfunctions.[22]

Cadmium (Cd) emissions have increased dramatically during the twentieth century, one reason being that Cd-containing products are rarely recycled, but often dumped together with household waste. Cigarette smoking is another major source of Cd exposure. In non-smokers, food is the most important source of intake. Data indicate that adverse health effects of Cd exposure may occur at lower levels than previously anticipated, primarily in the form of kidney damage, but possibly also bone effects and fractures.

The primary environmental exposure to mercury is via food, with fish being a major source of methyl mercury intake, and dental amalgam. Populations with high fish consumption may attain blood levels sufficient for mild neurological damage to adults, due to the methyl mercury contamination. Since there is a risk to the foetus, pregnant women should avoid a high intake of certain predatory fish, such as shark, swordfish, and tuna.

Environmental exposure to lead is mainly from air and food, but contaminated water can be an issue, especially due to old lead piping. Lead-based paints and old batteries are other sources. During the last century, Pb release to the ambient air has resulted in considerable pollution, mainly due to emissions from leaded petrol. Children are particularly susceptible to Pb exposure, due to their high gastrointestinal uptake and permeable blood–brain barrier. Hence, there is the proposal that accepted safe blood levels in children should be reduced considerably below current levels, with recent data indicating that neurotoxic effects occur at quite low levels of exposure.

Although Pb in petrol has dramatically decreased over the last decades, thereby reducing environmental exposure, soil contamination near highways can still cause significant exposure due to breathing in dust.

Exposure to inorganic arsenic is mainly via intake of food and drinking water, food being the larger source in most populations (especially from contaminated rice). Seafood and seaweed contain organic As, which is not toxic. Long-term exposure to As in drinking-water (mainly ground water) is related to increased risk of skin cancer (but also some other cancers), as well as other skin lesions such as hyperkeratosis and pigmentation changes. Occupational exposure to As, primarily by inhalation, is causally associated with lung cancer.

7.2.6 Air pollution

In terms of the capacity to cause detrimental health effects, air pollution levels are significantly high in many parts of the world. Recent data from the WHO demonstrated that 9 out of 10 people in the world breathe air containing unacceptable levels of pollutants.[23] The WHO estimates that every year around 7 million people die just from exposure to fine particles ($PM_{2.5}$) in polluted air that penetrate deep into the lungs and cardiovascular system, causing diseases such as stroke, heart disease, lung cancer, asthma, chronic obstructive pulmonary diseases, and respiratory infections, including pneumonia. Yet virtually no one has air pollution mentioned as the cause of death on their death certificate.[24]

$PM_{2.5}$ can be made of black carbon, nitrates, sulphates, ammonia, or mineral dust. Most are produced by burning wood or fossil fuels. Nitrogen dioxide, produced by diesel vehicles, not only reacts to form particles, but is now known to cause harm when breathed as a gas (see also oxides of nitrogen below).[25]

Globally, it is estimated that carbon monoxide is emitted into the atmosphere in amounts as high as 2,600 million tons each year, of which 60% is from human activities, mainly the incomplete burning of carbonaceous materials. The largest amount of these emissions is from automobiles with petrol engines. Other common sources comprise different industrial processes, waste incineration, and power plants using coal.

Oxides of nitrogen are gases produced mainly by human activity such as combustion of fossil fuels in motor vehicles and stationary sources (heating, power generation). Sulfur dioxide, one of the most prevalent and dangerous air pollutants, is released from natural sources such as volcanoes or anthropogenically from the burning of fossil fuel and biomass at large industrial plants, such as oil refineries and power stations.[26]

7.2.7 Fungal toxins

Fungal toxins (mycotoxins) are fungal secondary metabolites produced by phytopathogenic fungi such as *Aspergillus, Penicillium, Fusarium,* and *Alternaria* species. In terms of both chemical structure and toxicological properties, mycotoxins are a highly diverse group of compounds. Their classification is a complex task, due to this diverse chemistry and biosynthetic origin and because they are produced by a great variety of fungal species. Moreover, the same mycotoxin can be produced by several fungal species – for example, ochratoxin A. Aflatoxins and ochratoxins (produced by *Aspergillus spp.* and *Penicillium spp.*), fumonisins, trichothecenes, and zearalenone (produced by *Fusarium spp.*), and patulin and citrinin (produced by *Penicillium spp.*) are the most commonly observed mycotoxins that pose serious health threats to humans and animals.[27]

Human exposure to mycotoxins takes place through the consumption of contaminated food such as cereals, spices, and herbal teas. It can also occur through the ingestion of products of animal origin, such as eggs and milk, if the animals have previously been fed with contaminated feed. Additionally, we can be exposed to mycotoxins by inhalation and dermal contact with contaminated dust or mould.[28]

Work and home mycotoxin exposure due to damp conditions is an increasing clinical phenomenon. For example, it was found that toxins produced by three different species of fungus growing indoors on wallpaper can become aerosolised and easily inhaled. These findings will likely have implications for "sick building syndrome". One author of this study noted: "There are almost no data on toxicity of mycotoxins following inhalation."[29]

7.2.8 Glyphosate

Glyphosate, introduced in 1974 by Monsanto Company under the commercial name Roundup, became the most extensively used herbicide worldwide. It has been reported to increase the risk of cancer and might be a factor in endocrine disruption, coeliac disease, autism, and leaky-gut syndrome, to name a few. The reclassification of glyphosate in 2015 as "probably carcinogenic" under Group 2A by the International Agency for Research on Cancer created huge controversy. Moreover, several investigations have suggested that the surfactant polyethoxylated tallow amine (POEA), contained in formulations of glyphosate like Roundup, is potentially responsible for adverse impacts on human and ecological health. After the development of genetically modified glyphosate-resistant crops and the general indiscriminate use of glyphosate in recent years, about 38 weed species have developed resistance to this herbicide. Consequently, its use has been either restricted or banned in about 20 countries.[30]

An impressive group of environmental health academics have published a consensus statement concerning the risks involved from exposure to glyphosate-based herbicides (GBH) as follows:[31]

1. GBHs are the most heavily applied herbicide in the world, and usage continues to rise.
2. Worldwide, GBHs often contaminate drinking water sources, precipitation and air, especially in agricultural regions.
3. The half-life of glyphosate in water and soil is longer than previously recognised.
4. Glyphosate and its metabolites are widely present in the global soybean supply.
5. Human exposures to GBHs are rising.
6. Glyphosate is now authoritatively classified as a probable human carcinogen.
7. Regulatory estimates of tolerable daily intakes for glyphosate in the United States and European Union are based on outdated science.

7.3 A focus on some specific health issues linked to environmental toxins

7.3.1 The role of environmental toxins in autoimmunity

How can toxins trigger autoimmunity? There are three main possible mechanisms. First, cells are damaged by the toxin and die necrotically, causing the release of self-antigens that the immune system would not otherwise be exposed to. In addition, the release of other components of these necrotic cells can act as danger signals that create a high state of alarm for the immune system; this is the danger theory of Polly Matzinger.[32] The third mechanism is where the toxin combines with a protein that naturally occurs in the body. This is then recognised by the immune system as foreign, and it attacks that protein plus the toxin (for this mechanism the toxin is acting as a hapten, like several drugs can do). But often the immune system attack is not sufficiently specific, and it mounts an offensive against the protein even if it does not have the toxin bound to it. In other words, an immune cross-reactivity occurs, leading to an attack on normal tissue.

Some of the toxins implicated in human autoimmunity are the following:

- heavy metals: mercury, especially from dental amalgam; nickel via body implants[33,34]
- organic solvents, such as chemicals used in nail polish[35,36]
- pesticides[37]
- BPA[38]
- chemical hair dyes[39]

Patients with autoimmune disorders will benefit from a detoxification program, applied as treatment module. What does such a detoxification program involve? It does not necessarily feature throughout the total course of such treatment for the autoimmune disease, but perhaps for 2–6 months. Then modular treatment can be switched to the bowel flora protocol or to a protocol that addresses stealth pathogens and persistent viruses. Using this modular feature of FHT, the patient is not overburdened with too many treatments at the one time. (Examples of detoxification treatment modules are provided in Sections 7.7.2, 7.8, and 7.9.)

7.3.2 Is autism triggered by environmental toxins?

As mentioned in Section 7.1, there is general agreement that the incidence of autism spectrum disorders (ASD) is increasing, but there is no consensus as to why. Mounting evidence suggests a key role for environmental toxins, especially coupled with reduced defences in genetically (and hence environmentally) vulnerable children.[40] Key issues appear to be heavy metal (HM), pesticide, and other organic chemical exposures, coupled with reduced defensive mechanisms such as methylation, sulfation, and glutathione production.

In terms of heavy metal exposure/susceptibility, a 2009 US study found increased urinary porphyrin metabolites, which are linked to mercury susceptibility/toxicity in autistic children.[41] A 2013 study from the same research team found higher levels of lead in red blood cells (RBCs) and higher urinary lead and thallium in 55 children with ASD aged 5–16 years.[42] There is also speculation that toxic metals may contribute to the severity of autism, in part because of a low GSH status (which is needed to counter the cellular impact of toxic metals). A higher body burden of toxic metals might be caused by increased exposure, increased absorption due to greater intestinal permeability, and/or decreased ability to excrete them (due to low GSH and abnormal gut bacteria as a result of increased oral antibiotic use).

Another 2009 US study found multiple positive correlations between autism severity and urinary excretion of HMs (after challenge with a chelating agent).[43] Children with autism had significantly higher levels of mercury in their baby teeth.[44] A study from Oman found higher hair levels of HMs.[45] Treatment with the oral chelating drug DMSA (dimercaptosuccinic acid) to remove HMs was followed by significant clinical improvement in 49 children with ASD.[46] Several studies have found HM levels to be correlated with depleted RBC GSH and poor sulfation status in ASD children (see Section 7.3.2).

Organic environmental chemicals are also implicated in ASD. A publication from the CHARGE study (Childhood Autism Risks from Genetics and Environment) found proximity to agricultural organophosphates was associated with a 60% increased risk.[47] In another study, mothers living closer to agricultural organochlorine use during pregnancy were 6 times more likely to have a child with ASD.[48] Air pollution exposure around the San Francisco Bay area has also been linked to an increased risk of ASD.[49]

Significantly lower plasma levels of GSH, sulfate, cysteine, and S-adenosylmethionine (SAMe) have been observed in children with ASD.[50] Several studies suggest that children with ASD have an abnormal sulfation chemistry, limited thiol (sulfur) availability, and decreased GSH reserve capacity.[51,52] These are often associated with higher heavy metal levels.[53,54] Consequences of these vulnerabilities include increased oxidative stress, decreased detoxification, decreased methylation, and mitochondrial dysfunction.[55] And there are many more studies, this is just a snapshot. (Note: GSH is a major non-protein cellular thiol – a source of reactive sulfur. It provides the fundamental antioxidant protection for cells and is also a signalling molecule in cell regulation and apoptosis, making it a key modulator of xenobiotic toxicity.[56])

As mentioned, mitochondrial dysfunction should be considered in ASD (see **Figure 7.2**).[57] In the figure, the ASD children are represented on the

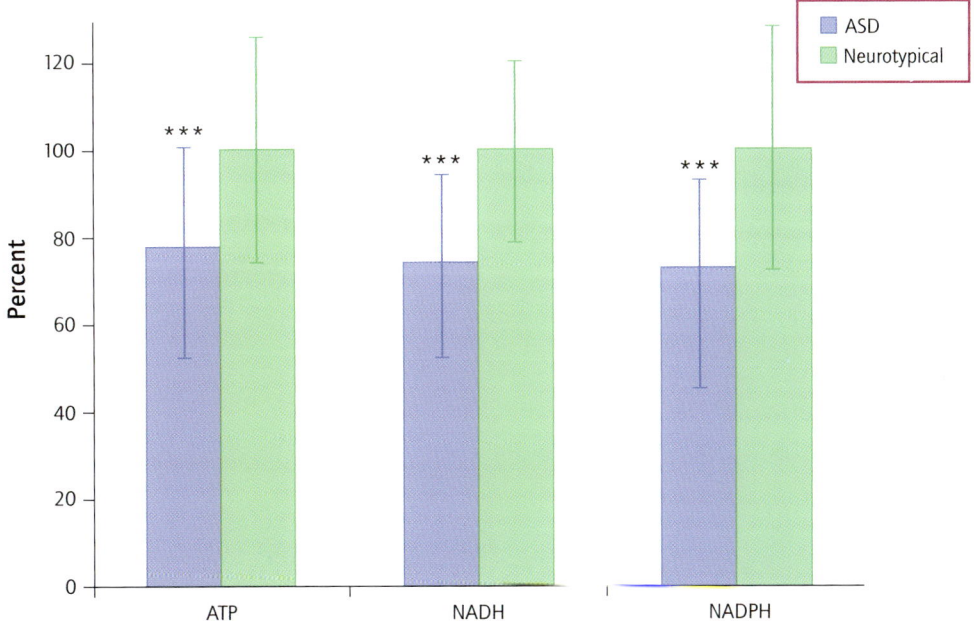

Figure 7.2 Mitochondrial dysfunction in autism spectrum disorders. [ATP = adenosine triphosphate; NADH = nicotinamide adenine dinucleotide+hydrogen; NADPH = nicotinamide adenine dinucleotide phosphate.]

left in blue, and what the authors refer to as neurotypical controls (children of the same age not exhibiting any symptoms of ASD) are on the right in green. ASD children exhibited much lower levels of plasma ATP and RBC levels of NADH (nicotinamide adenine dinucleotide+hydrogen); and NADPH (nicotinamide adenine dinucleotide phosphate), which are cofactors in mitochondrial metabolism (36–51% of the ASD group had levels below the neurotypical reference range). Environmental toxins are known to negatively impact mitochondrial function.[58] Exposure to toxic air pollutants (specifically dioxins) was linked to an increased risk of developing autism, according to a study of Chinese children during their first three-years of life. Mitochondrial dysfunction was suggested as a key pathway for this impact.[59]

7.3.3 Endocrine disruption

The Environmental Working Group published their "dirty dozen" endocrine disruptors in 2013:[60]

1. BPA
2. dioxin
3. atrazine
4. phthalates
5. perchlorate
6. fire retardants
7. lead
8. arsenic
9. mercury
10. perfluorinated chemicals (PFCs)
11. organophosphate pesticides
12. glycol ethers

Endocrine disruption can contribute to a range of chronic health problems, including type 2 diabetes, reduced fertility (in both men and women), poor development in children, and obesity. For example, PCB exposure from a waste incinerator was found to adversely impact thyroid function in children.[61]

The pseudoPOPs BPA and phthalates have been the subject of considerable recent research. For example, one study found that maternal BPA levels were associated with a high risk of first-trimester miscarriage.[62] A recent review concluded that, while current exposures to BPA have not shown marked or consistent results, there are sufficient data to raise concerns regarding negative impacts on ovarian function.[63] BPA has been reported to be associated with female infertility. Indeed, it is more frequently detected in infertile women. In addition, in procedures of medically assisted reproduction, BPA exposure has been found to be negatively associated with peak serum oestradiol levels during gonadotropin stimulation, number of retrieved oocytes, number of normally fertilised oocytes, and implantation success.[64]

In terms of male fertility, another review concluded that, despite some inconsistencies across different phthalates, results support the contention that phthalate exposure at levels seen in human populations may exert adverse male reproductive effects.[65]

Endocrine disruptors do not just impact sex hormonal function, they might also act on the pancreas and cause insulin resistance (IR); on the thyroid leading to obesity; on the adrenal glands leading to an abnormal stress response; and on the parathyroids impacting calcium metabolism, with possible implications for osteoporosis.[66] In fact, all major endocrine organs are vulnerable to endocrine disruption by environmental chemicals.

One fascinating example of endocrine disruption has recently emerged for the POPs and their role in the disruption of insulin effects, leading to IR, metabolic syndrome, and type 2 diabetes (see Chapter 11). In a surprising new finding, research also links outdoor air pollution, even at levels deemed safe, to an increased risk of diabetes globally. Overall, the researchers estimated that air pollution contributed to 3.2 million new diabetes cases globally in 2016, about 14% of all the new cases that year. They also estimated that 8.2 million years of healthy life were lost in 2016 due to air pollution-linked diabetes.[67]

7.3.4 Effects on cardiovascular and bone health

Heavy metal and POP exposure have both been linked to a higher risk of cardiovascular disease and osteoporosis. Possible mechanisms behind this are illustrated in **Figure 7.3**.

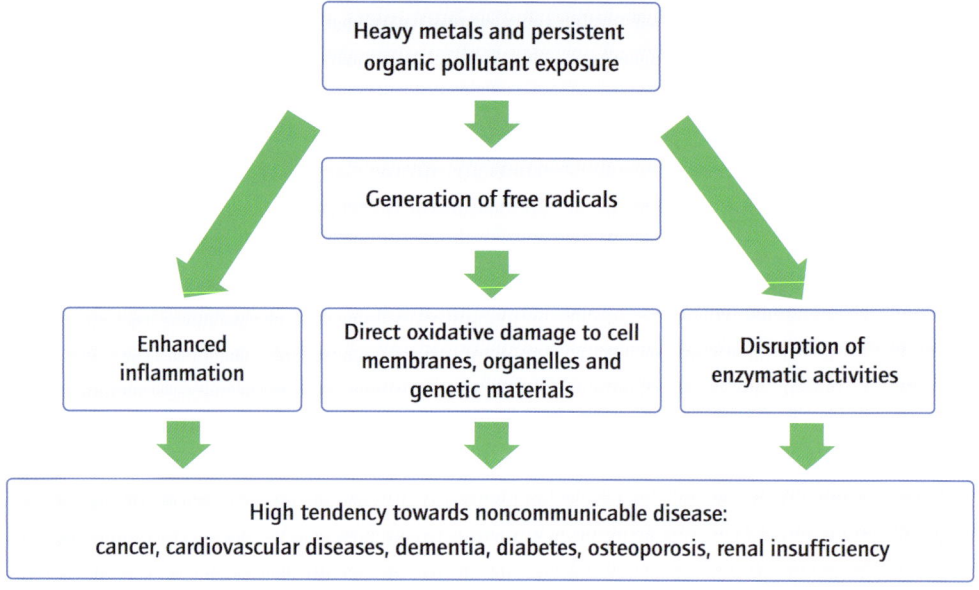

Figure 7.3   Effects on the body of heavy metals and persistent organic pollutants.[68]

Mercury seems to particularly affect the cardiovascular system. A significant increase in heart muscle HMs (assessed by biopsy) was found in patients with idiopathic dilated cardiomyopathy.[69] A high dietary intake of methyl mercury from fish was shown to increase the risk of coronary artery disease,[70] although results were variable. The association between Hg exposure and hypertension was described as "convincing" in one review.[71]

In terms of the POPs, serum levels of PCBs were found to correlate with blood pressure, which was independent of BMI or age.[72] A rapid rise in atmospheric NO levels within 24 hours increases the short-term risk of a heart attack. Such dynamic changes in concentrations of air pollutants are not covered by current statutory limits.[73]

One study demonstrated that consuming a canned beverage, and the consequent increase in BPA exposure, acutely increased blood pressure.[74] Systolic blood pressure (adjusted for daily variance) increased by about 4.5 mm Hg after consuming two canned beverages relative to consuming two glass-bottled beverages, and the difference was statistically significant.

Cadmium (Cd) exposure is linked to poor bone health. A link between Cd and skeletal damage was first reported from Japan in the 1950s due to

Cd-contaminated water used for irrigation of rice fields (itai-itai disease). This is now thought to be a re-emerging problem in some parts of China.[75]

However, during recent years, new data have emerged suggesting that relatively low Cd exposure may give rise to osteoporosis and fractures.[76] The US Occupational Safety and Health Administration (OSHA) minimum safety standard for urinary Cd (U-Cd) is 3 µg/g. But US women are at risk of developing osteoporosis at U-Cd levels 3–6 times less than this OSHA safety standard. Around 20% of the osteoporosis prevalence among women older than 50 years of age may be attributable to Cd body burden in the United States.[77]

7.4 How we are exposed

Our main pathways for encountering environmental toxins can be summarised as follows:

- air and smoking
- water, drinks, and drink packaging
- food and food packaging
- skin contact, clothes, and hand-oral transfer
- personal care products
- dental fillings and body implants
- in utero

Elaborating on the fourth point, we can be exposed to toxins through skin contact and hand-oral transfer. For example, these days if we touch a computer keyboard, that keyboard contains plasticisers, fire retardants, and many other chemicals, and we pick these up on our fingers. If we then eat afterwards, or just put our hands into our mouth (which many people do) we are transferring these toxins into our system by hand-oral transfer.

But in some cases, hand-oral transfer is not needed. Free BPA is applied to the outer layer of thermal receipt paper in very high quantities (~20 mg BPA/g paper) as a print developer. Not considered when assessing thermal paper as a source of BPA exposure is that some commonly used hand sanitisers, as well as other skin-care products, contain mixtures of dermal penetration enhancing chemicals that can increase by up to 100-fold the skin absorption of lipophilic compounds such as BPA. A research team found that when men and women held thermal receipt paper immediately after using a hand sanitiser containing penetration-enhancing chemicals, significant free BPA was transferred through the skin on their hands and also on to French fries that were then eaten. This combination of dermal and oral BPA absorption led within 90 minutes to a rapid and dramatic average maximum increase of unconjugated (bioactive) BPA of ~7 ng/mL in serum and ~20 μg total BPA/g creatinine in urine. The scientists noted the default method used by regulatory agencies to test for hazards posed by chemicals is intra-gastric gavage. For BPA this approach results in less than 1% of the administered dose being bioavailable in blood. But this safety standard ignores dermal absorption and sublingual absorption in the mouth, which both avoid first-pass liver metabolism.[78]

7.5 Managing our toxic burden

The **four pillars** for managing the toxic burden of modern life are:

1. avoid
2. protect
3. repair
4. eliminate

We can identify six key strategies to achieve this:

1. **Reduce exposure by avoidance**, including eating organic foods, especially animal products such as eggs, dairy, meat, and fish, as they can accumulate significant levels of POPs in the fat they contain.

    For pseudo-POPs, limiting exposure is the most relevant strategy, since they are readily excreted by the body. This includes avoiding packaged food and drinks (unless in glass), carefully screening personal care products (to avoid undesirable chemicals), and washing hands before eating (to minimise transfer from touched surfaces).

For heavy metals, reducing exposure includes eating minimal amounts of large predatory fish (such as shark, tuna, swordfish) and avoiding dental amalgam, jewellery containing nickel, and metal joint implants.

2. **Improve detoxification and excretion pathways:** one simple technique is to ensure adequate fluid intake to assist the flushing of pseudo-POPs from our tissues. The Nrf2 pathway is critical here (see Chapter 6). (FHT to achieve this strategy is described in Sections 7.7.2, 7.8, and 7.9.)

3. **Compensate for genetic weaknesses** in methylation, sulfation, and GSH production using herbs and supplements.

4. **Increase cellular protection:** toxins such as pseudoPOPs are transient in the body, so the best strategy is to ensure our cells are well protected against their negative impact (see cytoprotection in Chapter 2).

5. **Increase protective dietary factors:** B vitamins, the amino acid components of GSH, ascorbic acid, fibre, and minerals are key examples. For example, mineral intake protects against heavy metal toxicity. Toxic metals hitchhike on the same transport proteins that the gut uses to absorb key minerals such as calcium, magnesium, zinc, and iron. If mineral intake is adequate, there will be less room to give the toxic metals a ride. Furthermore, iron deficiency upregulates these transport proteins and thereby increases heavy metal uptake by the body. Dietary fibre can bind toxins and assist with their excretion.

6. **Increase cellular damage repair mechanisms:** GSH is the key factor here (discussed in Section 7.8.1). Again, this is a major strategy for pseudo-POPs, as regular exposure is the most important issue, rather than any problem with their elimination (although enhancing their elimination is still a worthwhile strategy).

Several studies support the use of avoidance measures. For example, exposure to individual flame retardants was reduced by about half (as measured by urinary excretion) by one week of increased hand washing, house cleaning to reduce dust, or combined activities.[79] Children have higher polybrominated diphenyl ether (PBDE) body burdens than adults, which may be related to hand-to-mouth behaviour. One study investigated associations between children's behaviour, including hand-to-mouth contacts, and markers of PBDE exposure.[80] More active children had higher levels of PBDEs on their hands and in their bodies. Children who licked their fingers while eating had higher serum PBDEs. Other behaviours were not consistently associated with serum levels. Playing with plastic toys was associated with higher hand levels of PBDEs, while frequent vacuuming decreased these. In a study in pregnant women, associations with serum PBDEs were observed with self-reported hand-to-mouth behaviours, including biting nails and licking fingers.[81] Serum levels of total PBDEs were also significantly higher in those individuals owning a large-screen television compared with those who did not.

In a population-based prospective cohort study among 68,946 French adults, high organic food intake scores were inversely associated with the overall risk of cancer (hazard ratio for quartile 4 vs quartile 1, 0.75; 95% CI, 0.63–0.88; $p = 0.001$).[82] An organic diet was associated with significant reductions in urinary excretion of several pesticide metabolites and their parent compounds.[83] The authors stated that their study adds to a growing body of literature indicating that an organic diet may reduce exposure to a range of pesticides in children and adults.

Summarising all of the guidelines for reducing toxin exposure and its impact (there is some overlap with the above):

- Eat organically when possible, especially eggs, meat, poultry, fish and dairy.
- Avoid large predatory fish: tuna, swordfish, shark.
- For non-organic vegetables and fruits, eat those that are less likely to be grown with excessive chemicals: for example, the EWG Clean 15 that includes avocados, mangos, cabbage, aubergine, and so on.
- Avoid canned (tinned) foods and plastic bottles and packaging.
- Personal care products and cosmetics should be natural; clothes should be made from natural fibres (organic if possible).
- Ensure adequate hydration and preserve good kidney function.
- Preserve good liver function and bile output.
- Dental fillings should not be amalgam.
- Say no to credit card receipts.

▷ Consider home water and air filters; vacuum and dust your house regularly.
▷ Use natural cleaning products at home, especially for washing clothes.
▷ Avoid household pesticides, air fresheners, and other aerosols.
▷ Always wash hands before eating (just use simple soap and water).
▷ Furnish with naturally treated furniture.
▷ Floors and carpet or rugs should not be treated with chemicals.
▷ Ensure the home and workplace is mould-free.
▷ Use protection during gardening, such as masks and gloves.

7.5.1 Clinical scenarios

Essentially there are four types of exposure scenarios that might need to be addressed in the clinic:

1. **Pervasive, insidious, and cumulative:** POPs and heavy metals. Here it is difficult to avoid some level of exposure, for example banned POPs are still consistently found in human breast milk. The main focus must be on elimination.
2. **Pervasive and cumulative,** but only have impact during the short time they are in the body: most pseudoPOPs. Repeated short-term impacts can eventually lead to physiological disruption and disease. The main focus must be on avoidance and protection.
3. **Exposure-related:** cause both immediate damage from acute and subacute exposures and cumulative damage with repeated exposure. Examples are air pollution, organophosphates, and biotoxins. The main focus must be on avoidance, protection, and repair.
4. **Developmental,** which can be any exposure of any of the above three types that lead to changes during development that might be permanent. The main focus will depend on the type of exposure, but repair of the damage, if possible, is key – or compensation for its effects if the damage is beyond repair.

In a recent editorial in the journal *Integrative Medicine,* Joseph Pizzorno wrote the following:[84]

Substantial research now shows that metal and chemical contamination of the environment has resulted in body loads of these toxicants at high enough levels to induce disease. The time has come to add screening for toxicant load to the **standard of care**. . . . Ideally, every patient should be screened annually for toxin load. Toxicity is now so common it must be considered in every patient, especially in those with chronic disease, known exposure or losing bone. . . . Could it be that the huge increase in disease burden as people age into the 50s and 60s is simply a reflection of cumulative damage from toxic exposure, accumulation of difficult to detoxify, new-to-nature chemicals (the human half-life of PCBs is 3–25 years!) and the added burden from toxins released from dissolving bones?

7.6 Evidence for key herbs

7.6.1 Green tea

Epigallocatechin gallate (EGCG) from green tea (GT) has been shown to prime Nrf2 responses in several *in vivo* models, and there are some indirect human data. In addition to *in vitro* testing, animal studies further confirm the beneficial effects of green tea extracts (GTE) against pesticide-induced toxicities, including oxidative damage in the liver, lungs, and nervous system. *In vitro* and *in vivo* studies also show protection against PCBs, aflatoxins, and arsenic. The protective activity of GT and its constituents on smoke-induced damage has been shown in cell culture, animal, and human studies (especially in terms of DNA protection for the human work).[85]

In terms of clinical trials:

- GT attenuated benzene-induced oxidative stress in pump workers (trial, $n = 60$)[86]
- RCT ($n = 123$): GTE improved metabolism of the carcinogenic mycotoxin fumonisin B1[87]
- RCT ($n = 35$): GT supplementation increased GSH and plasma antioxidant capacity in adults with metabolic syndrome[88]
- crossover RCT ($n = 16$): GT reduced lymphocyte DNA damage and increased DNA repair[89]

▸ RCT ($n = 43$ people with T2D): GT for 12 weeks was clearly associated with lowered DNA damage (15%), increased 8-oxoguanine glycosylase (hOGG1, a DNA repair enzyme) activity (50%), and higher HO-1 (haem oxygenase-1) protein levels (40%).[90]

7.6.2 Garlic

Without doubt, garlic is the key herbal heavy metal antidote. Garlic contains sulfur compounds that can bind to heavy metals (as do GSH and metallothioneins), increasing their excretion. Garlic primes the Nrf2/ARE pathway and increases H_2S production. Numerous laboratory studies have confirmed the protective action of garlic against HM toxicity.

Activity against lead (Pb) toxicity has been confirmed in two RCTs. Allicin is highly active in this regard, implying the superiority of allicin-releasing products or raw garlic.[91,92]

A clinical study compared the effect of a standardised garlic preparation with the chelating drug penicillamine in male workers exposed to lead at a car battery factory. They were randomised to receive garlic tablets (equivalent to 6 g/day of fresh bulb) or penicillamine (750 mg/day) for 4 weeks. The garlic tablets were said to release allicin, providing 3.6 mg/day. The double-blind trial included workers who were exhibiting signs and symptoms of mild to moderate lead poisoning. These signs and symptoms (elevated blood pressure, tendon reflex, and headache) improved only in the garlic group, possibly due to increased Nrf2 activity augmenting repair pathways. Blood lead decreased in both groups: by 18.5% for garlic versus 24.4% for the drug.[93]

In an earlier trial, the effect of garlic on workers in a lead smelter at risk of chronic lead poisoning was investigated in the 1960s in Europe.[94] Testing over 1–3 months showed that the number of workers already exhibiting signs of early lead toxicity (damaged RBCs and porphyrin in the urine) fell by 83% after treatment with garlic. The amount of porphyrin remaining in the urine was decreased, and there was a statistically significant increase RBCs and haemoglobin. Of the workers who were not showing signs of early lead toxicity at the beginning of the trial, 28% of those in the control group developed signs after three months, compared to only 3% in the group given garlic.

7.6.3 Turmeric/curcumin

In an open trial ($n = 14$), curcumin (500 mg/day for 15–30 days) attenuated urinary excretion of albumin in T2D patients, accompanied by an enhanced Nrf2 response – specifically, NQO-1, together with other antioxidative enzymes in patients' blood lymphocytes – and repressed inflammatory signalling efficacies.[95]

Curcumin (1,000 mg/day plus piperine for 3 months) protected against DNA damage in a chronically arsenic-exposed population of West Bengal. The chronic exposure to As was also found to significantly deplete activities of the antioxidant enzymes catalase ($p < 0.001$), SOD ($p < 0.001$), GST ($p < 0.001$), GSH reductase ($p < 0.001$), and GSH peroxidase ($p < 0.005$), as well as GSH levels ($p < 0.005$). Curcumin treatment also retarded ROS generation and lipid peroxidation and, over time, raised the depleted levels of these antioxidant enzymes and GSH (RCT, $n = 286$).[96]

7.6.4 Schisandra

Schisandra has been traditionally used to support the detoxification of alcohol and as a tonic and adaptogen. Key components are the dibenzocyclooctene lignans. It enhances phase I/II hepatic metabolism in experimental models and, most importantly, induces phase I enzymes without harmful bioactivation (see Section 7.7.1) and exerts anticarcinogenic activity.[97] Clinically, the herb has decreased drug side effects and lowered mildly elevated liver enzymes in some patients.[98]

7.6.5 Broccoli sprouts

Broccoli sprouts (BS) are a clinically validated primer of the Nrf2 response and its outcomes. These beneficial Nrf2 effects of BS may be amplified by noxious cell stressors, meaning it acts best when it is needed most. The herb is a clinically proven upregulator of detoxification pathways (via Nrf2), and it also exerts DNA and epigenetic benefits. BS might also act via increasing hydrogen sulfide (H_2S), with ensuing benefits, and there is some suggestion it may enhance proteostasis (possibly via Nrf2).

7.6.5.1 Clinical Nrf2 and detoxification activities of broccoli sprouts

A placebo-controlled dose escalation trial (n = 65, healthy volunteers) investigated the clinical impact of BS-containing sulforaphane (SFN) on the phase II enzymes GSTM1 (glutathione-S-transferase M1), GSTP1 (glutathione-S-transferase P1), NQO-1, and HO-1. Marked effects were observed: increases in enzyme expression in nasal lavage cells ranged from 101% for GSTP1 to 199% for NQO1 at the highest dose. All the phase II enzymes tested were increased, consistent with the understanding that BS acts by a common mechanism to induce these as a group, namely by activating Nrf2.[99]

Eight healthy women were given a single dose of BS (35.4 mg of SFN) approximately 50 minutes prior to the start of surgery (reduction mammoplasty). Upregulated gene transcripts of NQO1 and HO-1, and NQO1 enzymatic activity, were detected in the breast tissue of all volunteers.[100]

Residents of Qidong, People's Republic of China, are at high risk for the development of hepatocellular carcinoma, in part due to consumption of aflatoxin-contaminated foods. A randomised, placebo-controlled chemoprevention trial (n = 200) tested whether hot water infusions of 3-day-old BS could alter the disposition of aflatoxins. An inverse association was observed for the excretion of SFN metabolites and aflatoxin-DNA adducts in individuals receiving BS (p = 0.002).[101]

7.6.5.2 Clinical epigenetic and genetic effects of broccoli sprouts

Evidence is mounting that SFN also acts through epigenetic mechanisms. SFN has been shown to inhibit histone deacetylase (HDAC) activity in human colon and prostate cancer lines. In humans, ingestion of BS inhibited HDAC activity in circulating peripheral blood mononuclear cells after consumption, with concomitant induction of histone acetylation in chromatin (indicating possible value in preventing cancer and inflammatory disease).[102]

After cooked broccoli consumption by young healthy smokers, the level of oxidised DNA lesions in peripheral blood mononuclear cells decreased by 41%, and resistance to peroxide-induced DNA strand breaks increased by 23%. A higher protection was observed in smokers with the GST M1-null genotype.[103]

7.6.5.3 Broccoli sprouts and air pollution protection

Two RCTs in China ($n = 291$ and $n = 50$) found that consumption of BS substantially and rapidly enhanced the detoxification of airborne pollutants such as acrolein, ethylene oxide, and benzene, suggesting a reduction in their associated health risks.[104,105]

In another RCT ($n = 45$), BS improved the bronchoprotective response in asthmatics through Nrf2-mediated gene pathways.[106]

An initial intranasal challenge with diesel exhaust particles (DEP) in 29 human subjects was followed 4 weeks later by the same test, but after BS had first been given for 4 days. Nasal white blood cells increased by 85% following DEP but, conversely, decreased by 54% when DEP challenge was preceded by BS ($p < 0.001$).[107]

7.6.5.4 Broccoli sprouts and autism

The hypothesis that improving Nrf2 will help people with autism by enhancing detoxification and cellular protective pathways has been put to the test clinically. An exploratory RCT over 18 weeks was undertaken in young men aged 13–27 years with moderate to severe ASD ($n = 44$). There was minimal change for placebo, whereas those on BS showed substantial and significant improvement in two behaviour scores. Also, for the Clinical Global Impression Improvement Scale (CGI-I), a significantly greater number of participants receiving BS had improvement in social interaction, abnormal behaviour, and verbal communication ($p = 0.015$–0.007 vs placebo). Upon discontinuation of BS, total scores on all scales rose towards pre-treatment levels.[108]

Children and young adults ($n = 15$) with ASD and related neurodevelopmental disorders participated in a 12-week, open-label study of BS and seed. There was a significant improvement seen for the Social Responsiveness Scale (SRS). The authors identified 77 urinary metabolites that were correlated with changes in symptoms, and they clustered into pathways of oxidative stress, amino acid/gut microbiome, neurotransmitters, hormones, and sphingomyelin metabolism.[109]

In a follow-up case series from the first trial, of the 14 SFN responders in the RCT whose parents/carers agreed to participate, 13 parents/carers thought that BS had significantly improved behaviour.[110] Comments included: "He (T) is still on it. It's amazing. . . . I don't know what it is. It's almost like voodoo or magic but he is definitely better, and he has made improvements." And: "R is now happier, has more control over his body, and overall is a positive child with a great attitude. He is more social and goes to concerts, movies, restaurants, vacations and family outings (all of which were not possible before the study)."

7.6.6 Korean ginseng

Korean ginseng (RCT, $n = 57$) (3 or 6 g/day for 8 weeks) significantly increased plasma SOD activity in both the low- and high-dose groups; plasma GPx (glutathione peroxidase) and catalase activities increased only after the high-dose supplementation. DNA tail length and tail moment were significantly reduced after both the low and high doses (indicating protective activity), as were plasma oxidised low-density lipoprotein (LDL) levels.[111]

Another RCT (single blind, $n = 22$ young women) found Korean ginseng (2.7 g/day for 2 weeks) decreased urinary BPA and oxidative stress levels ($p < 0.05$) and alleviated "menstrual irregularity", "menstrual pain", and "constipation" ($p < 0.05$).[112]

7.7 Detoxifying organic pollutants

7.7.1 Overview

The liver plays a primary role in detoxification, both of ingested molecules (xenobiotics) and internal metabolites and agents such as hormones. There are two phases involved in this hepatic "biotransformation" of toxins. During phase I, enzymatic-induced oxidation, reduction, or hydrolysis generates a reactive site on the substrate toxin molecule. In phase II, a water-soluble (hydrophilic) group is conjugated with this reactive site to make the molecule more polarised (or electrically charged) and thus more able to be excreted by the body via the urine or bile.

The danger is phase I can create potentially toxic reactive oxygen intermediates with free radical activity, for which antioxidant protection is required. This phase is launched primarily by the cytochrome P450 enzyme family, which recognises and initiates biotransformation of a wide diversity of toxins (substrates). Excessive phase I activity can in fact generate more dangerous toxic intermediates. This might happen, for example, during fasting or other sudden losses of adipose tissue, where the stored fat-soluble toxins are released. The same challenge may occur if there is a reduction in antioxidant capacity, such as in heavy smoking, with exposure to industrial pollutants (which can also induce excessive phase I activity as well), or with chronically deficient diets.

Phase II reactions should quickly step in to neutralise the transformed toxins, reducing the toxic burden and relieving antioxidant defences. These reactions involve conjugation with glucuronic acid, sulfate, glutathione, glycine, or other amino acids, acetylation, or methylation. The onset of chronic diseases, notably cancer, has been often linked to an imbalance between phase I and phase II.

Herbs can help reduce our toxic burden by shifting the phase I/II balance towards the latter, by stimulating cleansing bile flow (phase III excretion) or by directly protecting the liver tissue itself from oxidant attack. Excessive phase I or cytochrome P-450 activity may lead to mutation, cancer or tissue necrosis, particularly of the liver with its high content of cytochrome P-450.[113] Hence the emphasis for FHT is to preferentially boost phase II, which is entirely consistent with activating the Nrf2 pathway.

7.7.2 FHT for detoxifying organic pollutants

Important FHT strategies that support the detoxification of organic pollutants include:[114]

- herbs that prime the Nrf2/ARE pathway: broccoli sprouts, turmeric, rosemary, green tea, garlic, turmeric, Korean ginseng

- herbs that boost phase II detoxification: as above plus Schisandra (Schisandra also appears to boost phase I)
- choleretic herbs (to improve bile flow), such as globe artichoke, dandelion root and milk thistle (silymarin) for phase III clearance

In addition, providing the amino acid components of GSH (e.g. via whey) and extra sulfate and potassium will help support phase II, as these are the substrates added to the toxin to assist its clearance from the body. Upregulating GSH production (via Nrf2/ARE priming) and methylation are also important core strategies.

7.8 FHT for detoxifying heavy metals

7.8.1 The critical role of glutathione in heavy metal detoxification

GSH is a major non-protein cellular thiol that provides fundamental antioxidant protection for cells.[115] It is also a signalling molecule in cell regulation and apoptosis, and a modulator of xenobiotic toxicity.

This reflects on the role of GSH in detoxifying heavy metals in the body.[116] GSH is in fact a key cellular detoxifier of heavy metals (HMs). The HM binds to the sulfur atoms in the tripeptide and is excreted via the bile. However, this causes cellular GSH depletion and a resultant increased risk of oxidative damage, which may impair, damage, or even kill the cell.

Cellular GSH levels can be increased using the following:

- herbs that prime the Nrf2/ARE pathway, including turmeric (curcumin), broccoli sprouts, garlic, rosemary, green tea, resveratrol
- the amino acid components: methionine, NAC and cysteine, glutamine, and glycine, or whey protein
- other cofactors: vitamins C, E, and especially selenium (Se)

7.8.2 Important herbs for heavy metal detoxification

Heavy metals are first absorbed into body fluids, such as the blood, and then are either excreted or stored in soft tissues, such as liver and kidney. Over time, long-term storage is rendered in hard tissue, namely bone and tooth.

To effectively lower the HM burden and impact in the body, a four-pronged strategy is needed, namely:

1. enhancement of intracellular GSH (as per above)
2. protection against toxic effects
3. preventing or minimising the gastrointestinal absorption of heavy metals by complexation or chelation in the gut lumen, possibly creating conversion to an insoluble and/or not absorbable form
4. complexing and promoting the excretion of heavy metals from the body

Complexation of HMs to remove them from the body reverses the storage pathway described above. In other words, removing HMs from body fluids will see a migration out of soft tissue and, eventually, from hard tissue.

In terms of key herbs, the critical role of garlic in HM protection and detoxification is noted above. It can achieve 1, 2, and 4 of the four-pronged strategy.

Milk thistle (*Silybum marianum*) fruit contains flavonolignans collectively referred to as silymarin. The major component of silymarin is silybin, which has pronounced metal chelating activity. Oral administration of silybin was shown to protect against iron-induced hepatic toxicity in rats.[117] A combination of ascorbic acid (10 mg/kg) and silymarin (10 mg/kg) ameliorated lead toxicity in the liver of rats.[118] In lead and cadmium poisoning in an experimental model, the structural and histochemical hepatic changes were significantly prevented by silymarin.[119] Supplementing milk thistle and silymarin ameliorated mortality, organ weights, spermatogenesis, and histopathological lesions in cadmium-induced toxicity in Japanese quails.[120]

The potent metal chelating capacity of milk thistle has been clinically investigated in the context of iron toxicity in beta-thalassaemia. Evidence is growing that the silymarin complex of flavonolignans from milk thistle can impact serum ferritin and iron overload in various clinical circumstances. This is demonstrated in two clinical trials of this extract in patients with beta-thalassaemia, mainly used in conjunction with the drug desferrioxamine.

Beta-thalassaemia is a relatively common genetic haemoglobin disorder that leads to severe chronic anaemia and requires regular blood transfusions, resulting in iron overload and very high serum ferritin levels. When the iron-binding capacities of transferrin and ferritin are exceeded, the excess iron also generates harmful free radicals and causes tissue and multi-organ damage.[121] Chelation therapy with the drug desferrioxamine is standard therapy for these iron-induced complications.

In the first trial, patients were treated with the combination of desferrioxamine and 420 mg/day silymarin ($n = 49$) or desferrioxamine and placebo ($n = 48$) for 9 months using a randomised, double-blind design.[122] Serum ferritin levels decreased significantly from the beginning to the end of silymarin treatment (3,028.8 ± 2,002.6 vs 1,972.2 ± 1,250.6 ng/mL); however, no significant change in serum ferritin was observed in the patients receiving placebo (2,249.0 ± 1,304.2 vs 2,015.6 ± 1,146.8 ng/mL).

The second trial was conducted over 6 months in 40 children (average age about 5 years) with beta-thalassaemia major and a serum ferritin level of more than 1,000 ng/mL.[123] Patients included in the study (group I) were divided into two subgroups (group IA and group IB) by simple random allocation. Group IA received a combination of oral desferrioxamine 20–40 mg/kg/day (supplied in orally dispersible tablets dissolved in water or juice and administered on an empty stomach), together with oral silymarin in the form of 140 mg tablets, one hour before each meal (in other words 3 times daily). Group IB received oral desferrioxamine 20–40 mg/kg/day and placebo. Group II included 20 healthy children matched in age and sex who served as a control group. Serum ferritin levels decreased markedly from baseline by around 67% in group IA compared with 43% for group IB ($p = 0.001$). However, levels were still well above those measured in the healthy control children. Serum iron was also reduced.

Based on the above research, milk thistle can achieve 2, 3, and 4 of the four-pronged strategy against HM toxicity.

Tannin-containing herbs such as hawthorn leaves (*Crataegus monogyna*) will bind to HMs in the gut lumen and impair their absorption. There is some suggestion that this herb will also enhance Nrf2 pathway responses.[124]

> **Summary FHT HM protocol:** Nrf2 herbs, especially garlic, green tea, bioavailable curcumin, and broccoli sprouts; together with milk thistle and hawthorn.

7.9 Comprehensive detoxification as an FHT treatment module

A combined protocol can be adopted as an FHT treatment module where a comprehensive detoxification strategy is needed. This will assist in the detoxification of both organic pollutants and HMs and also reduce their cellular impact via invoking the four **R**s of cellular protection noted in Chapter 2: **R**esist, **R**esolve, **R**epair, and **R**estore.

The key elements are as follows:

> broccoli sprouts and phase II conjugators
> garlic
> turmeric (either the herb or bioavailable curcumin, as dictated by the case)
> milk thistle (silymarin), Schisandra, and rosemary
> *optional:* Korean ginseng, green tea

References

1. Calderón-Garcidueñas L, Torres-Jardón R, Kulesza RJ, et al. Alzheimer disease starts in childhood in polluted Metropolitan Mexico City. A major health crisis in progress. *Environ Res.* 2020; **183**: 109137. doi:10.1016/j.envres.2020.109137.
2. Whyatt RM, Rundle AG, Perzanowski MS, et al. Prenatal phthalate and early childhood bisphenol A exposures increase asthma risk in inner-city children. *J Allergy Clin Immunol.* 2014; **134**(5): 1195–1197.e2. doi:10.1016/j.jaci.2014.07.02.
3. Zhou Z, Zhang J, Jiang F, Xie Y, Zhang X, Jiang L. Higher urinary bisphenol A concentration and excessive iodine intake are associated with nodular goiter and papillary thyroid carcinoma. *Biosci Rep.* 2017; **37**(4): BSR20170678. doi:10.1042/BSR20170678.
4. von Ehrenstein OS, Ling C, Cui X, et al. Prenatal and infant exposure to ambient pesticides and autism spectrum disorder in children: population-based case-control study. *BMJ.* 2019; **364**: l962. doi:10.1136/bmj.l962.
5. https://www.express.co.uk/news/uk/88705/Charles-hit-by-dodgy-detox-quackery-row
6. Vermeulen R, Schymanski EL, Barabási AL, Miller GW. The exposome and health: where

chemistry meets biology. *Science*. 2020; **367**(6476): 392–396. doi:10.1126/science.aay3164. [p 392]
7. Vermeulen R, Schymanski EL, Barabási AL, Miller GW. The exposome and health: where chemistry meets biology. *Science*. 2020; **367**(6476): 392–396. doi:10.1126/science.aay3164.
8. www.ewg.org/research/body-burden-pollution-newborns
9. www.ewg.org/research/flame-retardants-2014
10. Escher BI, Stapleton HM, Schymanski EL. Tracking complex mixtures of chemicals in our changing environment. *Science*. 2020; **367**(6476): 388–392. doi:10.1126/science.aay6636.
11. https://www.sciencedaily.com/releases/2020/02/200226080620.htm
12. Kumar SS, Ghosh P, Malyan SK, Sharma J, Kumar V. A comprehensive review on enzymatic degradation of the organophosphate pesticide malathion in the environment. *J Environ Sci Health C Environ Carcinog Ecotoxicol Rev*. 2019; **37**(4): 288–329. doi:10.1080/10590501.2019.1654809.
13. https://www.ewg.org/research/overexposed-organophosphate-insecticides-childrens-food
14. Hertz-Picciotto I, Sass JB, Engel S, et al. Organophosphate exposures during pregnancy and child neurodevelopment: Recommendations for essential policy reforms. *PLoS Med*. 2018 Oct 24; **15**(10): e1002671. doi:10.1371/journal.pmed.1002671.
15. Adeyinka A, Pierre L. Organophosphates. In: *StatPearls*. StatPearls Publishing, Treasure Island, FL, 2020.
16. https://en.wikipedia.org/wiki/Organophosphate
17. Hertz-Picciotto I, Sass JB, Engel S, et al. Organophosphate exposures during pregnancy and child neurodevelopment: recommendations for essential policy reforms. *PLoS Med*. 2018 Oct 24; **15**(10): e1002671. doi:10.1371/journal.pmed.1002671.
18. Jokanović M. Neurotoxic effects of organophosphorus pesticides and possible association with neurodegenerative diseases in man: a review. *Toxicology*. 2018; **410**: 125–131. doi:10.1016/j.tox.2018.09.009.
19. Filardi T, Panimolle F, Lenzi A, Morano S. Bisphenol A and phthalates in diet: an emerging link with pregnancy complications. *Nutrients*. 2020 Feb 19; **12**(2): 525. doi:10.3390/nu12020525.
20. Gonsioroski A, Mourikes VE, Flaws JA. Endocrine disruptors in water and their effects on the reproductive system. *Int J Mol Sci*. 2020 Mar 12; **21**(6): 1929. doi:10.3390/ijms21061929.
21. Järup L. Hazards of heavy metal contamination. *Br Med Bull*. 2003; **68**: 167–182. doi:10.1093/bmb/ldg032.
22. *Ibid*.
23. https://www.who.int/news-room/detail/02-05-2018-9-out-of-10-people-worldwide-breathe-polluted-air-but-more-countries-are-taking-action
24. https://www.theguardian.com/environment/2018/nov/05/air-pollution-everything-you-should-know-about-a-public-health-emergency
25. *Ibid*
26. Almetwally AA, Bin-Jumah M, Allam AA. Ambient air pollution and its influence on human health and welfare: an overview. *Environ Sci Pollut Res Int*. 2020 May 3 [published online ahead of print]. doi:10.1007/s11356-020-09042-2.
27. Arce-López B, Lizarraga E, Vettorazzi A, González-Peñas E. Human biomonitoring of mycotoxins in blood, plasma and serum in recent years: a review. *Toxins* (*Basel*). 2020 Feb 27; **12**(3): 147. doi:10.3390/toxins12030147.
28. *Ibid*.
29. https://www.news-medical.net/news/20170623/Fungal-toxins-become-easily-aerosolized-leading-to-potential-indoor-health-risk.aspx

30. Meftaul IM, Venkateswarlu K, Dharmarajan R, et al. Controversies over human health and ecological impacts of glyphosate: is it to be banned in modern agriculture? *Environ Pollut.* 2020 Mar 14 [published online ahead of print]; **263**(Pt A): 114372. doi:10.1016/j.envpol.2020.114372.
31. Myers JP, Antoniou MN, Blumberg B, et al. Concerns over use of glyphosate-based herbicides and risks associated with exposures: a consensus statement. *Environ Health.* 2016 Feb 17; **15**: 19. doi:10.1186/s12940-016-0117-0.
32. Matzinger P. The evolution of the danger theory. Interview by Lauren Constable, Commissioning Editor. *Expert Rev Clin Immunol.* 2012; **8**(4): 311–317. doi:10.1586/eci.12.21.
33. Napier MD, Poole C, Satten GA, Ashley-Koch A, Marrie RA, Williamson DM. Heavy metals, organic solvents, and multiple sclerosis: an exploratory look at gene–environment interactions. *Arch Environ Occup Health.* 2016; **71**(1): 26–34. doi:10.1080/19338244.2014.937381.
34. Hybenova M, Hrda P, Procházková J, Stejskal V, Sterzl I. The role of environmental factors in autoimmune thyroiditis. *Neuro Endocrinol Lett.* 2010; **31**(3): 283–289.
35. Björk A, Mofors J, Wahren-Herlenius M. Environmental factors in the pathogenesis of primary Sjögren's syndrome. *J Intern Med.* 2020; **287**(5): 475–492. doi:10.1111/joim.13032.
36. Schmid M, Grolimund Berset D, Krief P, Zyska Cherix A, Danuser B, Rinaldo M. Should systemic sclerosis be recognised as an occupational disease in Switzerland?. *Swiss Med Wkly.* 2020 Feb 21; **150**: w20193. doi:10.4414/smw.2020.20193.
37. Mostafalou S1, Abdollahi M. Pesticides and human chronic diseases: evidences, mechanisms, and perspectives. *Toxicol Appl Pharmacol* 2013; **268**(2): 157–177.
38. Kharrazian D. The potential roles of bisphenol A (BPA) pathogenesis in autoimmunity. *Autoimmune Dis.* 2014; **2014**: 743616. doi:10.1155/2014/743616.
39. Kouroumalis E. Environmental agents involved in the cause of primary biliary cirrhosis. *Dis Markers.* 2010; **29**(6): 329–336. doi:10.3233/DMA-2010-0769.
40. Herbert MR. Contributions of the environment and environmentally vulnerable physiology to autism spectrum disorders. *Curr Opin Neurol.* 2010; **23**(2): 103–110. doi:10.1097/WCO.0b013e328336a01f.
41. Geier DA, Kern JK, Garver CR, et al. Biomarkers of environmental toxicity and susceptibility in autism. *J Neurol Sci.* 2009; **280**(1–2): 101–108.
42. Adams JB, Audhya T, McDonough-Means S, et al. Toxicological status of children with autism vs. neurotypical children and the association with autism severity. *Biol Trace Elem Res* 2013; **151**(2): 171–180.
43. Adams JB, Baral M, Geis E, et al. The severity of autism is associated with toxic metal body burden and red blood cell glutathione levels. *J Toxicol.* 2009; **2009**: 532640. doi:10.1155/2009/532640.
44. Adams JB, Romdalvik J, Ramanujam VM, Legator MS. Mercury, lead, and zinc in baby teeth of children with autism versus controls. *J Toxicol Environ Health A.* 2007; **70**(12): 1046–1051.
45. Al-Farsi YM, Waly MI, Al-Sharbati MM, et al. Levels of heavy metals and essential minerals in hair samples of children with autism in Oman: a case-control study. *Biol Trace Elem Res.* 2013; **151**(2): 181–186.
46. Adams JB, Baral M, Geis E, et al. Safety and efficacy of oral DMSA therapy for children with autism spectrum disorders: part B—behavioral results. *BMC Clin Pharmacol.* 2009 Oct 23; **9**: 17. doi:10.1186/1472-6904-9-17.
47. Shelton JF, Geraghty EM, Tancredi DJ, et al. Neurodevelopmental disorders and prenatal residential proximity to agricultural pesticides: the CHARGE study. *Environ Health Perspect.* 2014; **122**(10): 1103–1109. doi:10.1289/ehp.1307044.
48. Roberts EM, English PB, Grether JK, et al. Maternal residence near agricultural pesticide

applications and autism spectrum disorders among children in the California Central Valley. *Environ Health Perspect*, 2007; **115**(10): 1482–1489.

49. Windham GC, Zhang L, Gunier R, et al. Autism spectrum disorders in relation to distribution of hazardous air pollutants in the San Francisco Bay area. *Environ Health Perspect*, 2006 Sep; **114**(9): 1438–1444.
50. Geler DA, Kern JK, Garver CR, et al. Biomarkers of environmental toxicity and susceptibility in autism. *J Neurol Sci*, 2009; **280**(1–2): 101–108.
51. Adams JB, Audhya T, McDonough-Means S, et al. Nutritional and metabolic status of children with autism vs. neurotypical children, and the association with autism severity. *Nutr Metab* (*Lond*). 2011; **8**(1): 34.
52. Kern JK, Haley BE, Geier DA, Sykes LK, King PG, Geier MR. Thimerosal exposure and the role of sulfation chemistry and thiol availability in autism. *Int J Environ Res Public Health*. 2013 Aug 20; **10**(8): 3771–3800. doi:10.3390/ijerph10083771.
53. Hodgson NW, Waly MI, Al-Farsi YM, et al. Decreased glutathione and elevated hair mercury levels are associated with nutritional deficiency-based autism in Oman. *Exp Biol Med* (*Maywood*). 2014; **239**(6): 697–706.
54. Mutter J, Naumann J, Schneider R, et al. Mercury and autism: accelerating evidence? *Neuro Endocrinol Lett* 2005; **26**(5): 439–446.
55. Rossignol DA, Frye RE. Evidence linking oxidative stress, mitochondrial dysfunction, and inflammation in the brain of individuals with autism. *Front Physiol*. 2014 Apr 22; **5**: 150. doi:10.3389/fphys.2014.00150.
56. Pizzorno JE, Katzinger JJ. Glutathione: physiological and clinical relevance. *J Restor Med* 2012; **1**(1): 24–37.
57. Adams JB, Audhya T, McDonough-Means S, et al. Nutritional and metabolic status of children with autism vs. neurotypical children, and the association with autism severity. *Nutr Metab* (*Lond*). 2011 Jun 8; **8**(1): 34. doi:10.1186/1743-7075-8-34.
58. Ko E, Choi M, Shin S. Bottom-line mechanism of organochlorine pesticides on mitochondria dysfunction linked with type 2 diabetes. *J Hazard Mater*. 2020; **393**: 122400. doi:10.1016/j.jhazmat.2020.122400.
59. Guo Z, Xie HQ, Zhang P, et al. Dioxins as potential risk factors for autism spectrum disorder. *Environ Int*. 2018; **121**(Pt 1): 906–915. doi:10.1016/j.envint.2018.10.028.
60. www.ewg.org/research/dirty-dozen-list-endocrine-disruptors
61. Osius N, Karmaus W, Kruse H, et al. Exposure to polychlorinated biphenyls and levels of thyroid hormones in children. *Environ Health Perspect*. 1999; **107**(10): 843–849.
62. Jukic AM, Calafat AM, McConnaughey DR et al. Urinary concentrations of phthalate metabolites and bisphenol A and associations with follicular-phase length, luteal-phase length, fecundability, and early pregnancy loss. *Environ Health Perspect*. 2016 Mar; **124**(3): 321–328.
63. Mathew H, Mahalingaiah S. Do prenatal exposures pose a real threat to ovarian function? Bisphenol A as a case study. *Reproduction*. 2019; **157**(4): R143–R157. doi:10.1530/REP-17-0734.
64. Pivonello C, Muscogiuri G, Nardone A, et al. Bisphenol A: an emerging threat to female fertility. *Reprod Biol Endocrinol*. 2020 Mar 14; **18**(1): 22. doi:10.1186/s12958-019-0558-8.
65. Radke EG, Braun JM, Meeker JD, Cooper GS. Phthalate exposure and male reproductive outcomes: a systematic review of the human epidemiological evidence. *Environ Int*. 2018; **121**(Pt 1): 764–793. doi:10.1016/j.envint.2018.07.029.
66. Schug TT, Janesick A, Blumberg B, Heindel JJ. Endocrine disrupting chemicals and disease susceptibility. *J Steroid Biochem Mol Biol*. 2011; **127**(3–5): 204–215. doi:10.1016/j.jsbmb.2011.08.007.
67. Bowe B, Xie Y, Li T, Yan Y, Xian H, Al-Aly Z. The 2016 global and national burden of

diabetes mellitus attributable to fine particulate matter air pollution. *The Lancet Planetary Health.* 2018 June 29.
68. Chung RT. Detoxification effects of phytonutrients against environmental toxicants and sharing of clinical experience on practical applications. *Environ Sci Pollut Res Int.* 2017 Apr; **24**(10): 8946–8956.
69. Frustaci A, et al. Marked elevation of myocardial trace elements in idiopathic dilated cardiomyopathy compared with secondary cardiac dysfunction. *J Am Coll Cardiol.* 1999; **33**(6): 1578–1583.
70. Järup L. Hazards of heavy metal contamination. *Br Med Bull.* 2003; **68**: 167–182.
71. Houston MC. The role of mercury and cadmium heavy metals in vascular disease, hypertension, coronary heart disease, and myocardial infarction. *Altern Ther Health Med.* 2007; **13**(2): S128–S133.
72. Kreiss K, Zack MM, Kimbrough RD, et al. Association of blood pressure and polychlorinated biphenyl levels. *JAMA.* 1981; **245**(24): 2505–2509.
73. Rasche M, Walther M, Schiffner R, et al. Rapid increases in nitrogen oxides are associated with acute myocardial infarction: a case-crossover study. *Eur J Prev Cardiol.* 2018; **25**(16): 1707–1716. doi:10.1177/2047487318755804.
74. Bae S, Hong YC. Exposure to bisphenol A from drinking canned beverages increases blood pressure: randomized crossover trial. *Hypertension.* 2015; **65**(2): 313–319. doi:10.1161/HYPERTENSIONAHA.114.04261.
75. Wang P, Chen H, Kopittke PM, Zhao FJ. Cadmium contamination in agricultural soils of China and the impact on food safety. *Environ Pollut.* 2019; **249**: 1038–1048. doi:10.1016/j.envpol.2019.03.063.
76. Järup L. Hazards of heavy metal contamination. *Br Med Bull.* 2003; **68**: 167–182.
77. Gallagher CM, Kovach JS, Meliker JR. Urinary cadmium and osteoporosis in U.S. Women > or = 50 years of age: NHANES 1988–1994 and 1999–2004. *Environ Health Perspect.* 2008; **116**(10): 1338–1343.
78. Hormann AM, Vom Saal FS, Nagel SC, et al. Holding thermal receipt paper and eating food after using hand sanitizer results in high serum bioactive and urine total levels of bisphenol A (BPA). *PLoS One.* 2014 Oct 22; **9**(10): e110509. doi:10.1371/journal.pone.0110509.
79. Gibson EA, Stapleton HM, Calero L, et al. Flame retardant exposure assessment: findings from a behavioral intervention study. *J Expo Sci Environ Epidemiol.* 2019; **29**(1): 33–48. doi:10.1038/s41370-018-0049-6.
80. Hoffman K, Webster TF, Sjödin A, Stapleton HM. Toddler's behavior and its impacts on exposure to polybrominated diphenyl ethers. *J Expo Sci Environ Epidemiol.* 2017; **27**(2): 193–197. doi:10.1038/jes.2016.11.
81. Buttke DE, Wolkin A, Stapleton HM, Miranda ML. Associations between serum levels of polybrominated diphenyl ether (PBDE) flame retardants and environmental and behavioral factors in pregnant women. *J Expo Sci Environ Epidemiol.* 2013; **23**(2): 176–182. doi:10.1038/jes.2012.67.
82. Baudry J, Assmann KE, Touvier M, et al. Association of frequency of organic food consumption with cancer risk: findings from the NutriNet-Santé Prospective Cohort Study [published correction appears in *JAMA Intern Med.* 2018 Dec 1; **178**(12):1732]. *JAMA Intern Med.* 2018; **178**(12): 1597–1606. doi:10.1001/jamainternmed.2018.4357.
83. Hyland C, Bradman A, Gerona R, et al. Organic diet intervention significantly reduces urinary pesticide levels in U.S. children and adults. *Environ Res.* 2019; **171**: 568–575. doi:10.1016/j.envres.2019.01.024.
84. Pizzorno, J. Time to change standard of care to include screening for common disease-

inducing toxicants. *Integrative Medicine: A Clinician's Journal.* 2019 Oct/Nov; **18**(5): 8–13. [pp 8, 10, 11]
85. Chen L, Mo H, Zhao L, et al. Therapeutic properties of green tea against environmental insults. *J Nutr Biochem.* 2017; **40**: 1–13. doi:10.1016/j.jnutbio.2016.05.005.
86. Emara AM, El-Bahrawy H. Green tea attenuates benzene-induced oxidative stress in pump workers. *J Immunotoxicol.* 2008; **5**(1): 69–80. doi:10.1080/15476910802019029.
87. Xue KS, Tang L, Cai Q, Shen Y, Su J, Wang JS. Mitigation of fumonisin biomarkers by green tea polyphenols in a high-risk population of hepatocellular carcinoma. *Sci Rep.* 2015 Dec 2; **5**: 17545. doi:10.1038/srep17545.
88. Basu A, Betts NM, Mulugeta A, Tong C, Newman E, Lyons TJ. Green tea supplementation increases glutathione and plasma antioxidant capacity in adults with the metabolic syndrome. *Nutr Res.* 2013; **33**(3): 180–187. doi:10.1016/j.nutres.2012.12.010.
89. Ho CK, Choi SW, Siu PM, Benzie IF. Effects of single dose and regular intake of green tea (*Camellia sinensis*) on DNA damage, DNA repair, and heme oxygenase–1 expression in a randomized controlled human supplementation study. *Mol Nutr Food Res.* 2014; **58**(6): 1379–1383. doi:10.1002/mnfr.201300751.
90. Choi SW, Yeung VT, Collins AR, Benzie IF. Redox-linked effects of green tea on DNA damage and repair, and influence of microsatellite polymorphism in HMOX–1: results of a human intervention trial. *Mutagenesis.* 2015; **30**(1): 129–137. doi:10.1093/mutage/geu022.
91. Najar-Nezhad V, Aslani MR, Balali-Mood M. Evaluation of allicin for the treatment of experimentally induced subacute lead poisoning in sheep. *Biol Trace Elem Res.* 2008; **126**(1–3): 141–147.
92. Shahsavani D, Baghshani H, Alishahi E. et al. Efficacy of allicin in decreasing lead (Pb) accumulation in selected tissues of lead-exposed common carp (*Cyprinus carpio*). *Biol Trace Elem Res.* 2011; **142**(3): 572–580.
93. Kianoush S. Balali-Mood M, Mousavi SR, et al. Comparison of therapeutic effects of garlic and d-Penicillamine inpatients with chronic occupational lead poisoning. *Basic Clin Pharmacol Toxicol* 2012; **110**(5): 476–481.
94. Petkov V. Bulgarian traditional medicine: a source of ideas for phytopharmacological investigations. *J Ethnopharmacol.* 1986; **15**(2): 121–132. doi:10.1016/0378-8741(86)90149-2.
95. Yang H, Xu W, Zhou Z, et al. Curcumin attenuates urinary excretion of albumin in type II diabetic patients with enhancing nuclear factor erythroid-derived 2-like 2 (Nrf2) system and repressing inflammatory signaling efficacies. *Exp Clin Endocrinol Diabetes.* 2015; **123**(6): 360–367. doi:10.1055/s-0035-1545345.
96. Biswas J, Sinha D, Mukherjee S, Roy S, Siddiqi M, Roy M. Curcumin protects DNA damage in a chronically arsenic-exposed population of West Bengal. *Hum Exp Toxicol.* 2010; **29**(6): 513–524. doi:10.1177/0960327109359020.
97. Liu GT. Hepato-pharmacology of fructus schizandrae. In: Chang HM, Yeung HW, Tso WW, et al (Eds). *Advances in Chinese Medicinal Materials Research.* World Scientific, Singapore, 1985: pp 257–267.
98. Chiu HF, Chen TY, Tzeng YT, Wang CK. Improvement of liver function in humans using a mixture of schisandra fruit extract and sesamin. *Phytother Res.* 2013; **27**(3): 368–373. doi:10.1002/ptr.4702.
99. Riedl MA, Saxon A, Diaz-Sanchez D. Oral sulforaphane increases Phase II antioxidant enzymes in the human upper airway. *Clin Immunol.* 2009; **130**(3): 244–251. doi:10.1016/j.clim.2008.10.007.
100. Cornblatt BS, Ye L, Dinkova-Kostova AT, et al. Preclinical and clinical evaluation of sul-

foraphane for chemoprevention in the breast. *Carcinogenesis.* 2007; **28**(7): 1485–1490. doi:10.1093/carcin/bgm049.
101. Kensler TW, Chen JG, Egner PA, et al. Effects of glucosinolate-rich broccoli sprouts on urinary levels of aflatoxin-DNA adducts and phenanthrene tetraols in a randomized clinical trial in He Zuo township, Qidong, People's Republic of China. *Cancer Epidemiol Biomarkers Prev.* 2005; **14**(11 Pt 1): 2605–2613. doi:10.1158/1055-9965.EPI-05-0368.
102. Clarke JD, Riedl K, Bella D, Schwartz SJ, Stevens JF, Ho E. Comparison of isothiocyanate metabolite levels and histone deacetylase activity in human subjects consuming broccoli sprouts or broccoli supplement. *J Agric Food Chem.* 2011; **59**(20): 10955–10963. doi:10.1021/jf202887c.
103. Riso P, Martini D, Møller P, et al. DNA damage and repair activity after broccoli intake in young healthy smokers. *Mutagenesis.* 2010; **25**(6): 595–602. doi:10.1093/mutage/geq045.
104. Kensler TW, Ng D, Carmella SG, et al. Modulation of the metabolism of airborne pollutants by glucoraphanin-rich and sulforaphane-rich broccoli sprout beverages in Qidong, China [published correction appears in *Carcinogenesis.* 2012 Mar; **33**(3):722]. *Carcinogenesis.* 2012; **33**(1): 101–107. doi:10.1093/carcin/bgr229.
105. Egner PA, Chen JG, Zarth AT, et al. Rapid and sustainable detoxication of airborne pollutants by broccoli sprout beverage: results of a randomized clinical trial in China. *Cancer Prev Res (Phila).* 2014; **7**(8): 813–823. doi:10.1158/1940-6207.CAPR-14-0103.
106. Brown RH, Reynolds C, Brooker A, Talalay P, Fahey JW. Sulforaphane improves the bronchoprotective response in asthmatics through Nrf2-mediated gene pathways. *Respir Res.* 2015 Sep 15; **16**(1): 106. doi:10.1186/s12931-015-0253-z.
107. Heber D, Li Z, Garcia-Lloret M, et al. Sulforaphane-rich broccoli sprout extract attenuates nasal allergic response to diesel exhaust particles. *Food Funct.* 2014; **5**(1): 35–41. doi:10.1039/c3fo60277j.
108. Singh K, Connors SL, Macklin EA, et al. Sulforaphane treatment of autism spectrum disorder (ASD). *Proc Natl Acad Sci USA.* 2014; **111**(43): 15550–15555. doi:10.1073/pnas.1416940111.
109. Bent S, Lawton B, Warren T, et al. Identification of urinary metabolites that correlate with clinical improvements in children with autism treated with sulforaphane from broccoli. *Mol Autism.* 2018 May 30; **9**: 35. doi:10.1186/s13229-018-0218-4.
110. Lynch R, Diggins EL, Connors SL, et al. Sulforaphane from broccoli reduces symptoms of autism: a follow-up case series from a randomized double-blind study. *Glob Adv Health Med.* 2017 Oct 26; **6**: 2164957X17735826. doi:10.1177/2164957X17735826.
111. Kim JY, Park JY, Kang HJ, Kim OY, Lee JH. Beneficial effects of Korean red ginseng on lymphocyte DNA damage, antioxidant enzyme activity, and LDL oxidation in healthy participants: a randomized, double-blind, placebo-controlled trial. *Nutr J.* 2012 Jul 17; **11**: 47. doi:10.1186/1475-2891-11-47.
112. Yang M, Lee HS, Hwang MW, Jin M. Effects of Korean red ginseng (Panax Ginseng Meyer) on bisphenol A exposure and gynecologic complaints: single blind, randomized clinical trial of efficacy and safety. *BMC Complement Altern Med.* 2014 Jul 25; **14**: 265. doi:10.1186/1472-6882-14-265.
113. Pessayre D. Cytochromes P450 and formation of reactive metabolites. Role in hepatotoxicity of drugs. *Therapie (Paris)* 1993; **48**(6): 537–548.
114. Bone KM, Mills SY. *Principles and Practice of Phytotherapy: Modern Herbal Medicine*, 2nd ed. Elsevier, UK, 2013.
115. Pizzorno JE, Katzinger JJ. Glutathione: physiological and clinical relevance. *J Restor Med.* 2012; **1**(1): 24–37.
116. Patrick L. Lead toxicity part II: the role of free radical damage and the use of antioxidants in the pathology and treatment of lead toxicity. *Altern Med Rev.* 2006 Jun; **11**(2):114–127.

117. Pietrangelo A, Borella F, Casalgrandi G, et al. Antioxidant activity of silybin in vivo during long-term iron overload in rats. *Gastroenterology.* 1995; **109**(6): 1941–1949. doi:10.1016/0016-5085(95)90762-9.
118. Shalan MG, Mostafa MS, Hassouna MM, El-Nabi SE, El-Refaie A. Amelioration of lead toxicity on rat liver with vitamin C and silymarin supplements. *Toxicology.* 2005; **206**(1): 1–15. doi:10.1016/j.tox.2004.07.006.
119. Barbarino F, Neumann E, Deaciuc I, et al. Effect of silymarin on experimental liver lesions. *Med Interne.* 1981; **19**(4): 347–357.
120. Saleemi MK, Tahir MW, Abbas RZ, et al. Amelioration of toxicopathological effects of cadmium with silymarin and milk thistle in male Japanese quail (*Coturnix japonica*). *Environ Sci Pollut Res Int.* 2019; **26**(21): 21371–21380. doi:10.1007/s11356-019-05385-7.
121. Moayedi B, Gharagozloo M, Esmaeil N, Maracy MR, Hoorfar H, Jalaeikar M. A randomized double-blind, placebo-controlled study of therapeutic effects of silymarin in β-thalassemia major patients receiving desferrioxamine. *Eur J Haematol.* 2013; **90**(3): 202–209. doi:10.1111/ejh.12061.
122. Moayedi B, Gharagozloo M, Esmaeil N, Maracy MR, Hoorfar H, Jalaeikar M. A randomized double-blind, placebo-controlled study of therapeutic effects of silymarin in β-thalassemia major patients receiving desferrioxamine. *Eur J Haematol.* 2013; **90**(3): 202–209. doi:10.1111/ejh.12061.
123. Hagag AA, Elfrargy MS, Gazar RA, El-Lateef AE. Therapeutic value of combined therapy with deferasirox and silymarin on iron overload in children with Beta thalassemia. *Mediterr J Hematol Infect Dis.* 2013 Nov 4; **5**(1): e2013065. doi:10.4084/MJHID.2013.065.
124. Yoo JH, Liu Y, Kim HS. Hawthorn fruit extract elevates expression of Nrf2/HO-1 and improves lipid profiles in ovariectomized rats. *Nutrients.* 2016 May 13; **8**(5): 283. doi:10.3390/nu8050283.

The FHT bowel flora protocol for dysbiosis management

This chapter outlines the evolution of the bowel flora protocol (BFP) as a technique for advancing a healthier microbiome. A balanced microbiome is now widely recognised as essential for good health, and FHT can play a valuable role in achieving a flourishing gut flora by working with a patient's intrinsic organisms. As outlined in Chapter 2, the BFP is primarily based on a cycle of weed and feed and is designed to gradually manipulate the microbiome to a better state over 6–10 cycles. It can then be stopped and reintroduced a few months later if needed. An appropriate diet is also essential, including a copious and diverse fibre intake, because this feeds beneficial bacteria.

In a sense the BFP uses the patient's existing gut microbiome as an "endogenous probiotic". By manipulating existing resident microflora, the changes in gut flora are more likely to be made permanent. All of the different prototypes of the BFP described below during its progressive development are viable therapeutic options.

While the theory of using a BFP was considered speculative and too radical by some 25 years ago, the concept of using medication to remodel an unhealthy gut microbiome profile to fight disease is now receiving serious research attention.[1] A recent review of this topic stated that:

> Empirical therapeutic modulation of the gut flora has been performed for thousands of years, for example implicitly in the use of traditional herbal medication or consciously by fecal microbiota transplantation.[2]

(The history of faecal microbiota transplantation dates back even to ancient China.[3])

8.1 The human microbiome

The human microbiome is composed of bacteria, archaea, viruses, and eukaryotic microbes (fungi, protozoa) that reside in and on our bodies, but especially in our gastrointestinal tract (GIT). The tremendous expansion of information collected on our microbiome in recent years is highlighted by data generated through several large-scale endeavours to characterise the human microbiome, namely the European Metagenomics of the Human Intestinal Tract (MetaHIT) and the NIH-funded Human Microbiome Project (HMP).[4] The number of microbiota in a person is estimated to be 10^{13}–10^{14} microbial cells, with an approximate 1:1 ratio of microbial cells to human cells.[5] However, with the genome of each bacterial strain harbouring thousands of genes, the collective bacterial genome contains about 100 times more genes than the human genome.

Our microbes have a tremendous potential to impact our physiology, both in health and in disease. They contribute to metabolic functions, protect against pathogens, educate the immune system, and, through these basic functions, affect directly or indirectly most of our biological functions. In turn, we supply them with the environment and nutrients to survive: a perfect symbiotic relationship.

Healthy adult humans each typically harbour more than a thousand species of bacteria belonging to relatively few known bacterial phyla, with *Bacteroidetes*, *Actinobacteria*, and *Firmicutes* being the dominant phyla.[6] The microbiota of the gut are quite diverse compared to other body sites, and there is considerable variation in the constituents of the gut microbiota among apparently healthy individuals.

The human digestive tract is a natural habitat for a large, diverse, dynamic population of micro-organisms (mainly bacteria) that have adapted to live on both mucosal surfaces or in the lumen. Native bacteria permanently colonise the digestive tract and are mainly acquired at birth and during the first year of life. Transient bacteria are continuously being ingested from the environment via food, water, and probiotics.[7]

The stomach and duodenum harbour very low numbers: around 10^3 colony-forming units (cfu) per g of contents. There is a progressive increase along the jejunum and ileum from 10^4–10^7 cfu/g. Gram-negative aerobes predominate in this part. In contrast, the large intestine is heavily populated by anaerobes with levels around 10^{12} cfu/g of luminal contents, encouraged by the slow transit time.[8]

While distinct detrimental changes to the gut microbiome composition – a state known as "dysbiosis" – have been described in various diseases, defining a "healthy" microbiome has been difficult, due to inter-individual variation.[9] One definition of dysbiosis from a mainstream medical journal was: "a breakdown in the balance between protective versus harmful intestinal bacteria"[10] The term was originally coined by Elie Metchnikoff (the first proponent of probiotics) in around 1907 to describe altered pathogenic bacteria in the gut.[11] Naturopathic thinking has refined the concept. Hence, according to Pizzorno and Murray, dysbiosis is "the state of disordered microbial ecology that causes disease".[12]

Predating the concept of dysbiosis is the bowel toxaemia theory (BTT). This extends as far back as Hippocrates, who stated: "Death sits in the bowel" and "Bad digestion is the root of all evil." Nineteenth-century proponents of the BTT include Metchnikoff as well as the naturopath Louis Khune. Their belief was that excess food intake or the wrong type of foods leads to production of toxins, often via fermentation. This could then lead to disease. More recently, the writings of chiropractor/naturopath Bernard Jensen maintained that poor bowel management was at the root of most people's health problems. Over time, the BTT eventually evolved into the intestinal dysbiosis hypothesis.[13]

The types of GIT dysbiosis can be classified as follows:

According to location
- *Helicobacter pylori* presence in the stomach (although some argue it is a commensal)
- small intestinal bacterial overgrowth
- colonic flora imbalance, which can include abnormal presence of parasites (protozoa) or yeasts (candida)

According to pattern (several patterns can coexist in a person)
1 **Putrefaction**
   - the classic Western degenerative disease pattern advanced by Metchnikoff
   - linked to higher fat and meat and lower fibre diets

> leads to higher *Bacteroidetes* and lower *Bifidobacteria spp.*, which induces bacterial enzymes such as urease and beta-glucuronidase

2 **Fermentation excess**
> carbohydrate intolerance induced by an overgrowth of endogenous bacteria in the stomach, small intestine, and caecum
> promoted by gastric hypochlorhydria
> symptoms include distension, flatulence, diarrhoea, constipation
> these patients typically react to psyllium (soluble fibre), fruits, and FODMAP foods
> can also be due to the excessive presence of yeasts (especially Candida)

3 **Deficiency**
> excessive antibiotics or a diet low in soluble fibre may create a deficiency of healthy flora, including Bifidobacteria and Lactobacillus
> has been linked to food intolerance and irritable bowel syndrome
> can occur in conjunction with putrefaction dysbiosis

4 **Sensitisation**
> abnormal responses to normal flora or excessive presence of pathogenic flora
> leads to deranged immune function, resulting in autoimmune disease or chronic skin disorders
> inflammatory bowel disease, spondyloarthropathies, other connective tissue disease, and skin disorders like psoriasis and acne are implicated[14]

8.1.1 Diseases linked to dysbiosis

As just flagged above, dysbiosis has been linked to an extraordinary range of chronic diseases. However, this large body of evidence seems to have had little impact on mainstream medical practice, despite being published in highly regarded and influential journals. **Figure 8.1** schematically summarises the role of the gut microbiota in health and disease, giving some examples of causes and effects.[15]

Dysbiosis has been particularly linked to autoimmunity,[16] and it was in that context the original BFP was developed. (Other examples of the link between gastrointestinal dysbiosis and chronic disease can be found in Chapters 11, 12, and 14.)

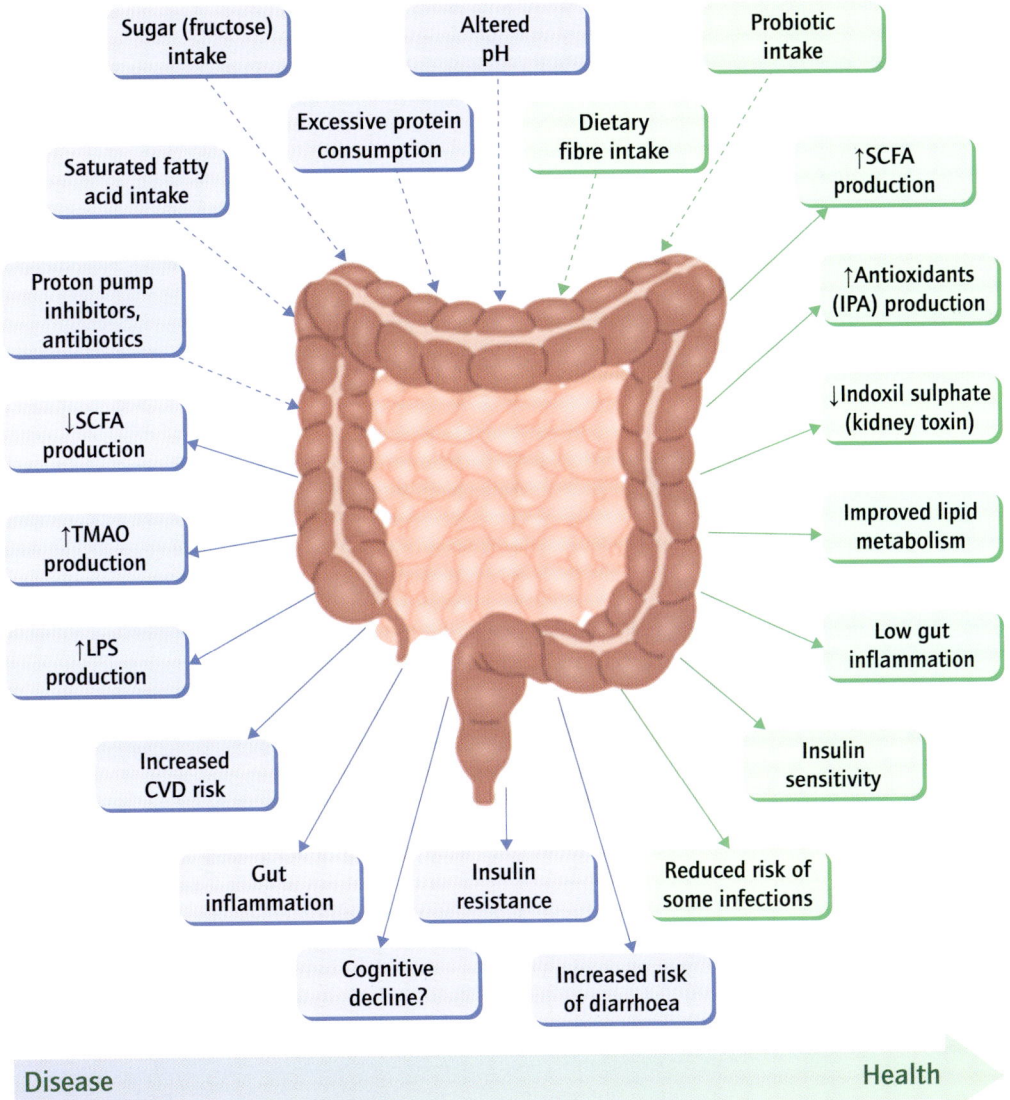

Figure 8.1 Schematic representation of the role of gut microbiota in health and disease. [CVD = cardiovascular disease; IPA = indolepropionic acid; LPS = lipopolysaccharide; SCFA = short chain fatty acids; TMAO = trimethylamine N-oxide.]

8.2 The original BFP (1970s)

Phytotherapist the late Hein Zeylstra (my principal herbal teacher) developed a highly successful treatment regime for inflammatory bowel disease (IBD). His approach originated from the naturopathic approach to Johne's disease in cattle, described by naturopath Roger Newman-Turner senior. Although Zeylstra provided no explanation as to why this protocol might work, it is my interpretation that the beneficial clinical outcomes observed were due to the regime having a favourable influence on bowel flora. A dysregulated microbiome is now widely recognised as a pathogenic contributor to IBD.[17]

His original regime is outlined in **Box 8.1**. Basically, the routine was to periodically fast, taking fresh garlic (*Allium sativum*) and slippery elm (*Ulmus rubra*). Pathogenic micro-organisms in the bowel lumen would be weakened by the fasting, since they rely on a ready source of nutrients. The garlic then reduces the population of all bacteria, fungi, and protozoa in the gut, and the slippery elm encourages only the growth of beneficial bacteria. This last aspect of the therapy occurs because favourable organisms such as Bifidobacteria can utilise the mucilaginous fibre in the slippery elm as a food source, whereas pathogenic bacteria cannot. If the routine is repeated several times

---

Box 8.1 The original BFP developed by Hein Zeylstra for IBD

Day	Protocol/dietary guidelines
Day 1	▹ Fast: no food, but water and medicines are allowed.
Days 2–3	▹ Continue as for Day 1. Twice during the day take one or two cloves of crushed fresh garlic with a copious quantity of water. This has the effect of flushing the fresh garlic quickly into the small intestine. ▹ At different times take 1–2 teaspoons of slippery elm powder with copious water.
Day 4	▹ Gradually introduce allowed foods; continue with medicines and slippery elm.
Days 5–14	▹ Follow exclusion diet; take medicines and slippery elm.

over a few months, a "normalisation" of bowel flora will result. According to Zeylstra the regime worked faster in Crohn's disease (CD) than ulcerative colitis, possibly because of the favourable effect of fasting on CD.

8.3 The interim adapted BFP (1990s)

Based on further clinical experience, this original programme was then adapted as follows. The main changes were the addition of other broad-spectrum antimicrobial herbs, such as golden seal (*Hydrastis canadensis*) and the use of green tea and grape seed extracts during the "feed" phase.

8.3.1 Step 1: Prepare and weed

8.3.1.1 Prepare – Day 1

In preparation for this BFP, it was ideal to have the patient fast for one day prior to commencement. For an optimal pre-protocol 24-hour fast, all food and beverages other than purified water were excluded. Vegetable juices and broths were acceptable in moderation – no more than 470 mL (16 oz) of juice during the day and, ideally, diluted with some purified water.

If the patient felt they could not go without food for 24 hours, they were permitted to include 1–2 servings of low-glycaemic vegetables, either raw or slightly steamed. It was essential to avoid foods containing yeast, sugar, and starches, including fruit, during this 24-hour period. No alcohol or caffeine was to be consumed during the fast and, ideally, during the BFP. If cravings for carbohydrates interfered with patient compliance, the addition of Gymnema tablets (2–3/day) or – even better – Gymnema liquid extract could help to alleviate this, as might bitter herbs.

8.3.1.2 Weed – Eradicate dysbiotic organisms (Days 2–3)

The main components of garlic are the sulfur compounds, including alliin. Allicin is produced from alliin via the action of the enzyme alliinase when garlic is crushed. Allicin is quite unstable and decomposes further, producing a range of compounds, including diallyl sulfides, ajoenes, and vinyldithiins.[18] Allicin and its decomposition products are thought to be the major antimicrobial factors in garlic.[19]

If fresh garlic was used in this protocol, it was crushed first and taken with enough water to flush the garlic through the stomach quickly, so the antimicrobial agents can act in the intestine. Alternatively, enteric-coated garlic tablets ensured the maximum potency of garlic was delivered to the site of dysbiosis.

Broad-spectrum antimicrobials are best for weeding, as they do not create imbalance in the microflora. Golden seal tablets or liquid extract equivalent to 2–3 g of golden seal root (in divided doses) was often added to this weeding protocol. Golden seal is broad-spectrum, due to the presence of berberine (see Chapter 9). Other broad-spectrum antimicrobial herbs could be included in the weeding phase (see Chapter 9). (Note: Phellodendron is now recommended in preference to golden seal, because of the cost of the former.)

8.3.2   Step 2: Feed (Days 4–15)

8.3.2.1   Step 2a: Feed the bowel flora with slippery elm powder

The growth of endogenous beneficial bowel flora can be encouraged by administering prebiotics. Prebiotics act as food for beneficial bowel flora, and include herbs and foods containing mucilages, polysaccharides, and fructooligosaccharides (FOS). The most common mucilage-containing herb historically used for gut disorders is slippery elm bark (*Ulmus rubra*). Its water-soluble polysaccharide is a linear chain of alternating D-galacturonic acid and L-rhamnose residues joined by alpha linkages with side branches of galactose or 3-O-methyl-galactose. The bark is demulcent, emollient, and nutrient and provides a simple mechanical soothing effect.[20]

Recent *in vitro* research supports the prebiotic activity of slippery elm.[21] Profiling of faecal cultures supplemented with licorice, slippery elm, or the Ayurvedic formula Triphala by 16S rDNA sequencing revealed profound changes in diverse taxa in human gut microbiota. Each herbal medicine promoted the formation of unique microbial communities. The relative abundance of approximately one-third of the 299 species profiled was altered by all three medicines, whereas additional species displayed herb-specific alterations. Herb supplementation increased the abundance of many beneficial bacteria, including *Bifidobacterium spp.*, *Lactobacillus spp.*, and *Bacteroides spp.* The herbs also resulted in the reduced relative abundance of many potential pathogens, such as *Citrobacter freundii* and *Klebsiella pneumoniae*. They specifically induced blooms of butyrate- and propionate-producing species, with slippery elm and Triphala significantly increasing the relative abundance of butyrate-producing bacteria, which is highly desirable.

8.3.2.2 Step 2b: Inhibit the regrowth of pathogenic flora

This involves the use of selective gastrointestinal antimicrobials to restore normal bowel flora, particularly green tea and grape seed extract. Polyphenols (oligomeric procyanidins, OPCs) from grape seed extract and green tea will selectively inhibit the regrowth of pathogenic bowel flora and encourage the growth of beneficial bacteria. The addition of these herbs to Step 2 of the protocol improved dysbiosis management and reduced flatulence and abdominal bloating.

There is experimental and clinical evidence to support these claims. A methanolic extract of green tea was found to moderately enhance the growth of certain Bifidobacteria and selectively inhibit the growth of pathogenic *Clostridia spp. in vitro*.[22] The polyphenols containing gallate (such as epigallocatechin gallate, EGCG) had the strongest activity.[23] A later *in vitro* study observed that faecal homogenates containing bacteria significantly catalysed tea phenolics, including epicatechin, catechin, 3-O-methyl gallic acid, gallic acid, and caffeic acid, to generate aromatic metabolites dependent on bacterial species.[24] Different strains of intestinal bacteria had varying degrees of growth sensitivity to the tea phenolics and metabolites. Growth of certain pathogenic bacteria, such as *Clostridium perfringens*, *Clostridium difficile*, and *Bacteroides spp.*, was significantly repressed by tea phenolics and their derivatives, while commensal anaerobes like *Bifidobacterium spp.* and probiotics such as *Lactobacillus spp.* were affected less severely. This indicates that tea phenolics exert significant effects on the intestinal environment by modulation of the intestinal bacterial population, probably by acting as "metabolic" prebiotics.

A small clinical study in Japan demonstrated that a green tea preparation was able to positively influence intestinal dysbiosis in nursing-home patients by raising levels of Lactobacilli and Bifidobacteria, lowering levels of Enterobacteriaceae, Bacteroidaceae, and Eubacteria, and decreasing odorous compounds. Levels of pathogenic bacterial metabolites were also decreased.[25,26] A further study found that supplementation with tea catechins produced favourable improvements in the participant's bowel condition, as evidenced by a reduction in faecal moisture, pH, ammonia, sulfide, and oxidation-reduction potential. In both trials the dose was 300 mg/day of tea catechins, which is equivalent to about 6 cups of green tea.[27]

Later clinical trials have confirmed that green tea increased proportions of Bifidobacteria.[28] For example, the effects on the gut microbiome of two weeks of green tea liquid (GTL) at 400 mL/day were investigated in healthy volunteers ($n = 12$).[29] An irreversible increase in the *Firmicutes:Bacteroidetes* ratio was seen, together with elevated SCFA-producing genera and a reduction of bacterial LPS synthesis in faeces. Another trial concluded that green tea consumption may act as a prebiotic and improve the colon environment by increasing the proportion of *Bifidobacterium spp.*[30]

Grape seed OPCs demonstrated a beneficial effect on caecal fermentation in rats. Caecal pH decreased, and fermentative activity was stimulated, without an increase in deleterious enzymatic activity.[31] There was a significant increment in the SCFA pool.

In healthy adults, faecal odour and the concentration of methyl mercaptan gas from faeces decreased significantly after 2 weeks of administration of grape seed extract (190 mg/day of OPCs). After a washout period, volunteers then took a green tea extract (providing 250 mg/day of catechins). The effect on these parameters was greater for grape seed than for green tea. In addition, compared to baseline, the number of Bifidobacterium increased significantly and the number of Enterobacteriaceae and putrefactive substances (such as ammonia and skatole) tended to decrease after 2 weeks of grape seed extract.[32]

The interim adapted BFP described and discussed above is summarised in **Box 8.2**.

Box 8.2 The interim adapted BFP

Day	Protocol	Dietary guidelines
Day 1	▷ Prescribed medicines and supplements are to be taken as normal if the patient is currently on a protocol	▷ Fasting: no food and plenty of water; if the patient cannot fast, recommend eating light, fresh meals of vegetables and salads only. ▷ No consumption of yeast, sugar, or starches is essential. This includes fruit. Vegetable juices and broths are acceptable. ▷ No alcohol or caffeine. ▷ If cravings for carbohydrates are interfering with patient compliance, add Gymnema liquid or tablets (3/day) into the protocol for blood sugar regulation.
Days 2–3	▷ Garlic: 1–2 fresh crushed cloves of garlic twice daily *or* 2 high-quality, enterically coated garlic tablets. If fresh garlic is used, it should be taken with a copious quantity of water. This has the effect of flushing the fresh garlic quickly into the small intestine. ▷ Golden seal could be taken here as well: 4 tablets containing at least 500 mg of root a day	▷ Fasting is ideal; if the patient cannot fast, recommend very light, fresh meals of vegetables and salads. ▷ Refraining from consumption of yeast, sugar, or starches is essential. This includes fruit and fruit juices. Vegetable juices and broths are acceptable. ▷ No alcohol or caffeine.
Days 4–14	▷ Slippery elm powder: 1–2 heaped teaspoons of slippery elm powder with copious (240 mL) water, to allow it to swell in the gut. ▷ Herbal antioxidant (green tea, grape seed extract, turmeric, rosemary): 2 tablets at night before bed or on an empty stomach, at least 2 hours away from food	▷ Gradually introduce clean, fresh foods, not from packets and largely comprising fresh fruits, vegetable and protein sources such as legumes, dairy and other animal protein. ▷ Daily consumption of green tea at 3–4 cups a day
Day 15	Repeat protocol for another 14-day cycle if desired	

8.4 The current BFP and its variants

Clinical experience with the interim adapted BFP described above revealed a few difficulties. The principal one was compliance with the fasting days. If a more aggressive weeding strategy is adopted, then this can do away with the need for fasting. Another difficulty was the 14-day cycle; hence a 7-day cycle was also adopted to improve compliance.

The key antimicrobial herbs to provide the weeding became oregano and anise oils, with Phellodendron for the berberine and (optionally) garlic and myrrh. These can be applied in quite high doses, as it is only for a short period. The weeding phase was shortened to 2 days, typically Saturday and Sunday (although in stubborn or severe cases it can be extended to 3–4 days). Slippery elm still provides the feeding treatment for the next 5 days, in conjunction with the grape seed and green tea. This should be combined with the appropriate diet (such as low sulfur, low starch, etc.) depending on the pattern of dysbiosis or the condition being treated. Optionally, an evidence-based probiotic can also be employed during this 5-day phase.

The current BFP is summarised in **Box 8.3.** Note that this protocol does not require fasting during the weeding phase.

It has become increasingly apparent that a disrupted gastrointestinal barrier, with resultant bacterial translocation through the gut wall, is a significant factor in the development of some, if not all, autoimmune diseases.[33] For this reason, a variant of the BFP that also stresses gut wall healing was developed. This is outlined in **Box 8.4**. The probiotic is no longer optional, and one that promotes the integrity of the gut wall barrier is preferred.

The bowel flora/barrier protocol is best combined with a high-fibre diet, full of vegetables, fruit, whole grains, legumes, and nuts and no gluten

---

Box 8.3   The current BFP

Weed

Saturday and Sunday (2 days)

- Andrographis: 2–3 g, twice a day
- oregano oil: 150–225 mg twice a day
- anise oil: 250–375 mg, twice a day
- Phellodendron: 3.2–4.8 g, twice a day
- myrrh: 1 g, twice a day
- garlic: one fresh crushed clove or tablet equivalent twice a day

Feed & Seed

Monday to Friday (5 days)

- slippery elm: 1.5 g, twice a day
- green tea: 4 g, twice a day
- grape seed: 6 g, twice a day
- probiotic: twice a day
- turmeric: 2 g, twice a day

One cycle (2 + 5) = 7 days. Repeat for 6–10 cycles.
Adapt as required for each patient: for example, Weed 3 or 4 days; Feed 4 or 3 days.

> **Box 8.4 BFP with a focus on gut wall healing**

Weed	Feed, Seed, & Heal
Saturday and Sunday (2 days)	Monday to Friday (5 days)
▸ oregano oil: 150–225 mg, twice a day ▸ anise oil: 250–375 mg, twice a day ▸ Phellodendron: 3.2–4.8 g twice a day ▸ myrrh: 1 g twice a day	*gut healing* ▸ meadowsweet: 2 g, twice a day ▸ licorice: 3 g, twice a day ▸ chamomile: 1.2 g, twice a day *probiotic* ▸ probiotic: twice a day ▸ slippery elm: 1.5 g, twice a day ▸ green tea: 4 g, twice a day ▸ grape seed: 6 g, twice a day

One cycle (2 + 5) = 7 days.
For best results, 6 to 10 cycles are recommended.
Base protocol can be adapted as per the needs of each patient.

(because of the negative effects of gluten on the gut barrier). Phellodendron and/or golden seal are recommended for weeding in children. The protocol is applied for 6–10 weeks and then either continued if progress is still ongoing or switched to a different treatment module.

8.5 Case history

The following case history illustrates the application of yet another interim form of the BFP that was based on a 7-day cycle but used garlic and golden seal for weeding.

A male patient aged 45 presented with acutely severe ulcerative colitis that had been diagnosed about 6 months previously. He was being treated with oral prednisone at 12 mg/day.

Herbal treatment for the first 6 months consisted of the following:

- tablets containing Boswellia, turmeric, celery seed, and ginger: 3 tablets per day
- tablets containing *Echinacea angustifolia* and *E. purpurea* roots: 2 tablets per day

- St John's wort tablets: 3/day
- slippery elm powder: 1–2 rounded teaspoons per day

A low-sulfur diet was also advised. This comprised the following:

- Intake of fats and complex carbohydrates was not curtailed.
- Patient was advised to completely avoid eggs, cheese, milk, ice-cream, mayonnaise, soy milk, mineral water, and sulfated drinks like wine.
- Other sulfur-containing additives, such as from dried fruit and processed foods, were to be avoided.
- Patient was also advised to avoid nuts and cruciferous vegetables.
- Intake of red meat was also reduced.

Progress was slow, and every time the prednisone was withdrawn, the patient experienced a severe relapse (debility, nausea, going to the toilet at least 20 times a day), which led to it being reinstated. Unfortunately, the patient was also not very compliant with the slippery elm powder treatment.

It was decided to place the patient on a version of the BFP (see **Box 8.5**) for at least 3 months and continue with the Boswellia combination tablets and Echinacea root tablets. Note that this BFP also included the use of capsules containing a combination of probiotic bacteria (3/day).

Box 8.5   Bowel flora protocol

Weed	**Feed & Re-seed**
Saturday and Sunday (2 days)	**Monday to Friday (5 days)**
- garlic tablets: 4 a day - golden seal tablets: 4 a day	*gut healing* - capsules containing slippery elm powder: 3 capsules, 2–3 times a day, with water - tablets containing the antioxidant herbs grape seed extract, turmeric, green tea, and rosemary: 2–3 tablets a day - capsules containing a combination of probiotic bacteria: 2–3 capsules a day, at a separate time (at least 2 hours away) from antioxidant herb tablets

One cycle (2 + 5) = 7 days.

After 2 months on this new regime, the patient was sufficiently stabilised so that he could go off prednisone and not require its reintroduction.

This was a particularly challenging autoimmune case, since oral steroids can interfere with natural treatments and create a dependency in the patient. Progress was triggered by the introduction of the BFP incorporating the probiotic bacteria and slippery elm powder capsules, with no requirement for fasting.

References

1. https://www.sciencedaily.com/releases/2019/08/190826092320.htm
2. Schmidt TSB, Raes J, Bork P. The human gut microbiome: from association to modulation. *Cell.* 2018; **172**(6): 1198–1215. doi:10.1016/j.cell.2018.02.044.
3. de Groot PF, Frissen MN, de Clercq NC, Nieuwdorp M. Fecal microbiota transplantation in metabolic syndrome: history, present and future. *Gut Microbes.* 2017; **8**(3): 253–267. doi:10.1080/19490976.2017.1293224.
4. Shreiner AB, Kao JY, Young VB. The gut microbiome in health and in disease. *Curr Opin Gastroenterol.* 2015; **31** (1): 69–75. doi:10.1097/MOG.0000000000000139.
5. Kho ZY, Lal SK. The human gut microbiome: a potential controller of wellness and disease. *Front Microbiol.* 2018 Aug 14; **9**: 1835. doi:10.3389/fmicb.2018.01835.
6. Shreiner AB, Kao JY, Young VB. The gut microbiome in health and in disease. *Curr Opin Gastroenterol.* 2015; **31** (1): 69–75. doi:10.1097/MOG.0000000000000139.
7. Guarner F. Enteric flora in health and disease. *Digestion.* 2006; **73**(Suppl 1): 5–12. doi:10.1159/000089775.
8. *Ibid.*
9. Ding RX, Goh WR, Wu RN, et al. Revisit gut microbiota and its impact on human health and disease. *J Food Drug Anal.* 2019; **27**(3): 623–631. doi:10.1016/j.jfda.2018.12.012.
10. Tamboli CP, Neut C, Desreumaux P, Colombel JF. Dysbiosis in inflammatory bowel disease. *Gut.* 2004; **53**(1): 1–4. doi:10.1136/gut.53.1.1.
11. Hawrelak JA, Myers SP. The causes of intestinal dysbiosis: a review. *Altern Med Rev.* 2004; **9**(2): 180–197.
12. Pizzorno JE, Murray MT (Eds). *A Textbook of Natural Medicine*, 2nd ed, Vol 1. Churchill Livingstone, Edinburgh, 1999, pp 110–111.
13. Hawrelak JA, Myers SP. The causes of intestinal dysbiosis: a review. *Altern Med Rev.* 2004; **9**(2): 180–197.
14. Elaborated from Galland L, quoted in: Pizzorno JE, Murray MT (Eds). *A Textbook of Natural Medicine*, 2nd ed, Vol 1. Churchill Livingstone, Edinburgh, 1999, pp 111–112.
15. Valdes AM, Walter J, Segal E, Spector TD. Role of the gut microbiota in nutrition and health. *BMJ.* 2018 Jun 13; **361**: k2179. doi:10.1136/bmj.k2179.
16. Anaya JM, Ramirez-Santana C, Alzate MA, Molano-Gonzalez N, Rojas-Villarraga A. The autoimmune ecology. *Front Immunol.* 2016 Apr 26; **7**: 139. doi:10.3389/fimmu.2016.00139.
17. Colquhoun C, Duncan M, Grant G. Inflammatory bowel diseases: host–microbial–environmental interactions in dysbiosis. *Diseases.* 2020 May 10; **8**(2): E13. doi:10.3390/diseases8020013.

18. British Herbal Medicine Association. *British Herbal Compendium*, Vol 1. BHMA, Bournemouth, 1992, pp 105–106.
19. Borlinghaus J, Albrecht F, Gruhlke MC, Nwachukwu ID, Slusarenko AJ. Allicin: chemistry and biological properties. *Molecules*. 2014 Aug 19; **19**(8): 12591–12618. doi:10.3390/molecules190812591.
20. British Herbal Medicine Association. *British Herbal Compendium*, Vol 1. BHMA, Bournemouth, 1992, p 204.
21. Peterson CT, Sharma V, Uchitel S, et al. Prebiotic potential of herbal medicines used in digestive health and disease. *J Altern Complement Med*. 2018; **24**(7): 656–665. doi:10.1089/acm.2017.0422.
22. Ahn YJ, Sakanaka S, Kim MJ, et al. Effect of green tea extract on growth of intestinal bacteria. *Microbial Ecology in Health and Disease*. 1990; **3**(6): 335–338. doi:10.3109/08910609009140256.
23. Ahn YJ, Kawamura T, Kim M, et al. Tea polyphenols: selective growth inhibitors of Clostridium spp. *Agric Biol Chem*. 1991; **55**(5): 1425–1426.
24. Lee HC, Jenner AM, Low CS, Lee YK. Effect of tea phenolics and their aromatic fecal bacterial metabolites on intestinal microbiota. *Res Microbiol*. 2006; **157**(9): 876–884. doi:10.1016/j.resmic.2006.07.004.
25. Hara Y. Influence of tea catechins on the digestive tract. *J Cell Biochem*. 1997; **27**: 52–58.
26. Goto K, Kanaya S, Nishikawa T, et al. Green tea catechins improve gut flora. *Ann Long-Term Care*. 1998; **6**: 1–7.
27. Goto K, Kanaya S, Ishigami T, Hara Y. The effects of tea catechins on fecal conditions of elderly residents in a long-term care facility. *J Nutr Sci Vitaminol*. 1999; **45**(1): 135–141.
28. Bond T, Derbyshire E. Tea compounds and the gut microbiome: findings from trials and mechanistic studies. *Nutrients*. 2019 Oct 3; **11**(10): 2364. doi:10.3390/nu1110236.
29. Yuan X, Long Y, Ji Z, et al. Green tea liquid consumption alters the human intestinal and oral microbiome. *Mol Nutr Food Res*. 2018; **62**(12): e1800178. doi:10.1002/mnfr.201800178.
30. Jin JS, Touyama M, Hisada T, Benno Y. Effects of green tea consumption on human fecal microbiota with special reference to Bifidobacterium species. *Microbiol Immunol*. 2012; **56**(11): 729–739. doi:10.1111/j.1348-0421.2012.00502.x.
31. Tebib K, Besancon P, Rouanet JM. Effects of dietary grape seed tannins on rat cecal fermentation and colonic bacterial enzymes. *Nutr Res*. 1996; **16**(1): 105–110.
32. Yamakoshi J, Tokutake S, Kikuchi M, et al. Effect of proanthocyanidin-rich extract from grape seeds on human fecal flora and fecal odor. *Microb Ecol Health Dis*. 2001; **13**(1): 25–31.
33. Segal AW. Making sense of the cause of Crohn's: a new look at an old disease. *F1000Res*. 2016 Oct 12; **5**: 2510. doi:10.12688/f1000research.9699.2.

9

Covert invaders: new FHT herbal defences against old foes

This chapter explores key strategies for dealing with stealth pathogens and presents effective herbal options to help manage their impact on chronic disease. It begins with a discussion of stealth pathogens as covert invaders, outlining a range of strategies they use to evade immune defences. Next, the contribution of medicinal plants to eliminating stealth pathogens from the body is discussed. Finally, key core strategies are outlined, including the essential role of using a combined antipathogen approach, together with immune support.

9.1 Introduction

Stealth pathogens: what are they and how do we deal with them? In the opinion of many experts, the threat to humanity of infectious diseases is on the rise. It has never been greater than today. The reasons for this relate to issues such as antibiotic resistance, climate change, increased travel, and increased transfer of infections from animals to humans via arthropods and other intermediate hosts. Even pollution is thought to play a role as well. It is not just the obvious infections that should concern us. Inadequate or inappropriate responses to hidden pathogens are now recognised to be a driver of many chronic diseases or lack of wellbeing.

Having the best evidence-based natural medicine approaches to deal with this complex clinical challenge is an absolute must for the functional clinician. Knowing the best herbal protocols for each type of pathogen is the key part of this. Some pathogens might even require the clinician to use different or unfamiliar herbs. Also, it should not simply be a matter of "killing our way back to health". Terrain and immune function are very important cornerstones of a comprehensive strategy.

9.2 Stealth pathogens as covert invaders

Stealth pathogens:

- are in your mouth
- shelter in your stomach
- hide in your brain
- circulate in your blood
- cling onto your lungs
- swim in your bladder
- lurk among your gut flora

The likely first reference to the concept of a stealth pathogen was by Radolf in 1994; when talking specifically about syphilis, he described the way the organism used strategies for immune evasion and concluded that it acted as a "stealth pathogen".[1] Hence, Radolf first coined the word "stealth" in the context of a pathogen. But the term was most likely given a wider audience by the late Lida Mattman. After Radolf, in 1994, Mattman added the subtitle "stealth pathogens" to her book (originally published in 1974) about cell-wall-deficient forms of bacteria (also known as mollicutes or L-forms).[2] Mattman specifically defined stealth pathogens as bacteria that can lose their cell wall and then infect intracellularly, hiding from the immune system inside cells. These L-forms are more difficult to kill with drugs, because many antibiotics are aimed at destroying the cell wall. If the bacterium no longer needs one, it cannot be readily killed by antibiotics that target this cellular structure. The list proposed by Mattman included Borrelia and other spirochaetes, Proteus,

Rickettsia, Mycobacteria, Chlamydia (Chlamydophila), Helicobacter, Streptococcus and Bartonella.[3] But now other organisms are – rightly – mentioned in this context.

In the modern context, a broader definition of a stealth pathogen is needed. A review in the prestigious journal *Nature* suggested that pathogenic microorganisms make use of two general strategies against their host: frontal assault and stealth assault. In frontal assaults the infecting pathogen rapidly replicates, causing marked symptoms, and finds a new host before the immune system fully engages. Stealth assaults, on the other hand, typically involve a slower infection process in which a pathogen subverts the host's immune system to set up a chronic or persistent infection.[4]

A new definition that best defines a stealth pathogen is: any pathogenic micro-organism that employs strategies to persist in the body by hiding from, evading, misdirecting, or even suppressing immune responses, leading to chronic disease or lack of wellbeing.

Stealth pathogens are controversially implicated in a range of diseases including autoimmune disease, chronic fatigue syndrome (CFS), fibromyalgia syndrome (FMS), chronic Lyme disease, and sarcoidosis. In contrast, the roles of certain chronic stealth viruses and bacteria in causing specific cancers is now widely acknowledged. Detrimental effects of stealth pathogens can be due either to the adverse consequences of immune camouflage (molecular mimicry) or otherwise via secreted toxins, microbial waste products, host cell necrosis (danger signals), or by driving chronic inflammation.

There might, in fact, be a considerable bioburden created by stealth pathogens. Studies have shown that more than one stealth organism might be driving chronic disease at any one time in a person. For example, a boy with an encephalopathy driven by autoantibodies had antibodies against *Mycoplasma pneumoniae* and human herpesvirus 7 in his cerebrospinal fluid.[5]

This new contention suggests a role for a broad-spectrum approach aimed across all types of pathogens, including viruses. It also highlights the limitations of specific pathogen testing when investigating any unknown causes of a chronic disease. Instead, a "test-by-treating" approach is advocated, applying the safe example protocols outlined below as treatment modules for a defined period.

9.3 Survival strategies used by stealth pathogens

Stealth mechanisms to escape detection and attack by the immune system are employed by most pathogens, including:

- helminths
- protozoa
- mycoplasma
- normal forms of bacteria
- even viruses

Viruses certainly employ stealth pathogen strategies for immune evasion. One example is the herpesviruses (HSV). When a cell is infected by a virus, normally it expresses MHC-I and other markers on the cell's outer surface to show the immune system that it has been infected. The immune system will then destroy that virus-infected cell. But if the infecting virus hinders that process, then the immune system will not know that the cell is infected. Due to this drastic reduction of cell surface MHC-I molecules by HSV, the signals that activate and recruit cytotoxic T lymphocytes (CTLs) to the infected cell are blocked. As a result, infected cells cannot be eliminated and thus become a reservoir for the sustained production and release of the virus.[6]

Epstein-Barr virus (EBV) uses a different mechanism. EBV is a large lymphotropic DNA virus that establishes life-long residency in the infected host and is associated with a number of human tumours. EBV has evolved to utilise selective DNA methylation (gene silencing) to maximise its persistence and cloak itself from immune detection.[7]

Hookworms employ yet another strategy. They suppress the host's immune response in the tissue surrounding their anchor point. One author suggested that this is achieved by the secretion of molecules that assist the parasite in a stealthy evasion of the host immune response by influencing regulatory T cell function.[8] Researchers are in the process of developing drugs from such factors for the treatment of autoimmunity.

When *Chlamydia trachomatis*, the bacterium that causes one of the most common sexually transmitted infections worldwide, enters a human cell, it hijacks parts of the host to build protective layers around itself, hiding from immune attack.[9]

Mycobacterium tuberculosis, the tuberculosis pathogen, escapes death in macrophages by fighting back. It releases a toxin that enzymatically hydrolyses NAD+, and this loss of NAD+ inside the macrophage leads to its necrotic cell death, releasing the *M. tuberculosis* bacterium to reproduce and infect more cells.[10]

A study in *Nature Microbiology* investigated how the malaria parasite, *Plasmodium falciparum*, evades the immune system. Once inside a red blood cell (RBC), the parasite releases proteins that are presented on the outside surface of the RBC. These proteins stick to other blood cells and blood vessel walls, so that infected cells no longer circulate around the body and pass through the spleen. This protects the malaria parasite from immune surveillance inside the spleen.[11]

The complete removal of acetic acid molecules from its chitin cell wall acts like an invisibility cloak, making a fungus invisible to the immune system. The fungal enzymes that can do this are known as chitin deacetylases. A particularly aggressive fungus, *Cryptococcus neoformans*, which can easily lead to fatal infection (especially in immunocompromised patients), has four genes that encode chitin deacetylases.[12]

9.4 Some important stealth pathogens

9.4.1 Helicobacter

Helicobacter pylori is a stealth pathogen so elusive that its role in causing gastric ulcers was missed for many decades. Only discovered in 1982 after much controversy, it employs elaborate means to hide from and subvert our immune response. *H. pylori* (Hp) releases a range of biotoxins (virulence factors) that ensure its survival, but also damage the host. As a direct consequence, it is implicated in or proven to initiate a wide range of chronic diseases, including peptic ulcers, cancers, food allergies, skin disorders, and multiple autoimmune and neurological diseases.[13]

Hp is characterised by an unusual capability to rearrange itself in both genotypic and phenotypic ways. Stressful conditions, including exposure to low levels of antimicrobial agents, facilitate a viable, but non-culturable, state in which its cells acquire the coccoid form. This morphotype is an important strategy for survival in unsuitable conditions and allows escape from the immune system. Hp is also capable of intracellular infection (another stealth strategy) and can form a biofilm outside and inside the host.[14]

9.4.2 Mycoplasmas

Mycoplasmas are the smallest – and have smallest genomes of – any free-living organism.[15] Since they lack a cell wall, they are in fact more evolved than bacteria. *Mycoplasma pneumoniae* (MP) is the most common pathogenic mycoplasma infecting humans, and there is a growing awareness that these stealth pathogens are more widespread and lurk in more biological niches than first thought.[16]

Figure 9.1 represents *Mycoplasma pneumoniae* at the site of the lung respiratory epithelium. The mycoplasma first shoot biotoxins at the cell and weaken it; then they latch on to the cell membrane, staying outside the cell, sucking the nutrients out of the cell. As also shown in this diagram, they eventually infect intracellularly and then penetrate deeper into the bloodstream and spread around the body.

Mycoplasma are very important stealth pathogens. Most antibiotics cannot harm them, because they lack a cell wall. There are certain antibiotics that do kill them, but even then there are difficulties with entirely eradicating the mycoplasma. Recent research has found that mycoplasma pathogens make DNA in a unique way that may protect them from our immune response.[17]

Many early studies have implicated mycoplasma species as stealth pathogen factors in autoimmune disease, especially rheumatoid arthritis (RA).[18] This has now been supported by a 13-year nationwide, population-based, retrospective cohort study from Taiwan on a population of 116,053 hospitalised patients diagnosed with MP. This cohort study demonstrated that patients with MP had a much higher risk of developing RA, especially in the first 2 years – where the risk (Hazard Ratio) was 4 times – and in those aged younger than 19 and over 65 years.[19]

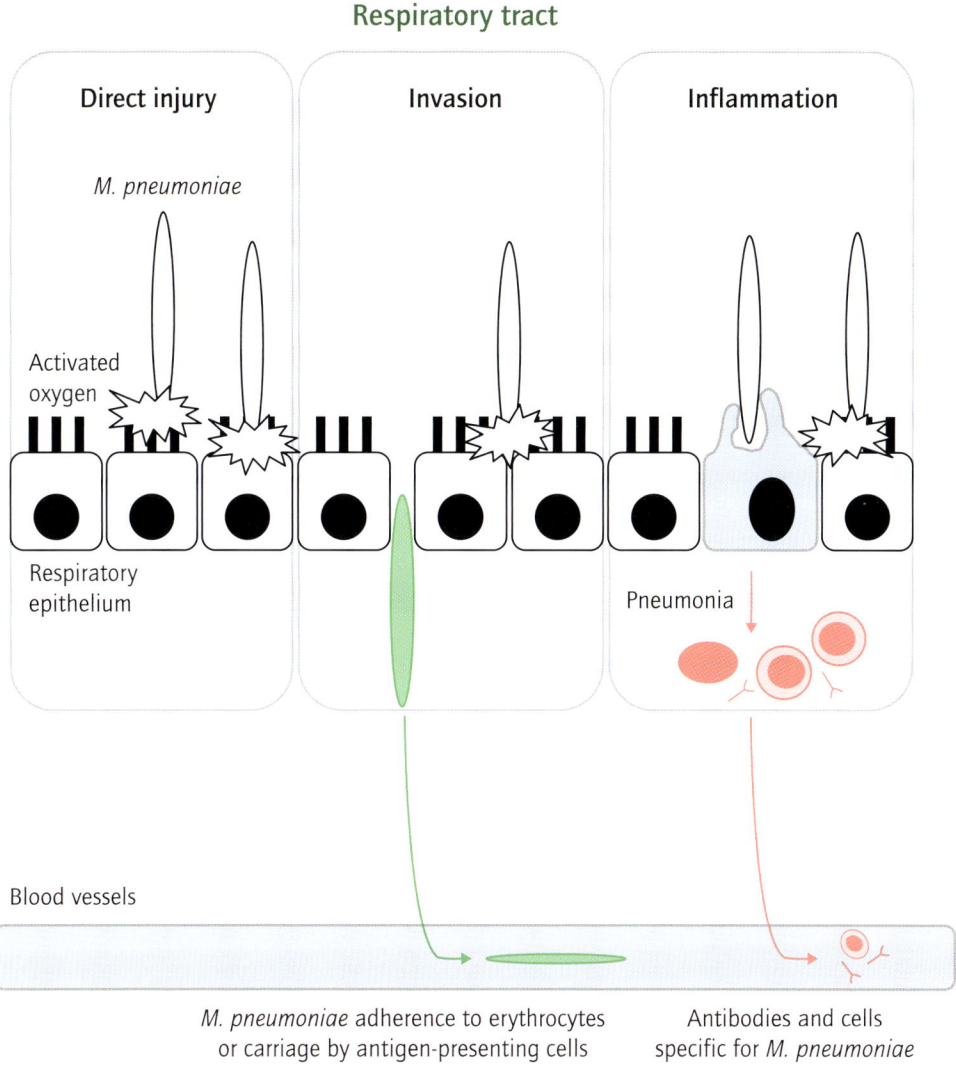

Figure 9.1 *Mycoplasma pneumoniae* impacting respiratory epithelium.

9.4.3 The syphilis spirochaete: "making a living as a stealth pathogen"[20]

Treponema pallidum, the syphilis spirochaete, has a poorly antigenic and non-inflammatory surface that forms part of its stealth strategy. There is also evidence that its capacity for ongoing antigenic variation contributes to its ability to evade host defences.[21] From a pathogenesis standpoint, this emerging picture of a wily, adaptive adversary makes sense. The complex natural history of syphilis clearly shows that the parasitic strategy of the spirochaete is ambitious. It is hard to imagine that the bacterium could implement such an agenda without invoking complex and versatile genetic programmes to achieve antigenic variability. Its phenomenal persistence as a stealth pathogen eventually leads to massive destruction of internal organs in its tertiary phase.

9.4.4   Zoonotic stealth pathogens: a growing threat

Zoonotic stealth pathogens are transferred from an animal to a human via a vector. That vector can be a mosquito, a tick, a louse, or a flea. Of 1,415 species of infectious organisms pathogenic to humans, 61% are zoonotic.[22] After an evaluation of the recent data, 175 pathogenic species were classed as "emerging". Zoonotic pathogens made up 75% of these emerging pathogens, and such pathogens were twice as likely to be associated with emerging diseases. Protozoa and viruses are particularly likely to emerge in this way.

9.4.4.1   Babesia

Babesia is a zoonotic protozoal stealth pathogen that is very persistent. It is a tick-transmitted haemoprotozoan that infects mammals and birds (see **Figure 9.2**).[23] Babesia have adapted over hundreds of millions of years, evolving into stealthy cryptic inhabitants within their vertebrate and invertebrate hosts. Nowadays, there is increasing identification and description of novel species in a great array of hosts. Coinfection with Borrelia is thought to increase the health impact of Babesia (specifically *B. microti*).[24]

In the United States, Babesia is transferred from a particular species of mouse via ticks. In Australia it is, instead, transferred via macropods (kangaroos and wallabies) and domestic cattle. *Babesia macrocarpus* can, indeed, kill macropods.[25] As Babesia also infects birds, presumably it might also be contracted from them.

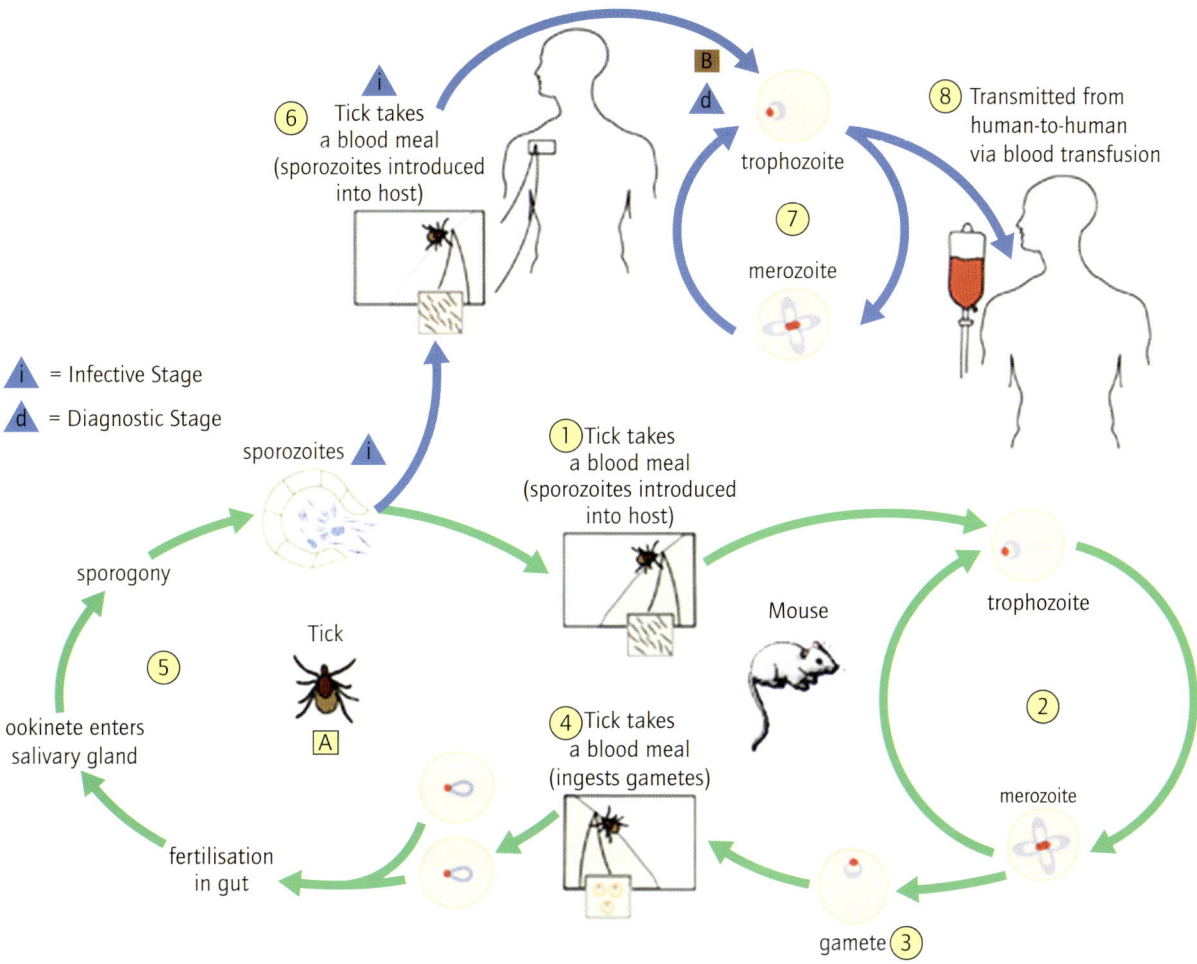

Figure 9.2 Babesia life cycle.

9.4.4.2 Bartonella

Bartonella spp. are gram-negative bacteria that are typically slow growing and facultative intracellular microbes.[26] This underlies their capacity to act as stealth pathogens. Bartonella is linked with a constantly increasing number of human diseases, and there are 13 known species that can infect humans. It can be contracted from cats: this infection is commonly known as "cat scratch fever". *Bartonella quintana* and *Bartonella bacilliformis* are the agents of trench fever and Oroya fever, respectively.

Humans can be infected with Bartonella from arthropod vectors such as fleas, ticks, and lice. Bartonella infections are often characterised by an intra-erythrocytic bacteraemia: in other words, they infect inside RBCs, like the malaria parasite. Hence, although they are bacteria, Bartonella are insidious organisms that behave to some extent like a parasite by infecting inside RBCs.

9.4.4.3 Borrelia

Lyme disease, caused by the spirochete *Borrelia burgdorferi*, has become a major worldwide epidemic. Studies show that in the United States more than 300,000 people are diagnosed each year with the acute syndrome known as Lyme disease. Up to two-thirds of infected individuals will not be helped by conventional 30-year-old antibiotic therapy. Animal and human evidence even suggests that sexual transmission of the Lyme spirochaete may occur.[27]

Chronic Lyme disease is said to occur when a person who is treated with antibiotic therapy for the disease continues to experience symptoms. The condition is also referred to as post-Lyme disease syndrome or post-treatment Lyme disease syndrome.[28] This can occur in 10–20% of people who contract acute Lyme disease.

The phenomenon of chronic Lyme disease has created a huge controversy, confounded by debate and uncertainty over the accuracy and relevance of various tests used to detect the pathogen long after acute infection has passed. The condition resembles a severe, protracted variant of chronic fatigue syndrome, with the distinguishing characteristic that it developed after an infected tick bite – the "not been well since" (NBWS) tick bite syndrome, see Section 9.9. It might even involve severe neurological and cardiovascular complications. Consequently, some clinicians are advocating 6 months of treatment with antibiotics, with the goal of eliminating any residual presence of the stealth pathogen.

On the other hand, there are those who maintain that chronic Lyme disease is unproven and that the symptoms are not due to persistent *Borrelia burgdorferi* infection requiring prolonged antibiotic therapy. In other words, chronic Lyme disease does not exist as a clinical entity.

Some middle ground might be emerging. Recently it has been proposed that the antibiotic-tolerant *Borrelia burgdorferi* detected *in vitro* are not clinically relevant. Hence post-treatment Lyme disease symptoms are most likely to be caused by persistent pharmacologically active remnants of *B. burgdorferi* cells, not by a persistent infection that is refractory to antibiotic therapy. Hence, other therapeutic approaches should be explored.[29]

Proposed coinfection with other tick-borne organisms, such as the parasite Babesia, further complicates the picture. A key implication of the current conundrum is that a gentle broad-based herbal approach to lowering stealth pathogen bioburden and supporting immune function might well be a safe and effective strategy for these patients – with due consideration for other relevant core strategies indicated by the FHT approach, such as supporting adrenal reserves (see Section 9.8).

9.4.5 Toxoplasma

Toxoplasma gondii is a highly prevalent stealth pathogen. It is thought that 30–50% of people are positive for *Toxoplasma gondii*. However, one study from France found that this percentage might be as high as 84%.

The Toxoplasma organism is capable of actually infecting the endothelial cells of the blood–brain barrier (BBB). When they reach a certain point of multiplication, they burst the endothelial cell. This means that *Toxoplasma gondii* can blast holes in the BBB, which would explain its link to neurological disease (see Section 9.4.5). Not only does it then infect the brain and cause damage there, but the resultant damage to the BBB also allows further traffic of other toxic substances into the brain. This is a very important, highly prevalent stealth pathogen to consider, especially in patients with neurological issues.

Although mild flu-like symptoms occasionally occur during the first few weeks following exposure, infection with *T. gondii* produces no readily observable symptoms in healthy human adults. This asymptomatic state is referred to as a latent infection and has recently been associated with numerous subtle adverse or pathological behavioural alterations in humans. In infants, HIV/AIDS patients, and others with weakened immunity, infection can cause a serious and occasionally fatal illness: toxoplasmosis.[30]

Domestic cats are a significant source of exposure for humans. Humans are only an intermediate host, and *T. gondii* needs to infect cats for its sexual reproduction.[31] Pet cats in Australia – and most probably elsewhere – are commonly infected with *T. gondii*. Feeding raw meat to cats, a common practice in

Australia, is associated with *T. gondii* infection, highlighting the need for education about the health implications for cats of a diet containing raw meat.[32]

In a meta-analysis of 50 studies, which considered data from tens of thousands of patients, it was found that antibodies against *Toxoplasma gondii* were linked to schizophrenia, to bipolar and obsessive-compulsive disorder (OCD), and to addiction.[33] Significant odds ratios (ORs) for IgG antibodies were found in schizophrenia (OR 1.81, $p < 0.00001$), bipolar disorder (OR 1.52), OCD (OR 3.4), and addiction (OR 1.91), but no link was found with major depression. Especially in patients with chronic brain disorders, autism, and other similar conditions, it is important to remember a potential role of *Toxoplasma gondii* as a stealth pathogen.

9.4.6 Other stealth pathogens

Other important stealth pathogens involved in chronic disease include:

- Epstein-Barr virus
- *Klebsiella pneumoniae*
- *Proteus mirabilis*
- *Mycobacterium spp.* (e.g. MAP)
- parvovirus B19

9.5 Important herbs for reducing the stealth pathogen bioburden

9.5.1 Qing Hao – *Artemisia annua*

The discovery and development of qinghaosu (artemisinin) as an antimalarial drug is a truly remarkable story. *Artemisia annua* (also known as sweet wormwood or Chinese wormwood) became the first medicinal plant to ever be recognised in a Nobel Prize for Medicine, which was shared in 2015 by Tu You You for her contribution to the discovery of artemisinin. Artemisinin and its derivatives were the first significant development for malaria treatment in decades.

In the 1960s the Chinese government started an antimalarial research programme to search for traditional Chinese medicinal plants to support the Vietnamese army. As a result, in 1972 artemisinin was identified as the active antimalarial constituent of *A. annua*.

Today, artemisinin and its derivatives (artemisinins) are widely used as antimalarials against drug-resistant *Plasmodium* strains, cerebral malaria, and malaria in children. In addition to the treatment of malaria, artemisinins have the potential to treat infection with *Schistosoma spp.*, *Pneumocystis carinii*, *Toxoplasma gondii*, human cytomegaloviruses (CMV), herpes simplex viruses, and hepatitis B and C.

The use of *A. annua* dates back to 168 BCE, when it was used for periodic fevers (what we now know as malaria). Traditional methods of preparation probably optimised artemisinin extraction.[34] Because of its structure, artemisinin is generally not stable in water or ethanol, so herbal liquid preparations such as teas or tinctures need to be consumed immediately after preparation or otherwise stabilised by drying into tablets or capsules.

The main artemisinin-related compounds in *A. annua* are artemisinin (ART), arteannuin B, and artemisinic acid. Up to 42% of ART is found in the upper leaves, in the glandular trichomes. The herb also contains flavonoids and essential oil.[35]

Figure 9.3 demonstrates the various actions and potential therapeutic roles for the various artemisinins.[36] The range is extraordinary and is not just restricted to antimalarial activity, as mentioned above. A notable absence is any significant antibacterial activity for these compounds.

A. annua is a potent antiparasitic,[37] of use in treatment of infestation by:

- *Leishmania spp.*
- *Trypanosoma spp.*
- *Toxoplasma gondii*
- *Cryptosporidium parvum*
- *Giardia lamblia*
- *Babesia spp.*

It was also demonstrated that artemisinins exhibited anthelmintic activity *in vivo* against Schistosoma and foodborne trematodes such as *Fasciola hepatica*, the common liver fluke.[38] These activities are supported in some instances by clinical trials.

Artemisia annua is also a promising antiviral herb. Artemisinin and its derivatives have exhibited potent activity against viruses *in vitro* and were effective against herpesviruses such as cytomegalovirus (CMV) and EBV (with human data for the former),[39] hepatitis viruses B and C, and human papilloma virus (HPV)-infected and -transformed cells and cervical cancer cells.[40]

The broad-spectrum of the antiviral activity of the artemisinins is illustrated in **Figure 9.4**.[41]

Figure 9.5 shows the chemical structure of artemisinin. The broad-based stealth-pathogen-killing activity of this phytochemical results from a specific

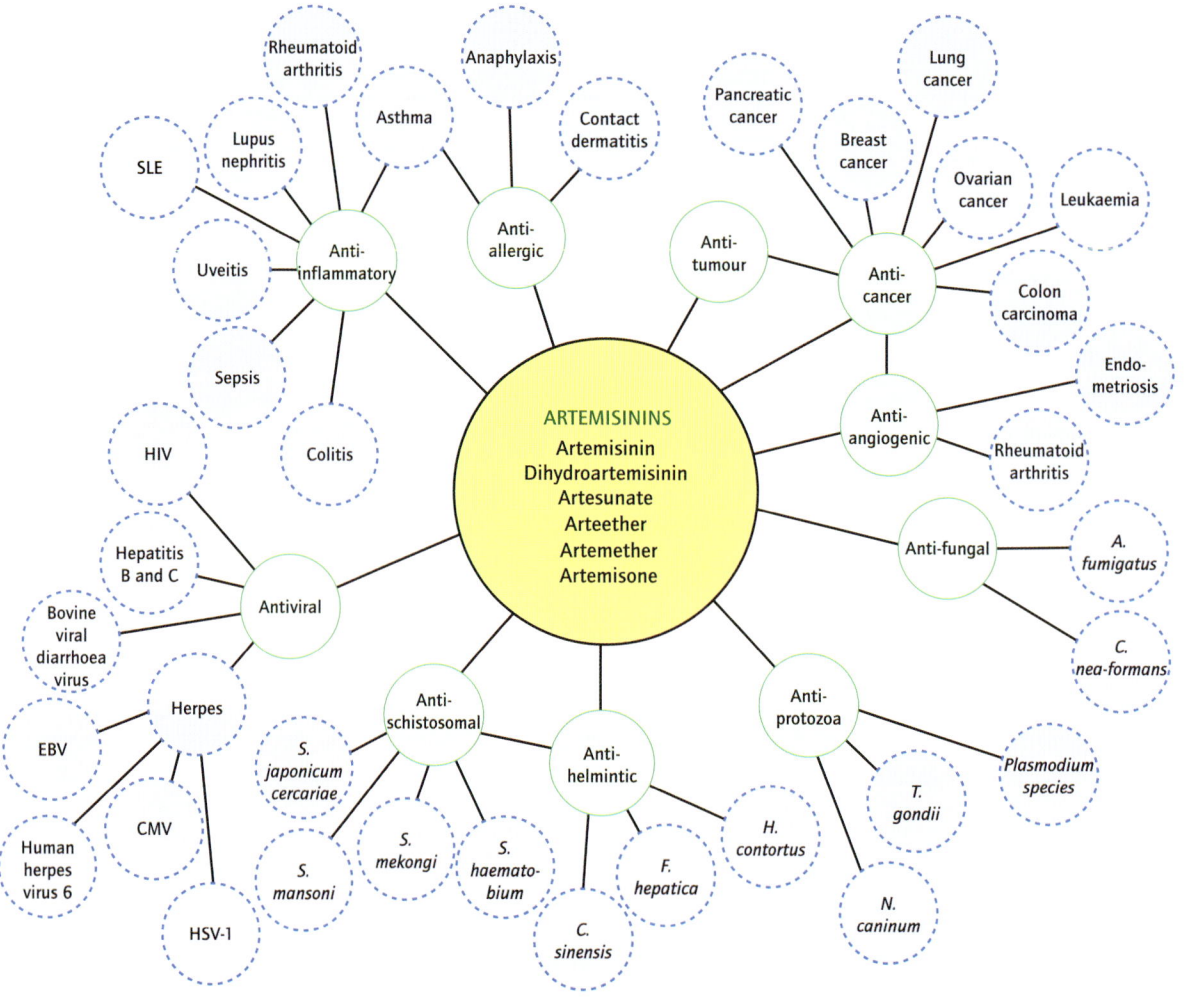

Figure 9.3 Therapeutic activity of artemisinins. [CMV = cytomegalovirus; EBV = Epstein-Barr virus; HSV-1 = herpes simplex virus; SLE = systemic lupus erythematosus.]

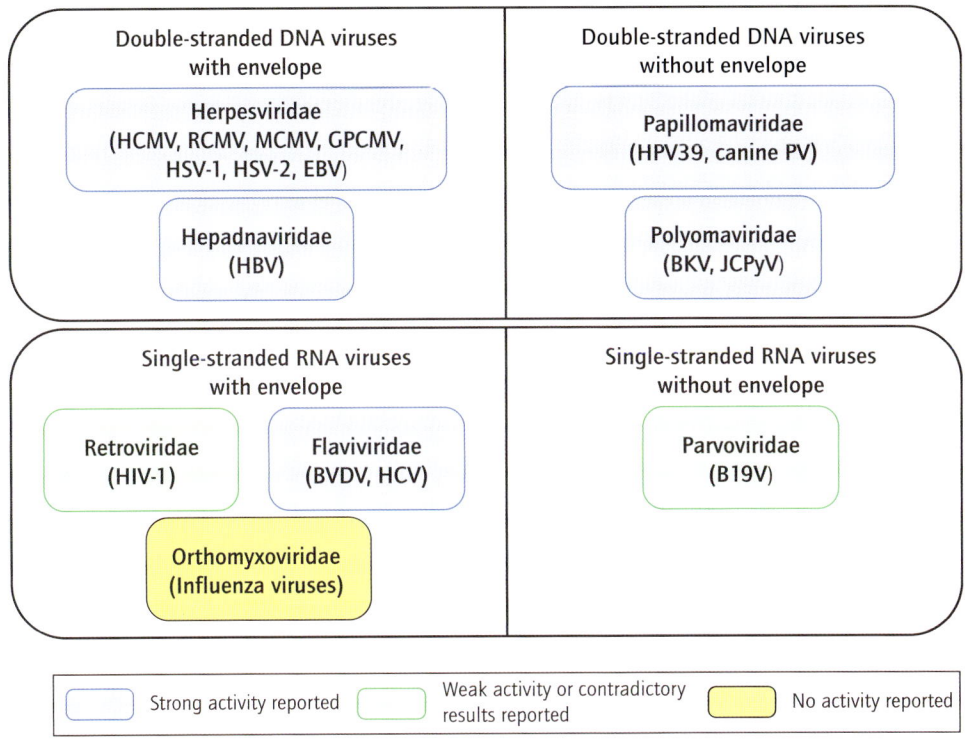

Figure 9.4 Synopsis of the antiviral activity of artemisinin-type agents *in vitro* towards diverse virus types. [GPCMV = guinea pig cytomegalovirus; HBV = hepatitis B virus; HCMV = human cytomegalovirus; HCV = hepatitis C virus; HIV-1 = human immunodeficiency virus type 1; HPV39 = human papilloma virus subtype 39; HSV-1 = herpes simplex virus 1; HSV-2 = herpes simplex virus 2; JCPyV = human polyomavirus; MCMV = mouse cytomegalovirus; PV = polycythaemia vera; RCMV = rat cytomegalovirus.]

part of its chemical structure: the bridge with the two oxygen atoms. This portion of the molecule is unstable and underlies artemisinin's high reactivity. The molecule can split at that oxygen–oxygen bond, forming two hydroxyl free radicals. These two free radicals enable it to inactivate and kill pathogens of virtually any class.

9.5.1.1 Clinical trials for *Artemisia annua*

An open RCT of *A. annua* in uncomplicated malaria led to quick resolution of parasitaemia and clinical symptoms, but with a high recrudescence rate.[42] Another RCT found that *A. annua* tea compared with sulfadoxine-pyrimethamine in uncomplicated falciparum malaria produced similar results.[43] A

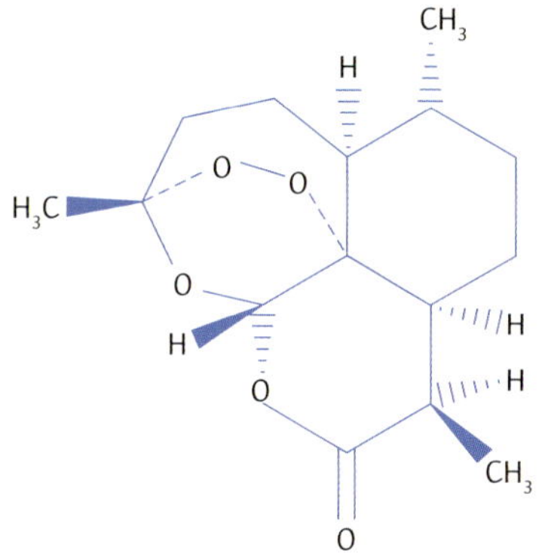

Figure 9.5 Artemisinin chemical structure.

12-week RCT of *A. annua* in osteoarthritis delivered promising results,[44] and these were maintained in a 6-month open label trial extension.[45] (Such continuous long-term use of the herb is, however, not advocated, and this particular product has been associated with idiopathic drug-induced liver injury, DILI).[46]

9.5.1.2 Why use the whole *A. annua* herb?

Whole *A. annua* slows the evolution of malaria drug resistance and overcomes resistance to artemisinin *in vivo*.[47] A single dose of *A. annua* (24 mg/kg artemisinin) reduced *in vivo* parasitaemia more effectively than a comparable dose of pure artemisinin, suggesting synergistic activity with other components in the herb (see also the clinical study below).[48] Artemisinin, which has a low bioavailability, is also substantially more bioavailable from the whole herb.[49] Again, a synergy between the other components of the whole plant may be responsible for this.

A fascinating clinical study from the Congo featured 16 cases, adults and children, who had failed to respond to conventional antimalarial therapy. The conventional antimalarial therapy given was either artemisinin combination therapy (ACT) or intravenous artesunate. A last resort treatment of these patients with severe, resistant malaria was initiated. For 5 days patients received tablets made from whole herb of *Artemisia annua*, delivering only 55 milligrams a day of artemisinin, a dose that, in terms of malaria, would be regarded as subtherapeutic, as normally 250–500 mg a day is used. Every patient was cured of the malaria. This is an extremely convincing demonstration of the value of using of the whole herb.[50]

9.5.1.3 Dosage considerations for *A. annua*

Pharmacokinetic studies of pure artemisinin have exhibited an unusual time dependency during a 7-day oral daily dose of 500 mg/day in 10 healthy adults.[51] Artemisinin areas under the plasma concentration-time curve (AUC) decreased to 34% (median) by Day 4, with a further decrease by Day 7 to only 24% of the first day. After a 2-week washout period, the artemisinin AUCs had almost normalised, demonstrating the reversibility of the liver enzyme induction. These results suggest that artemisinin exhibits an auto-inductive effect on its metabolism of an unusual magnitude. Several key drug-metabolising enzymes were involved.

For this reason, *A. annua* should only be administered continuously for no more than 7 days and then followed by a 7-day break before starting again. This will also mitigate against any (low) risk of DILI (flagged in Section 9.5.1.1). Hence, this is a herb that should be included in protocols as pulsed dosing.

Other important anti-parasitic herbs include:

- myrrh (discussed in Section 9.5.2)
- Stemona
- wormwood
- cloves
- tannin herbs

9.5.2 Myrrh – a promising new agent against stealth pathogens

Myrrh is the oleo-gum resin from the stem of various species of *Commiphora* growing in north-east Africa and Arabia. It is mentioned in the Bible in writings as old as the Psalms. Several clinical studies have been published, suggesting that high-dose myrrh represents a significant advance in the treatment of parasites. Myrrh appears to be active against parasites that infest deeper into the body than the gut, such as the liver and bladder, indicating a distinct capacity for dealing with pathogens that hide in the deeper recesses of the body.[52]

Myrrh contains an essential oil (2–10%) largely composed of sesquiterpenes. It also contains an alcohol-soluble resin (25–40%) with commiphoric acids. The key actions of myrrh are antimicrobial, antiparasitic, anti-inflammatory, and vulnerary, and it is probably also immune enhancing. The resin components are most likely more important for the immunological and immune-enhancing effects. On the other hand, the resin can also trigger a marked allergic reaction, highlighting its capacity to galvanise and up-regulate the immune response – and, indeed, sometimes agitate it.[53]

The way myrrh works against pathogens is not entirely understood, but it can probably have a direct toxic effect where there is good access to the pathogen. Otherwise, as per above, it most probably acts by stimulating natural immune resistance and overcoming stealth defences. In a clinical trial of 35 patients with chronic fascioliasis treated with myrrh, IL-4 (interleukin 4) was found to be significantly lower than controls before therapy ($p = 0.04$), probably due to immune suppression induced by the parasite. After myrrh treatment, IL-4 levels increased significantly ($p < 0.001$), to reach control levels, suggesting an enhancement of immune cell cytokine release.[54]

The clinical studies summarised here are open-label studies, all with oral doses. There are at least 6 positive trials for fascioliasis. Results are mixed for schistosomiasis, but with several positive trials. Individual trials with positive results include for lanceolate fluke, *Heterophyes heterophyes* flukes, dwarf tape worms, and vaginal trichomoniasis (given orally).[55]

9.5.2.1 Dosage considerations for myrrh

- Pulsed dosing is recommended, short term, as per the trials.
- The reason for short-term pulsed dosing is that it reduces risk of an allergic response and does not allow the stealth pathogen to adapt to the myrrh.
- It can be taken for 3–9 consecutive days on an empty stomach.
- The patient then takes a break for 4–14 days, and then the myrrh is repeated.
- The daily dose should approximate that used in the trials: this corresponds to approximately 2–3 g/day of herb or 10–15 mL/day of a 1:5 tincture.

9.5.3 Antiviral herbs

At this point it is worth discussing an unfortunately common misinterpretation of herbal research that applies especially to potential antimicrobial activity. We can call this *in vitro non veritas*: in other words, test-tube research – on herbs in particular – has a limited capacity to lead to the truth. There are some important exceptions to this, but in general we should be highly cautious about extrapolating the findings of *in vitro* herbal research to clinical situations.

By way of illustration, when we mix a diluted herbal extract with a collection of cells in an *in vitro* experiment, all the many phytochemicals in the extract will have equal access to those cells, resulting in a range of effects that can be measured.

But after oral doses in the human body, the phytochemicals in a herbal extract will exhibit one or more of three behaviours:

1. They will be absorbed in varying amounts, but often leading to body cell exposure that is much less than that reflected in the *in vitro* model.
2. They will not be absorbed and pass out of the digestive tract largely unchanged.
3. They will be changed by the digestive process, especially the gut flora, leading to metabolites that can be absorbed to a greater or lesser extent.

Consequently, the resultant effects in most cases will be quite different from those seen in the *in vitro* model. For this main reason, extrapolation of *in vitro* research on herbs needs to be done **with great caution**.

One way to overcome this limitation is to model only those phytochemical constituents of a herb that have good oral bioavailability. But even then, considerations such as hepatic metabolism, tissue access, target access, and relevance of the model used will still limit the clinical value of any findings, unless they are appropriately accommodated in any interpretation of the latter.

Applying these considerations to herbs with potential antiviral activity, for this finding to be clinically relevant, the following criteria should ideally be met:

- antiviral activity demonstrated *in vitro*, preferably broad-based
  and
- identified antiviral active phytochemicals (or metabolites) with known bioavailability (or can be enhanced)
  and
- *in vivo* activity demonstrating reduced viral loads
  and
- clinical trial activity demonstrating reduced viral loads and improved clinical outcomes

There are currently no herbs that meet these criteria fully, although *Artemisia annua* (reviewed in Section 9.5.1) goes close, as does St John's wort (briefly reviewed in Section 9.5.3.2). Given this, and the fact that herbal antiviral activity is likely to be mild, antiviral herbs should **always** be combined with immune herbs. In addition to *Artemisia annua*, there are other key clinically relevant antiviral herbs.

9.5.3.1 Licorice

Multiple studies show *in vitro* antiviral activity for licorice and glycyrrhizin and its aglycone.[56]

These include activity principally against enveloped viruses, such as HIV, SARS, and vaccinia virus.

Reduced mortality and antiviral activity were observed for *in vivo* models of herpes simplex virus encephalitis and influenza A viral pneumonia. A 2008 review noted that RCTs have clearly demonstrated that intravenous treatment with glycyrrhizin can reduce hepatocellular damage in patients with chronic hepatitis B and C.

9.5.3.2 St John's wort (SJW)

Hypericin has a significant *in vitro* antiviral activity against enveloped viruses and was originally researched as an agent for HIV infection.[57] These trials failed, due largely to phototoxicity induced by the phytochemical, something that might be reduced by using the whole herb extract. Hypericin and pseudohypericin have demonstrated activity against a wide range of enveloped viruses *in vitro*, including vesicular stomatitis virus, herpes simplex virus types 1 and 2, parainfluenza virus, vaccinia virus, murine cytomegalovirus, duck hepatitis B virus, bovine viral diarrhoea virus (BVDV), influenza virus type A, parainfluenza virus type 3, radiation leukaemia virus, Moloney murine leukaemia virus, Friend leukaemia virus, vesicular stomatitis virus, Sendai virus, Sindbis virus, equine infectious anaemia virus, bovine immunodeficiency virus, and human cytomegalovirus.

Antiviral activity for SJW has also been demonstrated in clinical trials. Two 90-day RCTs of SJW for recurrent orofacial herpes (94 patients) and genital herpes (110 patients) were conducted. Doses used were 900 mg/day of a dry 6:1 extract (0.3% hypericins) during symptom-free periods and 1,800 mg/day during skin outbreaks. The average symptom scores were 20.3 for SJW versus 32.1 for placebo for the first trial, and 15.6 vs 29.4 for the second trial. There were also fewer outbreaks in the SJW groups, hence a clear clinical benefit from taking the SJW was seen in both trials.

The antiviral activity of hypericin is substantially intensified by exposure to visible light, although activity has also been demonstrated in the absence of light. Efficacy in the facial herpes trial above may have been enhanced, as this part of the body has access to light. On the other hand, it is known that light can penetrate quite deep into the skin, and it is possible that sunlight exposure might activate hypericin circulating in the bloodstream, which can then exert the augmented antiviral activity wherever the circulation takes it.

9.5.3.3 Turmeric (curcumin)

Several *in vitro* studies have indicated antiviral activity for curcumin, but because it has limited bioavailability as such, this is only likely to have clinical relevance if curcumin with significantly enhanced bioavailability is used. Activity against HIV was recently reviewed, indicating extensive research on this topic (see **Figure 9.6**).[58] Recent activity has been found against other viruses (enveloped and naked) *in vitro*, including influenza A virus (IAV),[59] hepatitis B virus (HBV)[60] and human norovirus.[61] Additionally, curcumin significantly increased the survival rate of mice infected with IAV and reduced lung inflammatory cytokines and lung IAV titre.[62]

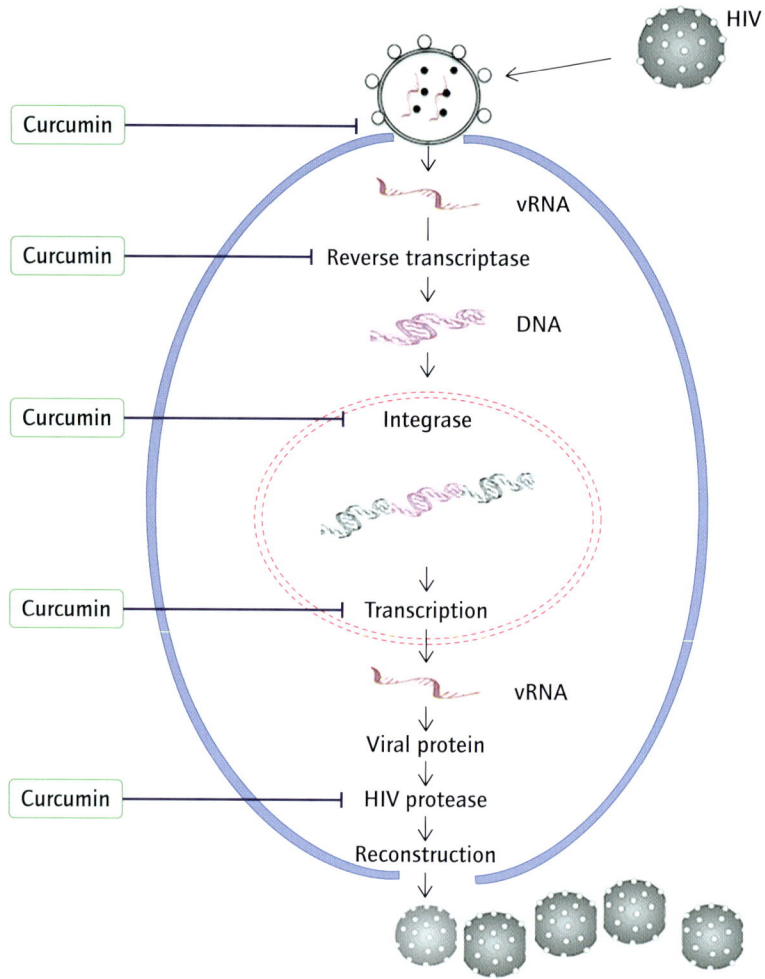

Figure 9.6 Multiple sites of activity for curcumin against HIV. [HIV = human immunodeficiency virus; vRNA = viral ribonucleic acid.]

9.5.4 Antibacterial herbs

The concept of *in vitro non veritas* is especially relevant to understanding the potential antibacterial activity of herbs. Whether the herbal actives can access the microbe in sufficient quantities is the key point here.

This begs the question, is there such a thing as a herbal antibiotic? The answer is **no**, in the sense of how we can take an oral antibiotic that is then absorbed, travels via the bloodstream to the site of an infection, and is still present in sufficient quantity to kill bacteria at that remote site. This key point seems to be widely misunderstood, based on my readings of "Dr Google". The under-recognised reality is that the herbal equivalent of an antibiotic is a herb that enhances immunity. In other words, oral doses of an immune herb can act against remote infections, but only indirectly, by enhancing the immune response in the infected tissue.

A key aspect of the *in vitro* versus *in vivo* discussion for antibacterial activity hinges on the type of model used. *In vitro* models test for either bacteriostatic or bactericidal activity, with the former test being most commonly used for herbal research. Bacteriostatic activity indicates only that the herb can inhibit the growth of bacteria, not that it will necessarily kill them. In general, bactericidal activity requires higher and more prolonged exposure than does bacteriostatic activity, and sometimes – depending on the organism – a bacteriostatic agent might never be bactericidal. However, the translation of these concepts to clinical outcomes can be complex.[63]

The reality is that herbs will best exhibit a bactericidal action when they can directly access the infection. This will be on body surfaces, in orifices, and in the gut. Since phytochemicals and their metabolites are often excreted via the urine, antibacterial activity can also be accomplished there – for example, in cystitis. There is the possibility that some volatile herbal components, such as of essential oils, can be exhaled by the lungs, exerting a mild antibacterial action in the process. But anyone who believes that a herb showing activity against a bacterial species in a test tube – however good it might seem – will then have clinical relevance for someone suffering from an infection with that organism, say, in their brain, needs a serious reality check.

Any use of antibacterial herbs will benefit immensely from the co-prescription of immune herbs to reinforce their activity. Combinations of antibacterial herbs often demonstrate synergy, so this strategy is also recommended.

Preferred antibacterial herbs include thyme, oregano, and tea tree, which are best used as their essential oils. Other key herbs in this category are the berberine-containing herbs, garlic (in forms that release allicin), sage, and myrrh. Most herbs that kill bacteria can also kill single-celled fungi and protozoa, and nearly all the herbs just listed share this feature.

Oregano and the berberine-containing herbs are briefly reviewed in Sections 9.5.4.1 and 9.5.4.2, in the context of bacteria, single-celled fungi, and protozoa.

9.5.4.1 Oregano

Oregano essential oil demonstrated growth inhibitory activity towards several human pathogens including *Candida albicans* and a range of bacterial pathogens when tested *in vitro*. The phenolic compounds carvacrol and thymol are important for such activity.[64] Oral administration of oregano oil for 30 days had a success rate of 80% *in vivo* against systemic candidiasis.[65]

In a study of the effects of oregano, 14 adults who tested positive for the enteric parasites *Blastocystis hominis*, *Entamoeba hartmanni*, and *Endolimax nana*[66] were treated for 6 weeks with emulsified oil of oregano (*Origanum vulgare*, 200 mg three times daily with meals). Parasites could no longer be detected in 10 of these patients, and 7 reported a reduction of symptoms. Parasite scores had decreased for the other 3 patients by follow-up. The recommended dose of oregano essential oil for parasites and stealth pathogens is 225–450 mg/day.

9.5.4.2 Berberine and berberine-containing herbs

Berberine exhibits broad-spectrum antimicrobial activity against fungi, bacteria, and protozoa. Most of any administered dose will remain in the gut, influencing the organisms there, so its poor absorption can be used to therapeutic advantage.[67] Berberine also inhibits pathogenic bacterial adherence to the gut wall. This degree of adherence to the wall is often proportional to bacterial virulence and pathogenicity.

Several controlled trials in the mid-1980s found that berberine, at a dose of around 400 mg/day, effectively treated acute infectious diarrhoea, for example from *E. coli*. Giardiasis patients aged 1–10 years were administered berberine (5 mg/kg/day for 6 days) and 68% became negative for the presence of Giardia cysts.

Berberine-containing herbs include barberry (*Berberis vulgaris*), *Coptis chinensis*, and golden seal (*Hydrastis canadensis*). The Chinese herb *Phellodendron amurense* is also a rich source of berberine. Phellodendron, for example in tablet form with a high berberine content, is a cost-effective way to exploit the antimicrobial effects of berberine.

9.5.4.3 What about biofilms?

Bacteria and fungi can form biofilms on body surfaces, and this is a significant self-protecting strategy that can result in resistance to antibiotics. But as per the discussion above, direct access to the biofilm by herbs is needed to effectively counter such biofilm defences. Therefore, while we can certainly deal with biofilms on the skin, in orifices, and in the gut and bladder, herbal biofilm-disrupting strategies are unlikely to be successful elsewhere in the body.

Anti-adhesive herbs such as cranberry and tannin-rich herbs can assist to break up biofilm coherence. Other herbs, including garlic, oregano oil,[68] and tannin herbs, can disrupt quorum sensing.[69] Quorum sensing is where bacteria communicate with each other to coordinate biofilm behaviour. Essential oils are also good biofilm disruptors, because the surface of biofilms is water-repellent and fat-loving, and essential oils are able to dissolve in fat-loving environments.

It is important to ensure that enough fibre and probiotics are consumed. Fibre in the colon[70] and probiotics[71] have been shown to be effective at disrupting gut biofilms.

We can use protease enzymes as well, but it is important to be gentle here. This preferentially involves prescribing bromelain, papain, and other plant-derived enzymes. Because many of the protective healthy organisms in our gut also exhibit biofilm behaviour, using aggressive biofilm strategies might actually weaken these body defences. Foods can be a useful source of gentle proteolytic enzymes. Protease activities are high in ginger, pineapple, pawpaw, and kiwi fruit. Persimmons, apricots, and peaches have high activity at an alkaline pH, making them suitable for further down the digestive tract. The most active vegetables in terms of proteolytic activity are garlic, onions, capsicum, asparagus, and kale, but leeks are also particularly active.[72]

Table 9.1 Key herbal categories for stealth pathogen classes

Pathogen	Key herbs
Chronic viruses	▹ licorice, Thuja, St John's wort, Echinacea root, Astragalus, *A. annua*, bioavailable curcumin, Eleutherococcus, cat's claw
Helminths	▹ myrrh, wormwood, Stemona, cloves, *A. annua*, garlic, Andrographis
Protozoa	▹ myrrh, Phellodendron (and other berberine-containing herbs), oregano oil, Andrographis, garlic
Bacteria	▹ myrrh, Phellodendron (and other berberine-containing herbs), oregano oil, garlic, thyme, sage, Echinacea root, Astragalus, cranberry, cat's claw
Fungi	▹ Phellodendron (and other berberine-containing herbs), oregano oil, anise oil, garlic, Echinacea root, cat's claw

9.6 Herb summary

The key immune herbs against stealth pathogens include:

- Echinacea root
- Astragalus
- cat's claw
- Eleutherococcus
- Andrographis (mainly for protozoa and helminths)

Table 9.1 summarises the main effective herbs (including immune herbs) to assist with the eradication of stealth pathogens, organised by class of pathogen.

Sage is effective for gut biofilms because it contains an essential oil and tannins, both of which disrupt biofilms.

9.7 Sample protocols for reducing the stealth pathogen bioburden

The various mechanisms stealth pathogens use to evade immune defences and standard treatment methods makes them difficult to eradicate, unless specific protocols are utilised. Also, we can only find the pathogens that we specifically look for, meaning that less common or currently unknown stealth pathogens might be missed in the patient. Hence a broad-spectrum "test-by-treating" approach is considered the best way to deal with reducing the stealth pathogen bioburden, noting that a single pill or quick-fix approach may not address all the aspects of what is required to eradicate these organisms. The sample treatment modules that follow have been developed with these objectives in mind. Furthermore, the pulsed dosing approach outlined should help to reduce any "die-off" effects and reduce the risk of adverse reactions.

9.7.1 A stealth-bioburden-reducing protocol aimed at parasites

- Protocol based on a 14-day treatment cycle (see **Box 9.1**).
- For the first 4 days, the two Artemisias (European wormwood and *Artemisia annua*) and Andrographis are prescribed in high doses: wormwood up to 2 g/day (e.g. 5 mL at 1:5); *A. annua* up to 32 g/day; Andrographis up to 12 g/day.
- For the next 5 days, myrrh and garlic are prescribed in high doses: myrrh up to 2 g/day; garlic up to the equivalent of 10 g of fresh cloves per day.
- During the final 5 days there is no treatment.

Box 9.1 The purge parasite (4-5-5) protocol.

Days 1–4 (4 days)	Days 5–9 (5 days)	Days 10–14 (5 days)
- *Artemisia annua*: 3 times a day - wormwood (*Artemisia absinthium*): 3 times a day - Andrographis: 3 times a day	- myrrh resin: 3 times a day - garlic, allicin releasing: twice a day	- zero herbs

One cycle (4 + 5 + 5) = 14 days. Repeat for 2–3 cycles.
Drink high-tannin teas: strong peppermint tea or green tea.
For dosages, see text above.

> **Box 9.2** A general stealth-bioburden-reducing protocol
>
> | Days 1–4 (4 days) | Days 5–14 (10 days) |
> |---|---|
> | ‣ myrrh: 3 times a day
‣ *Artemisia annua*: 3 times a day
‣ Andrographis: 3 times a day | ‣ Echinacea root: 2–3 times a day
‣ Thuja: 3 times a day
‣ St John's wort: 3 times a day
‣ licorice: 3 times a day
‣ bioavailable curcumin: twice a day |
>
> One cycle (4 + 10) = 14 days. Repeat for 3–6 cycles.
> Base protocol can be adapted as per the needs of each patient.
> Combine with bowel flora protocol, as required.
> For dosages, see Sections 9.5 and 9.7.1.

‣ These steps are repeated for 2–3 cycles, and then the situation is assessed.
‣ It is recommended that the patient drink 3–4 cups/day of high-tannin herbal teas (e.g., strong peppermint or green tea) throughout this protocol.

9.7.2 A general stealth-bioburden-reducing protocol

Another 14-day sample treatment module aimed at both viruses and parasites is shown in **Box 9.2**. If gastrointestinal pathogenic bacteria and fungi are also of concern, then berberine-containing herbs can be added on Days 1–4 and garlic (allicin-releasing) on Days 5–14. Should dysbiosis need correcting, this protocol can be readily combined with a 14-day version of the bowel flora protocol (4 days of weeding and 10 days of feeding – see Chapter 8.)

9.8 FHT treatments for chronic Lyme disease

For a patient with diagnosis of chronic Lyme disease, many other FHT strategies need consideration as part of the overall treatment plan. These are outlined in **Table 9.2**.

Table 9.2 Additional considerations for chronic Lyme disease

Symptom	Treatment
For depleted energy	▹ adrenal support is essential: licorice and/or Rehmannia ▹ Rhodiola, Korean ginseng, Schisandra ▹ Rhodiola, Korean ginseng are best for instant energy and/or where mood is low ▹ Withania (ashwagandha) for parasympathetic dominance or where patient is sleeping long hours
Address neuroinflammation as a factor	▹ Boswellia ▹ turmeric as bioavailable curcumin ▹ omega-3 fatty acids
Treating for immune depletion is paramount	▹ Echinacea, Astragalus, Eleuthero
Support the nervous system, sleep, and cognition	▹ kava ▹ valerian, passionflower ▹ St John's wort, saffron
Manage pain and inflammation	▹ Corydalis, Californian poppy, Jamaica dogwood ▹ St John's wort, ▹ willow bark ▹ Boswellia and bioavailable curcumin

9.9 Case history: "not been well since" (NBWS) tick bite, an Australian story

As discussed above, chronic Lyme disease is a controversial topic in the United States and elsewhere. For example, the US Centers for Disease Control and Prevention (CDC) states the following on their website:

> The term "chronic Lyme disease" (CLD) has been used to describe people with different illnesses. While the term is sometimes used to describe illness in patients with Lyme disease, in many occasions it has been used to describe symptoms in people who have no evidence of a current or past infection with *Borrelia burgdorferi*.

In Australia, there is a further layer to the controversy, as *Borrelia burgdorferi* is not regarded as endemic, leading to certain therapists describing the syndrome they witness in some patients after tick bite as a "chronic Lyme-like" illness. This debate is not in the interest of patients, who have clearly become unwell following their exposure to a tick bite. On the one hand, they might be told that there is nothing wrong with them, as CLD does not exist. On the other, they might be offered radical treatments as their only hope, sometimes involving high doses of antibiotics over a prolonged period.

Perhaps a way forward is to focus less on whatever specific organism(s) might have led to the patient's ill health (while still acknowledging that micro-organisms are involved) and to remove the controversial terminology by stating the obvious: these people are not well, and it all started with them being bitten by a tick. The following is a case of exactly this, which I will refer to simply as NBWS tick bite, probably a preferable title for this condition.

The patient was a 61-year-old male school teacher, who was bitten by a tick while bush-walking in October 2016. He tested positive for rickettsial infection, but not for Lyme, and he was treated with doxycycline for 14 days. Following this, he became so unwell that he had to take early retirement from his teaching position. Even then, with less stress in his life, he remained in poor health, so in May 2017 he sought natural treatments, as no other options were offered to help him out of his predicament.

When he presented for treatment, the patient was needing to sleep 10–11 hours a day and was suffering with aches and pains all over, but especially in his joints, and with recurrent headaches and brain fog. But the worst problem was his disabling fatigue, especially in the late afternoon, which meant he could only do a fraction of what he used to do in a day.

The decision was made to support his stress response and immune system with a "baseline therapy" before targeting treatments at any pathogens. Hence, he was prescribed the following:

- Echinacea root tablets, 3/day
- Rehmannia/Hemidesmus/Bupleurum/feverfew tablet combination, 3/day
- Rhodiola and Korean ginseng tablets, 4/day (2 mornings and 2 evenings)

After 6 weeks, he felt a noticeable improvement. His sleep was of better quality, although he still needed 10 hours a day. Headaches and joint pain diminished, but there were occasional relapses. A stealth parasite bioburden-reduction protocol was then initiated (in addition to the baseline therapy above) as per Section 9.7.1, for 3 cycles, then a one-week break, followed by another 3 cycles.

By early October 2017, the patient reported that he was now 80% better. He had started swimming again. Another 3 rounds of the stealth parasite protocol were commenced. In late November, when he had completed this, the patient reported he was still at 80%, and felt he had plateaued. So, 6 rounds of the following 10-day protocol were initiated (still with baseline therapy):

- for 5 days: myrrh, 5 tablets twice a day
- for the next 5 days: an antiviral combination of St John's wort/licorice/Thuja, 2 tablets twice a day

By February 2018, the patient reported that he was feeling very well: much stronger, with fewer symptoms, and more energetic. By April he commented that on some days he was 100%, though on others around 80–90%. He reported that he was now quite active, living a normal life; he had packed and moved to a new house without any adverse effects and was back to relief teaching. Treatment was continued with:

- Echinacea root, 3 tablets a day
- Astragalus/Eleutherococcus/Echinacea combination, 2 tablets twice daily
- Rhodiola and Korean ginseng, 2 tablets a day (mornings)
- Mexican valerian for sleep when needed

He has continued this until the present time (April 2021) and remains well.

It is not unusual for someone experiencing the health circumstances described above to suffer debilitating symptoms for many years, with little hope from conventional medical treatments. The fact that this patient responded so fully and quickly underlines the key role that herbs can play in helping people to recover from the effects of a NBWS tick bite.

References

1. Radolf JD. Role of outer membrane architecture in immune evasion by *Treponema pallidum* and *Borrelia burgdorferi*. *Trends Microbiol* 1994; **2**(9): 307–311.
2. Mattman, LH. *Cell Wall Deficient Forms: Stealth Pathogens* 3rd ed. CRC Press, Boca Raton, FL, 2000.
3. Astrauskiene D, Bernotiene E. New insights into bacterial persistence in reactive arthritis. *Clin Exp Rheumatol*. 2007; **25**(3): 470–479.
4. Merrell DS, Falkow S. Frontal and stealth attack strategies in microbial pathogenesis. *Nature*. 2004; **430**(6996): 250–256. doi:10.1038/nature02760.
5. Venâncio P, Brito MJ, Pereira G, et al. Anti-N-methyl-D-aspartate receptor encephalitis with positive serum antithyroid antibodies, IgM antibodies against mycoplasma pneumoniae and human herpesvirus 7 PCR in the CSF. *Pediatr Infect Dis J*. 2014; **33**(8): 882–883. PMID: 25222311.
6. Huang T, Osterrieder N. The herpesvirus stealth program. *Oncotarget*. 2015; **6**(26): 21761–21762. doi:10.18632/oncotarget.5261.
7. Tao Q, Robertson KD. Stealth technology: how Epstein-Barr virus utilizes DNA methylation to cloak itself from immune detection. *Clin Immunol*. 2003; **109**(1): 53–63. doi:10.1016/s1521-6616(03)00198-0.
8. Pearson MS, Tribolet L, Cantacessi C, et al. Molecular mechanisms of hookworm disease: stealth, virulence, and vaccines [published correction appears in *J Allergy Clin Immunol*. 2012 Oct; **130**(4): 852 (Valerio, Maria Adela corrected to Valero, Maria Adela)]. *J Allergy Clin Immunol*. 2012; **130**(1): 13–21. doi:10.1016/j.jaci.2012.05.029.
9. Pruneda JN, Bastidas RJ, Bertsoulaki E, et al. A Chlamydia effector combining deubiquitination and acetylation activities induces Golgi fragmentation. *Nat Microbiol*. 2018; **3**(12): 1377–1384. doi:10.1038/s41564-018-0271-y.
10. Pajuelo D, Gonzalez-Juarbe N, Tak U, Sun J, Orihuela CJ, Niederweis M. NAD$^+$ depletion triggers macrophage necroptosis, a cell death pathway exploited by mycobacterium tuberculosis. *Cell Rep*. 2018; **24**(2): 429–440. doi:10.1016/j.celrep.2018.06.042.
11. Davies H, Belda H, Broncel M, et al. An exported kinase family mediates species-specific erythrocyte remodelling and virulence in human malaria. *Nat Microbiol*. 2020 Apr 13 [published online ahead of print]; **5**: 848–863. doi:10.1038/s41564-020-0702-4.
12. Hembach L, Bonin M, Gorzelanny C, Moerschbacher BM. Unique subsite specificity and potential natural function of a chitosan deacetylase from the human pathogen *Cryptococcus neoformans*. *Proc Natl Acad Sci USA*. 2020; **117**(7): 3551–3559. doi:10.1073/pnas.1915798117.
13. Chmiela M, Gonciarz W. Molecular mimicry in *Helicobacter pylori* infections. *World J Gastroenterol*. 2017; **23**(22): 3964–3977. doi:10.3748/wjg.v23.i22.3964.
14. Cellini L. *Helicobacter pylori*: a chameleon-like approach to life. *World J Gastroenterol*. 2014; **20**(19): 5575–5582. doi:10.3748/wjg.v20.i19.5575.
15. Clark J. Mycoplasmas: identifying hosts for a stealth pathogen. *Vet J*. 2005; **170**(3): 273–274. PMID: 16266841.
16. Chaudhry R, Ghosh A, Chandolia A. Pathogenesis of *Mycoplasma pneumoniae*: an update. *Indian J Med Microbiol*. 2016; **34**(1): 7–16. PMID: 26776112.
17. Srinivas V, Lebrette H, Lundin D, et al. Metal-free ribonucleotide reduction powered by a DOPA radical in Mycoplasma pathogens. *Nature*. 2018; **563**(7731): 416–420. doi:10.1038/s41586-018-0653-6.

18. Schaeverbeke T, Gilroy CB, Bébéar C, Dehais J, Taylor-Robinson D. Mycoplasma fermentans, but not M penetrans, detected by PCR assays in synovium from patients with rheumatoid arthritis and other rheumatic disorders. *J Clin Pathol*. 1996; **49**(10): 824–828. doi:10.1136/jcp.49.10.824.
19. Chu KA, Chen W, Hsu CY, Hung YM, Wei JC. Increased risk of rheumatoid arthritis among patients with Mycoplasma pneumonia: a nationwide population-based cohort study in Taiwan. *PLoS One*. 2019 Jan 14; **14**(1): e0210750. doi:10.1371/journal.pone.0210750.
20. Radolf JD, Deka RK, Anand A, Šmajs D, Norgard MV, Yang XF. Treponema pallidum, the syphilis spirochete: making a living as a stealth pathogen. *Nat Rev Microbiol*. 2016; **14**(12): 744–759. doi:10.1038/nrmicro.2016.141.
21. Radolf JD, Desrosiers DC. Treponema pallidum, the stealth pathogen, changes, but how?. *Mol Microbiol*. 2009; **72**(5): 1081–1086. doi:10.1111/j.1365-2958.2009.06711.x.
22. Taylor LH, Latham SM, Woolhouse ME. Risk factors for human disease emergence. *Philos Trans R Soc Lond B Biol Sci*. 2001; **356**(1411): 983–989. PMID: 11516376.
23. Schnittger L, Rodriguez AE, Florin-Christensen M, et al. Babesia: a world emerging. *Infect Genet Evol*. 2012; **12**(8): 1788–1809. PMID: 22871652.
24. Knapp KL, Rice NA. Human coinfection with Borrelia burgdorferi and Babesia microti in the United States. *J Parasitol Res*. 2015; **2015**: 587131. doi:10.1155/2015/587131. PMID: 26697208.
25. Donahoe SL, Peacock CS, Choo AY, et al. A retrospective study of Babesia macropus associated with morbidity and mortality in eastern grey kangaroos (Macropus giganteus) and agile wallabies (Macropus agilis). *Int J Parasitol Parasites Wildl*. 2015 Feb 28; **4**(2): 268–276. doi:10.1016/j.ijppaw.2015.02.002.
26. Regier Y, O'Rourke F, Kempf VA. Bartonella spp.: a chance to establish One Health concepts in veterinary and human medicine. *Parasit Vectors*. 2016; **9**(1): 261. doi:10.1186/s13071-016-1546-x. PMID: 27161111.
27. Stricker RB, Johnson L. Lyme disease: the promise of Big Data, companion diagnostics and precision medicine. *Infect Drug Resist*. 2016 Sep 13; **9**: 215–219. doi:10.2147/IDR.S114770.
28. https://www.healthline.com/health/lyme-disease-chronic-persistent
29. Baker PJ. A review of antibiotic-tolerant persisters and their relevance to posttreatment Lyme Disease symptoms. *Am J Med*. 2020; **133**(4): 429–431. doi:10.1016/j.amjmed.2019.12.007.
30. https://en.wikipedia.org/wiki/Toxoplasma_gondii
31. Desmettre T. Toxoplasmosis and behavioural changes. *J Fr Ophtalmol*. 2020; **43**(3): e89–e93. doi:10.1016/j.jfo.2020.01.001.
32. Brennan A, Hawley J, Dhand N, et al. Seroprevalence and risk factors for *Toxoplasma gondii* infection in owned domestic cats in Australia. *Vector Borne Zoonotic Dis*. 2020; **20**(4): 275–280. doi:10.1089/vbz.2019.2520.
33. Sutterland AL, Fond G, Kuin A, et al. Beyond the association. Toxoplasma gondii in schizophrenia, bipolar disorder, and addiction: systematic review and meta-analysis. *Acta Psychiatr Scand*. 2015; **132**(3): 161–179. PMID: 25877655.
34. de Ridder S, van der Kooy F, Verpoorte R. Artemisia annua as a self-reliant treatment for malaria in developing countries. *J Ethnopharmacol*. 2008; **120**(3): 302–314. doi:10.1016/j.jep.2008.09.017.
35. *Ibid.*
36. Ho WE, Peh HY, Chan TK, et al. Artemisinins: pharmacological actions beyond antimalarial. *Pharmacol Ther*. 2014; **142**(1): 126–139. PMID: 24316259.
37. *Ibid.*

38. Loo CS, Lam NS, Yu D, Su XZ, Lu F. Artemisinin and its derivatives in treating protozoan infections beyond malaria. *Pharmacol Res.* 2017; 117: 192–217. doi:10.1016/j.phrs.2016.11.012.
39. *Ibid.*
40. Goodrich SK, Schlegel CR, Wang G, et al. Use of artemisinin and its derivatives to treat HPV-infected/transformed cells and cervical cancer: a review. *Future Oncol.* 2014; **10**(4): 647–654. PMID: 24754594.
41. Efferth T. Beyond malaria: the inhibition of viruses by artemisinin-type compounds. *Biotechnol Adv.* 2018; **36**(6): 1730–1737. doi:10.1016/j.biotechadv.2018.01.001.
42. Mueller MS, Runyambo N, Wagner I, et al. Randomized controlled trial of a traditional preparation of *Artemisia annua* L. (Annual Wormwood) in the treatment of malaria. *Trans R Soc Trop Med Hyg.* 2004; **98**(5): 318–321. PMID: 15109558.
43. Blanke CH, Naisabha GB, Balema MB, et al. Herba *Artemisiae annuae* tea preparation compared to sulfadoxine-pyrimethamine in the treatment of uncomplicated falciparum malaria in adults: a randomized double-blind clinical trial. *Trop Doct.* 2008; **38**(2): 113–116. PMID: 18453510.
44. Stebbings S, Beattie E, McNamara D, et al. A pilot randomized, placebo-controlled clinical trial to investigate the efficacy and safety of an extract of *Artemisia annua* administered over 12 weeks, for managing pain, stiffness, and functional limitation associated with osteoarthritis of the hip and knee. *Clin Rheumatol.* 2016; **35**(7): 1829–1836. PMID: 26631103.
45. Hunt S, Stebbings S, McNamara D. An open-label six-month extension study to investigate the safety and efficacy of an extract of *Artemisia annua* for managing pain, stiffness and functional limitation associated with osteoarthritis of the hip and knee. *NZ Med J.* 2016; **129**(1444): 97–102. PMID: 27806033.
46. Savage RL, Hill GR, Barnes J, Kenyon SH, Tatley MV. Suspected hepatotoxicity with a supercritical carbon dioxide extract of *Artemisia annua* in grapeseed oil used in New Zealand. *Front Pharmacol.* 2019 Dec 20; **10**: 1448. doi:10.3389/fphar.2019.01448.
47. Elfawal MA, Towler MJ, Reich NG, et al. Dried whole-plant *Artemisia annua* slows evolution of malaria drug resistance and overcomes resistance to artemisinin. *Proc Natl Acad Sci USA.* 2015; **112**(3): 821–826. PMID: 25561559.
48. Elfawal MA, Towler MJ, Reich NG, et al. Dried whole plant *Artemisia annua* as an antimalarial therapy. *PLoS One.* 2012; **7**(12): e52746. doi:10.1371/journal.pone.0052746. PMID: 23289055.
49. Weathers PJ, Elfawal MA, Towler MJ, et al. Pharmacokinetics of artemisinin delivered by oral consumption of *Artemisia annua* dried leaves in healthy vs. Plasmodium chabaudi-infected mice. *J Ethnopharmacol.* 2014; **153**(3): 732–736. PMID: 24661969.
50. Daddy NB, Kalisya LM, Bagire PG, Watt RL, Towler MJ, Weathers PJ. *Artemisia annua* dried leaf tablets treated malaria resistant to ACT and i.v. artesunate: case reports. *Phytomedicine.* 2017; **32**: 37–40. doi:10.1016/j.phymed.2017.04.006.
51. Ashton M, Hai TN, Sy ND, et al. Artemisinin pharmacokinetics is time-dependent during repeated oral administration in healthy male adults. *Drug Metab Dispos.* 1998; **26**(1): 25–27.
52. Bone KM, Mills SY. *Principles and Practice of Phytotherapy: Modern Herbal Medicine*, 2nd ed. Elsevier, UK, 2013, pp 753–759.
53. *Ibid.*, pp 753–759.
54. *Ibid.*, pp 753–759.
55. *Ibid.*, pp 753–759.
56. *Ibid.*, pp 719–741.
57. *Ibid.*, pp 826–860.

58. Prasad S, Tyagi AK. Curcumin and its analogues: a potential natural compound against HIV infection and AIDS. *Food Funct.* 2015 Nov; **6**(11): 3412 3419. doi:10.1039/c5fo00485c. PMID: 26404185.
59. Dai J, Gu L, Su Y, Wang Q, et al. Inhibition of curcumin on influenza A virus infection and influenzal pneumonia via oxidative stress, TLR2/4, p38/JNK MAPK and NF-κB pathways. *Int Immunopharmacol.* 2018 Jan; **54**: 177–187. doi:10.1016/j.intimp.2017.11.009. PMID: 29153953.
60. Wei ZQ, Zhang YH, Ke CZ, et al. Curcumin inhibits hepatitis B virus infection by down-regulating cccDNA-bound histone acetylation. *World J Gastroenterol.* 2017 Sep 14; **23**(34): 6252–6260. doi:10.3748/wjg.v23.i34.6252. PMID: 28974891.
61. Yang M, Lee G, Si J, et al. Curcumin shows antiviral properties against norovirus. *Molecules.* 2016 Oct 20; **21**(10). pii: E1401. PMID: 27775614.
62. Dai J, Gu L, Su Y, Wang Q, et al. Inhibition of curcumin on influenza A virus infection and influenzal pneumonia via oxidative stress, TLR2/4, p38/JNK MAPK and NF-κB pathways. *Int Immunopharmacol.* 2018 Jan; **54**: 177–187. doi:10.1016/j.intimp.2017.11.009. PMID: 29153953.
63. Pankey GA, Sabath LD. Clinical relevance of bacteriostatic versus bactericidal mechanisms of action in the treatment of Gram-positive bacterial infections. *Clin Infect Dis.* 2004; **38**(6): 864 870. doi:10.1086/381972.
64. Hammer KA, et al. Antimicrobial activity of essential oils and other plant extracts. *J Appl Microbiol.* 1999; **86**(6): 985–990.
65. Manohar V, et al. Antifungal activities of origanum oil against *Candida albicans*. *Mol Cell Biochem.* 2001; **228**(1–2): 111–117.
66. Force M, et al. Inhibition of enteric parasites by emulsified oil of oregano in vivo. *Phytother Res.* 2000; **14**(3): 213–214.
67. Bone KM, Mills SY. *Principles and Practice of Phytotherapy: Modern Herbal Medicine*, 2nd ed. Elsevier, UK, 2013, pp 399–418.
68. Alibi S, Ben Selma W, Ramos-Vivas J, et al. Anti-oxidant, antibacterial, anti-biofilm, and anti-quorum sensing activities of four essential oils against multidrug-resistant bacterial clinical isolates. *Curr Res Transl Med.* 2020; **68**(2): 59–66. doi:10.1016/j.retram.2020.01.001.
69. Vattem DA, Mihalik K, Crixell SH, McLean RJ. Dietary phytochemicals as quorum sensing inhibitors. *Fitoterapia.* 2007; **78**(4): 302–310. doi:10.1016/j.fitote.2007.03.009.
70. Kleessen B, Blaut M. Modulation of gut mucosal biofilms. *Br J Nutr.* 2005; **93**(Suppl 1): S35–S40. doi:10.1079/bjn20041346.
71. Barzegari A, Kheyrolahzadeh K, Hosseiniyan Khatibi SM, Sharifi S, Memar MY, Zununi Vahed S. The battle of probiotics and their derivatives against biofilms. *Infect Drug Resist.* 2020 Feb 26; **13**: 659–672. doi:10.2147/IDR.S232982.
72. Sun Q, Zhang B, Yan QJ, Jiang ZQ. Comparative analysis on the distribution of protease activities among fruits and vegetable resources. *Food Chem.* 2016; **213**: 708–713. doi:10.1016/j.foodchem.2016.07.029.

10

FHT for relieving anxiety and boosting healthy sleep

This chapter examines the role of herbs in relieving anxiety and boosting healthy sleep. In terms of FHT, helping with sleep and anxiety can be clinical end goals in themselves, or they can form part of a larger strategy to treat a different health problem, when they are considered to be contributing factors that need to be addressed.

Due to the pressures of modern living, the incidences of chronic pain, addiction syndromes, depression, anxiety, and sleep disorders are all on the rise. Healthy sleep is the universal panacea that can assist with these issues and improve wellbeing, immunity, body weight, and energy, just to name a few extra benefits. Anxiety often occurs when the nervous system is stressed and overstimulated. Promoting restful sleep can therefore assist greatly with relieving anxiety.

In this chapter we first review a recent definition of anxiety; we then explore the evidence for and clinical application of herbs for this disorder. Next, some exciting developments in sleep science are outlined, together with a brief discussion of how good sleep hygiene can be achieved. Finally, evidence-based FHT protocols for improving sleep are provided.

There is a reasonable evidence base supporting the gentle option of using herbal treatments for anxiety and insomnia. Unlike conventional medications, such herbs do not impair cognitive function and reaction times at normal doses. As part of the FHT principles outlined in this book, they should be adapted to the individual needs and responses of the patient.

10.1 A modern definition of anxiety

New classifications of anxiety according to the *DSM-5* are as follows:[1]

1. **Anxiety disorders:** separation anxiety disorder, selective mutism, specific phobia, social phobia, panic disorder, agoraphobia, and generalised anxiety disorder
2. **Obsessive-compulsive disorders:** obsessive-compulsive disorder, body dysmorphic disorder, hoarding disorder, trichotillomania, and excoriation disorder
3. **Trauma and stressor-related disorders:** reactive attachment disorder, disinhibited social engagement disorder, post-traumatic stress disorder (PTSD), acute stress disorder, and adjustment disorder

Generalised anxiety disorder (GAD) is a relatively common presentation and might be missed during a consultation unless the patient specifically raises it as an issue. It is therefore good practice to assess the anxiety level of all patients using a simple questionnaire. One example is the GAD-7 (**Box 10.1**). Its application can help the clinician to determine objectively the extent of a patient's anxiety.[2]

10.1.1 Drug medication for anxiety

A recent analysis based on 89 trials included 25,441 patients randomly assigned to 22 different active drugs or to a placebo.[3] The primary outcomes assessed were efficacy (mean difference [MD] in change in the Hamilton Anxiety Scale Score above the placebo change) and acceptability (discontinuations for any cause). The authors used network meta-analyses to analyse the data.

Four drugs demonstrated the best evidence: duloxetine (MD −3.13), pregabalin (MD −2.79), venlafaxine (MD −2.69), and escitalopram (MD −2.45) were more efficacious than placebo, with a relatively good level of acceptability. Quetiapine (MD −3.60) had the largest effect but was poorly tolerated, and paroxetine and benzodiazepines were also poorly tolerated.

Box 10.1 The GAD-7 survey

GAD-7 Anxiety

Over the *last two weeks*, how often have you been bothered by the following problems?	Not at all	Several days	More than half the days	Nearly every day
1 Feeling nervous, anxious, or on edge	0	1	2	3
2 Not being able to stop or control worrying	0	1	2	3
3 Worrying too much about different things	0	1	2	3
4 Trouble relaxing	0	1	2	3
5 Being so restless that it is hard to sit still	0	1	2	3
6 Becoming easily annoyed or irritable	0	1	2	3
7 Feeling afraid, as if something awful might happen	0	1	2	3

0–4: minimal anxiety; 5–9: mild anxiety; 10–14: moderate anxiety; 15–21: severe anxiety.

The perspective of many herbal clinicians is that while they might often have side effects, drugs are quite strong. But is that the case? Are current drugs necessarily that effective for anxiety over and above placebo? This high-level, well-regarded study by esteemed scientists published in a major journal (*The Lancet*) implies that they are not. The full Hamilton Anxiety Scale score totals 56 (14 questions rated 0 to 4). The study found that modern drugs improve anxiety over and above placebo by only around three points on that scale.

We can suggest a bold proposal based on this high-level evidence from a top medical journal: that conventional drugs for anxiety have limited additional benefits over placebo, and many carry high side-effect risks. This begs the question of why more research is not being undertaken into herbal medicines for this disorder.

10.2 Evidence and clinical application of key herbs for anxiety

10.2.1 European valerian

10.2.1.1 European valerian and OCD

Valerian was shown to benefit patients with obsessive-compulsive disorder (OCD) in a small randomised controlled trial.[4] A total of 31 patients took either a valerian dried extract (765 mg/day) or a placebo for 8 weeks. This relatively high dose was extracted from 5.5 g of dried root. There was a significant reduction in the Yale-Brown OCD symptom score compared to the placebo ($p < 0.05$) (see **Figure 10.1**).

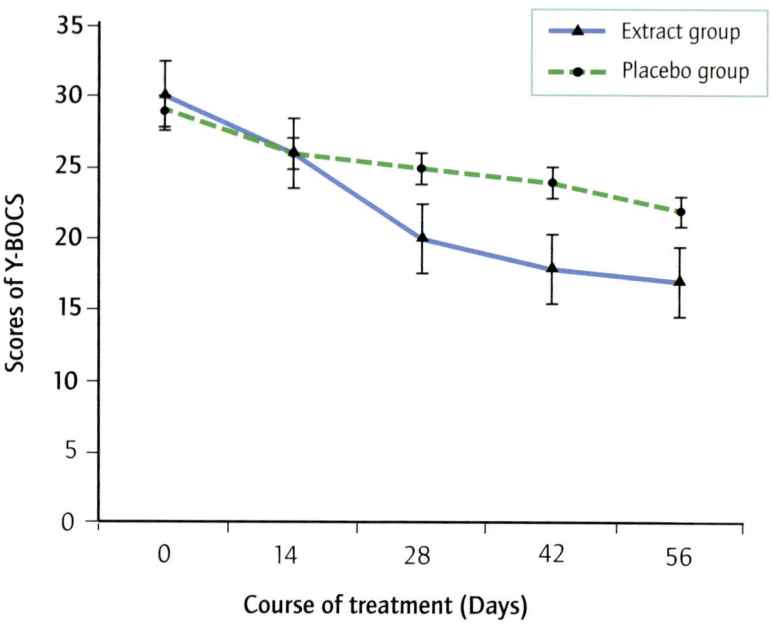

Figure 10.1 Clinical effect of valerian on OCD score. Each point represents mean for 15–16 patients. [*$p < 0.05$ compared to placebo (Student's t-test).] (Y-BOCS = Yale–Brown Obsessive-Compulsive Scale.)

10.2.1.2 European valerian and anxiety

Some early clinical trials investigated the use of a combination of European valerian (*Valeriana officinalis*) and St John's wort (*Hypericum perforatum*) for the treatment of depression and/or anxiety.[5] In an RCT on 100 patients suffering from moderate anxiety, after 2 weeks a combination (at a dose containing 0.3–0.6 mg/day total hypericin and 450–900 mg valerian dried extract) was significantly more effective than diazepam. Fewer side-effects were observed in the herbal treatment group (4%) than in the group treated with diazepam (14%). A comparable reduction in symptoms of fear and depressive mood was observed for a valerian–St John's wort combination compared with amitriptyline.

Patient anxiety is commonly encountered by dentists and is recognised as one of the main factors that can negatively affect treatment outcomes. Conscious sedation using drugs such as benzodiazepines is an option but often causes undesirable side effects. A group of dentists in Brazil evaluated the efficacy of valerian for control of anxiety during impacted lower third molar surgery. A double-blind, crossover RCT was used, meaning that each patient underwent two dental procedures. A single oral dose of either valerian (100 mg, presumably a dried concentrated extract) or placebo was randomly administered one hour before each surgical procedure to 20 volunteers between 17 and 31 years of age.[6] Their anxiety level was rated by physiological parameters (blood pressure and heart rate) and the observation of clinical signs, assessed by a researcher and the dental surgeon. There was good agreement between the assessment of anxiety performed by the researcher and the surgeon (concordance index = 0.85). Based on the researcher's assessment, patients medicated with valerian were calmer and more relaxed (85%) in comparison to those medicated with the placebo (45%) ($p = 0.022$). A similar trend was found for the surgeon's assessment, but the difference did not quite achieve statistical significance ($p = 0.102$).

When the volunteers were asked about their preference for one of the surgical procedures at the end of the experiment, 11 (55%) reported greater comfort during the procedure when valerian was employed, 5 (25%) preferred the procedure with the placebo, and the remaining 4 (20%) had no preference. There was no significant impact of valerian on systolic blood pressure and heart rate. From their overall findings, the authors suggested that valerian was more effective at controlling anxiety than a placebo. Results might have been more marked if a higher dose of valerian had been used.

10.2.1.3 Valerian alters brain connectivity

In a recent RCT featuring 64 non-clinical volunteers suffering from psychological stress, significant responses from baseline in depression and anxiety scores were seen after 4 weeks of 300 mg / day of valerian extract, but there was no difference for the placebo.[7] Compared to placebo, valerian effected significantly greater *increases* in EEG frontal brain region alpha coherence (associated with neurophysiological integration, cognitive flexibility, and information processing) across four electrode pairs, and these changes were significantly correlated with anxiolysis. Significantly greater *decreases* in theta coherence across another four electrode pairs were also seen for the valerian treatment group.

The authors concluded that:

> The relationship between strengthened connectivity and anxiolysis implies that valerian-induced increases in cortical information exchange can relieve anxiety in stressed individuals.

If you were to perhaps ask your average medical practitioner: "What do you think of the herb valerian?", what would their response most probably be? The most likely reply would be that it is just an expensive placebo. (Mind you, we should be happy to play the game "my placebo is better than yours", but that is not the point here). If one can correlate a reduction in a person's feelings of anxiety with objective changes on an electroencephalograph, how can that be due to a placebo effect? Consequently, this is, in fact, groundbreaking work.

When the scientists measured electrode pairs across the front of the brain, they found a significant increase in alpha coherence. This means that the person was more alert but also relaxed – like, for example, the effect of a mild form of meditation. The observed decreases in theta coherence mean they also were not sedated, the way they might be from a drug. Mental functioning was fully there, so a person taking valerian can deal with the issues of life and not just cotton-wool them: they are relaxed but alert. This is a real effect happening in the brain that can be objectively demonstrated.

10.2.2 Passionflower

In Western herbalism one of the key herbs used for anxiety is the vine of the medicinal species of passionflower (*Passiflora incarnata*). Its unusual name is not a reference to earthly passions. It comes, rather, from the Christian symbolism (Christ's passion) seen in the flower by the Spanish conquistadores when they first encountered the vine growing in South America. Clinical trials suggest that it can be fast acting in relieving anxiety, as demonstrated by effects seen before surgical procedures.

10.2.2.1 Passionflower and pre-surgical anxiety

Many patients suffer from anxiety before surgery, but any premedication must be sufficiently anxiolytic while not causing undue sedation or interacting with general anaesthesia. One clinical study found that a single dose of passionflower prior to outpatient surgery reduced anxiety without increasing sedation.

In a double blind RCT, 60 patients received either 500 mg of passionflower (probably as the dried herb) as a tablet or a matching placebo for premedication 90 minutes before surgery.[8] The passionflower tablet was standardised to contain 1.01 mg of benzoflavone. A numerical rating scale of 1–10, with 10 being the worst possible anxiety, was used to assess anxiety and sedation before and 10, 30, 60, and 90 minutes after the premedication. Psychomotor function was assessed upon arrival in the operating theatre and 30 and 90 minutes after tracheal extubation.

Anxiety scores were similar for both groups at baseline, being 4.6 ± 1.7 for the passionflower group and 5.1 ± 2.0 for the control group. After 90 minutes these had changed to a remarkable 0.97 for the herbal treatment versus 3.88 for a control treatment, a significant difference ($p < 0.001$). There were no significant differences between the groups in the level of sedation before surgery and the recovery of psychomotor function after surgery. Discharge times were also similar, and no side effects were observed.

This study provides useful information on a number of levels. Most significantly, it has shown that a single, relatively low dose of passionflower acts as an effective short-term anxiolytic without causing undue sedation. The study also demonstrates that herbal premedication can be a safe and beneficial option to manage the significant apprehension or anxiety in patients that can precede general anaesthesia and surgery. Unfortunately, such a proposition would be viewed as too radical in most hospitals.

In another similar RCT ($n = 60$), passionflower suppressed the increase in anxiety before spinal anaesthesia without changing psychomotor function test results, sedation level, or haemodynamics.[9] In a third RCT ($n = 30$), a single dose of passionflower or midazolam prior to molar extraction demonstrated comparable anxiolytic effects.[10]

10.2.2.2 Passionflower and anxiety

In a pilot RCT ($n = 36$), passionflower extract was as efficacious as oxazepam (a benzodiazepine drug) for the management of GAD and resulted in a lower incidence of impaired job performance.[11]

In another small RCT ($n = 12$), a single dose of passionflower extract (equivalent to about 7 g of dried herb) demonstrated a calming effect in healthy female volunteers, using a self-rating scale for alertness.[12]

Passionflower helped with drug withdrawal symptoms in an RCT ($n = 65$), which was a 14-day trial that compared clonidine plus passionflower extract against clonidine plus placebo in the outpatient detoxification of opiate addicts.[13] Passionflower showed additional superiority over clonidine alone in terms of the management of mental symptoms.

10.2.3 Withania and anxiety

A perhaps surprising recent development is the good clinical evidence that has emerged this century for ashwagandha (*Withania somnifera*) as a treatment for anxiety. This was well illustrated by a 2014 systematic review that located five clinical trials.[14] Three studies compared several dosage levels of Withania extract with placebos using versions of the Hamilton Anxiety Scale, with two demonstrating a significant benefit of Withania versus placebo, and the third demonstrating beneficial effects that approached, but did not quite achieve, significance ($p = 0.05$). A fourth study compared naturopathic care with Withania versus psychotherapy by using Beck Anxiety Inventory (BAI) scores as the outcome. BAI scores decreased by 56.5% in the Withania group versus 30.5% for psychotherapy ($p < 0.0001$). A fifth study measured changes in Perceived Stress Scale (PSS) scores for Withania against placebo; there was a 44.0% reduction in PSS scores in the Withania group versus a 5.5% reduction in the placebo group ($p < 0.0001$). Due to the heterogeneous design of the trials, a meta-analysis was not deemed to be appropriate. The authors did advise some caution due to potential bias and variations in study design, but they nonetheless concluded Withania was found to improve anxiety and stress in all studies undertaken to date.

10.2.4 Zizyphus seed and anxiety

Suanzaorentang is a traditional Chinese formula containing Zizyphus seeds (45.5%).[15] At a dose of 750 mg / day, Suanzaorentang demonstrated almost the same anxiolytic effect as diazepam (6 mg / day) in a short-term RCT. Suanzaorentang, but not diazepam, also improved mental performance during the daytime as well as anxiety symptoms. In patients with anxiety and heart symptoms, treatment with Suanzaorentang demonstrated an anxiolytic effect in an uncontrolled trial.[16]

10.2.5 Melissa and anxiety

There are a few clinical trials of the herb lemon balm (*Melissa officinalis*), either alone or in combination, for various aspects of anxiety. For example, in a double blind RCT, 80 patients with chronic stable angina (CSA) were divided randomly into two groups (taking 3 g Melissa or placebo daily for 8 weeks).[17] Supplementation with Melissa decreased depression, anxiety, stress, and sleep disorders in these patients with CSA.

10.2.6 Lavender essential oil and anxiety

There is high-level clinical evidence that lavender essential oil (80–160 mg / day) can reduce anxiety. A meta-analysis of five clinical studies found lavender oil to be significantly superior to placebo in ameliorating anxiety symptoms, independent of diagnosis.[18] Interestingly, there was a tendency for a greater clinical effect with GAD patients than with all other diagnoses. In addition, lavender oil was as effective as the active comparator drug (lorazepam) in the pooled analysis.

10.2.7   Chamomile for GAD

In a significant RCT, 93 GAD responders to chamomile were enrolled and given either chamomile (1,500 mg / day extract = 6 g of water-extracted herb) or a placebo.[19] The relapse rates over 6 months were 25.5% for the placebo versus 15.2% for chamomile (not quite significant). Mean times to relapse were 11.4 ± 8.4 weeks for chamomile versus 6.3 ± 3.9 weeks for placebo. Chamomile participants also maintained significantly lower GAD symptoms than did those taking a placebo ($p = 0.0032$). The limited sample size and lower than expected rate of placebo group relapse probably contributed to the non-significant primary outcome finding. The significance of this trial is two-fold: first, chamomile tea can readily be added to a patient's regime to help alleviate their anxiety, and, second, its long-term nature (6 months) in diagnosed GAD affords it a high level of evidence.

10.2.8   Saffron and comorbid anxiety

In a placebo-controlled RCT ($n = 54$, type 2 diabetes) in patients with mild to moderate comorbid depression and anxiety (CDA), anxiety, and sleep disturbance, but not depression alone, were relieved significantly in the saffron group ($p < 0.05$).[20] In another RCT ($n = 60$ with CDA), saffron treatment had a significant effect on anxiety and depression scores compared to placebo at the 12-week time-point ($p < 0.001$).[21] In a third RCT ($n = 66$ with CDA), saffron treatment had the same effect on anxiety and depression scores as citalopram at the 6-week time-point ($p = 0.984$).[22]

In yet another RCT, the administration of a standardised saffron extract for 8 weeks improved anxiety and depressive symptoms in young people aged 12–16 years with mild-to-moderate symptoms, at least from the perspective of the adolescent.[23] However, these beneficial effects were inconsistently corroborated by parents. Based on the self-reports, saffron was associated with greater improvements in overall internalising symptoms ($p = 0.049$), separation anxiety ($p = 0.003$), social phobia ($p = 0.023$), and depression ($p = 0.016$). Total internalising scores decreased by an average of 33%, compared to 17% in the placebo group ($p = 0.029$).

10.2.9 The resurgence of kava

Towards the end of the last century, the herb kava (*Piper methysticum*) was emerging as a serious player in the battle against anxiety and insomnia. Several clinical trials confirmed its efficacy and the experience of herbal clinicians was that it worked well in real life. But then concerns began to emerge about kava causing liver toxicity in a few users, not because it was toxic to the liver itself, but because it triggered a rare response in the immune system. This reaction caused the immune cells of some users to attack their livers, apparently resulting in severe damage in some cases. The phenomenon, known as drug-induced liver injury (DILI), occurs at varying frequencies for most orthodox medications.

Under political pressure over this issue, the German health authority decided in June 2002 to ban the therapeutic use of kava – even though an extensive analysis suggested that the incidence of DILI from kava use was lower than the rate from the use of conventional sedative drugs, such as the benzodiazepines.[24] One by one, international authorities in Europe, Canada, and Japan moved to stop the sale of kava products.

However, a group of scientists in Australia, led by Prof Jerome Sarris, decided to test out the efficacy and safety of a kava water (aqueous) extract. Ironically, they undertook the very first clinical trials on this ancient – and potentially safer – way of taking kava, leading to its resurgence as a safe and effective herbal treatment. Since then, the original decision by the German health authorities has been overturned in court.[25]

10.2.9.1 Kava and anxiety

In earlier trials, kava was shown to be as effective as the anxiolytic drugs buspirone and opipramol for the treatment of GAD in an 8-week randomised, double blind trial involving 129 patients.[26] The administered dose was 400 mg / day of a kava extract standardised for 30% kava lactones (120 mg / day lactones). A lower than normal dose of kava extract (150 mg vs 300 mg) was still effective for neurotic anxiety compared to placebo in a 4-week double blind, placebo-controlled trial involving 141 patients.[27]

In the most significant trial by Sarris and co-workers, a total of 75 participants with GAD and no comorbid mood disorder were enrolled in a 6-week double blind trial of an aqueous extract of kava (120 / 240 mg of kavalactones per day, depending on response) versus placebo.[28] Gamma-aminobutyric acid (GABA) and noradrenaline transporter polymorphisms were also analysed as potential pharmacogenetic markers of response. Reductions in anxiety were measured using the Hamilton Anxiety Rating Scale (HAMA) as the primary outcome. After an initial 1-week placebo run-in phase, intention-to-treat analysis was performed on 58 participants who met inclusion criteria. Results revealed a significant reduction in anxiety for the kava group compared with the placebo group, with a moderate effect size ($p = 0.046$). Among participants with moderate to severe *DSM*-diagnosed GAD, this effect was larger ($p = 0.02$).

At the end of the control phase, 26% of the kava group were classified as remitted (HAMA ≤ 7) compared to 6% of the placebo group ($p = 0.04$). Within the kava group, GABA transporter polymorphisms rs2601126 ($p = 0.021$) and rs2697153 ($p = 0.046$) were associated with the HAMA reduction. Kava was well tolerated, and aside from more headaches reported in the kava group ($p = 0.05$), no other significant differences between groups occurred for any other adverse effects, nor for liver function tests.

10.3 FHT for anxiety: goals, actions, and herbs

- Calming or anxiolytic herbs (sometimes incorrectly referred to as herbal sedatives) are the key part of any herbal treatment. The main herbs with this property are valerian, Mexican valerian (see Section 10.7.7), kava, chamomile, passionflower, Zizyphus seed, lavender oil, and hops
- Other anxiolytic herbs include: Californian poppy, Corydalis (various species), lemon balm (Melissa), and ashwagandha (Withania)

- Nervine tonic herbs also have a role (these herbs are anxiolytic, but also lift mood) in the treatment of anxiety; they include St John's wort, saffron, American skullcap, Schisandra, and Bacopa.
- Cramp bark, lemon balm, and chamomile may be useful for any visceral symptoms associated with anxiety, and hawthorn can be prescribed where there are cardiac symptoms such as palpitations.
- Anxious patients stress their bodies and deplete their adrenal reserves. This can create a vicious cycle. Hence adrenal tonics (licorice and Rehmannia) and adaptogenic herbs (especially Withania) may be required.
- Any associated sleep disturbance should be treated with a separate formula or tablet(s) at night. (For a full discussion of herbs for sleep see Section 10.7.)

10.4 The basic science of sleep

There are three basic states of awareness: wakefulness, REM (rapid eye movement) sleep, and non-rapid eye movement (NREM) sleep.[29] REM sleep is an active period of sleep marked by intense brain activity, where brain waves are fast and desynchronised, like those in the waking state.

NREM sleep consists of three stages:

- *N1* (formerly "stage 1"): a time of drowsiness or transition from being awake to falling asleep
- *N2* (formerly "stage 2"): a period of light sleep during which eye movements stop; brain waves become slower, with occasional bursts of rapid waves (called sleep spindles)
- *N3* (formerly "stages 3 and 4"): also called slow wave sleep (SWS), this is characterised by the presence of very slow brain waves, called delta waves, interspersed with smaller, faster waves

10.4.1 Brain waves

- **Beta waves** occur during daily wakefulness; they have the highest frequency and the lowest amplitude, compared to other waves.

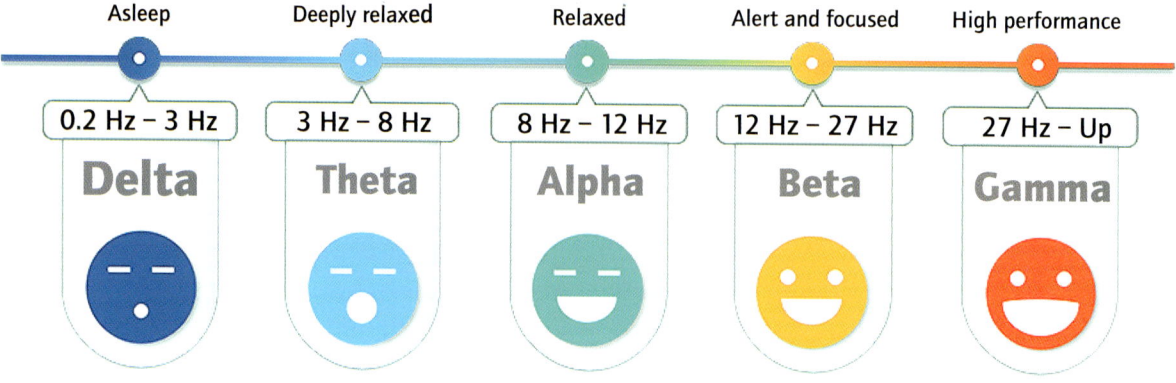

Figure 10.2 Types of brain waves.

- **Alpha waves** occur during wakefulness and periods of relaxation (including meditation); they are slower, and have less amplitude and variability than beta waves.
- **Theta waves** occur during N1 and N2 and are slower in frequency and greater in amplitude than alpha waves; as a person moves from N1 to N2 sleep, theta wave activity continues.
- **Delta waves** occur during N3 sleep; they are the slowest waves with the highest amplitude.

Figure 10.2 depicts different types of brain waves.[30]

10.4.2 Why do we sleep?

Scientists have discovered a revolutionary new treatment that makes you live longer. It enhances your memory, makes you more attractive. It keeps you slim and lowers food cravings. It protects you from cancer and dementia. It wards off colds and flu. It lowers your risk of heart attacks and stroke, not to mention diabetes. You'll even feel happier, less depressed, and less anxious. Are you interested?[31]

So writes Matthew Walker in *Why We Sleep: Unlocking the Power of Sleep and Dreams*.

Human beings are the only species that deliberately deprive themselves of sleep for no apparent gain.[32]

Matthew Walker goes on to assert:

> In terms of our natural sleeping tendencies, people can be divided into two broad groups, or "chronotypes": morning larks and night owls. Each group operates along different circadian lines, and there is pretty much nothing owls can do to become larks – which is tough luck, because work and school scheduling overwhelmingly favour early risers. Owls are often forced to burn the proverbial candle at both ends. Greater ill health caused by a lack of sleep therefore befalls owls, including higher rates of depression, anxiety, diabetes, cancer, heart attack and stroke.[33]

Dr Michael J. Breus gives a dire warning concerning sleep deprivation: "Populations are at greater risk for a number of chronic diseases and mental health disorders, as well as challenges to daily life and relationships. These are dangerous and expensive problems."[34] Hence, from the perspective of FHT, improving sleep quality should not be regarded just as an end in itself. Restoring healthy sleep forms an important core strategy for many health problems, as listed above.

During NREM sleep, we move information from short-term in the hippocampus into long-term memory. It frees up space in short-term memory for the next day and allows us to have access to past knowledge in the future.

During REM sleep we now take this new knowledge and compare it to our total catalogue of past experiences and knowledge. This allows us to make connections between things learnt in the past and this new knowledge.

Plus, another rather extraordinary thing happens: the area of our brain dedicated to rational thought goes offline. This allows us to make seemingly unrelated connections that consolidate our knowledge base and boost creative thinking.[35]

During the night, as we sleep, we move between REM and NREM sleep several times, a phenomenon that can be recorded by polysomnography. The resultant pattern is termed sleep architecture.

10.5 Improving sleep naturally might save lives!

In a widely publicised 2012 article, a group of US scientists found a strong association between the use of modern hypnotic drugs (sleeping pills) and increased risk of death. The study's principal author, Dr Daniel Kripke, had been interested in this association for more than a decade, after he and colleagues found an increased mortality hazard with prescription hypnotics in a 1998 analysis that used earlier data from the American Cancer Society (ACS) Cancer Prevention Study II. In fact, as Kripke points out in the 2012 article, Study I of the ACS also found that both hypnotic use and cigarette smoking were associated with excessive deaths, but the hypnotic findings were discounted as the study was not designed to investigate these drugs.

Since then, at least 24 published studies have examined mortality linked to hypnotic consumption, with 18 ($p < 0.05$) reporting significant positive associations.[36] The analysis of these by Kripke and co-workers was a matched cohort study to compare mortality and cancer risk of modern sleeping drugs (short-acting benzodiazepine agonists such as zolpidem, zaleplon, and eszopiclone) with controls and older hypnotics.

Their results were both surprising and alarming. Participants (mean age 54 years) were 10,529 patients who received hypnotic prescriptions and 23,676 matched controls with no hypnotic prescriptions, followed for an average of 2.5 years between January 2002 and January 2007. Data were adjusted for age, gender, smoking, body mass index, ethnicity, marital status, alcohol use, and prior cancer. Hazard ratios (HRs) for death were computed from Cox proportional hazards models controlled for risk factors and using up to 116 strata, which matched cases and controls exactly by 12 classes of comorbidity (so that any confounding effect of a pre-existing health condition was controlled for).

Patients prescribed any hypnotic had substantially elevated hazards of dying compared to those prescribed no hypnotics. For groups prescribed up to 18, 18–132, and greater than 132 doses/year, HRs (95% CI [confidence intervals]) were 3.60 (2.92–4.44), 4.43 (3.67–5.36), and 5.32 (4.50–6.30), respectively, demonstrating a dose–response association. HRs were elevated in separate analyses for several common hypnotics, including zolpidem, temazepam, eszopiclone, zaleplon, other benzodiazepines, barbiturates, and sedative antihistamines. Hypnotic use in the upper third was also associated with a significant risk of cancer; HR = 1.35 (95% CI 1.18–1.55). Results were robust within groups suffering each comorbidity, indicating that the death and cancer hazards associated with hypnotic drugs were not attributable to pre-existing disease. Particularly disturbing was the finding that hypnotic prescriptions were associated with a greater than threefold increased hazard of death, even when prescribed at fewer than 18 pills/year. This association held in separate analyses for several commonly used hypnotics and for newer shorter-acting drugs.

While it should be stressed that cohort studies such as this one do not necessarily imply causality, it is possible that the use of hypnotic drugs is responsible for millions of early deaths worldwide each year. Certainly, in Kripke's opinion, the risks of the use of such drugs now outweigh the benefits:

> The recommended doses objectively increase sleep little if at all, daytime performance is often made worse, not better, and the lack of general health benefits is commonly misrepresented in advertising. Treatments such as the cognitive behavioral treatment of insomnia and bright light treatment of circadian rhythm disorders might offer safer and more effective alternative approaches to insomnia.[37]

Clearly, it is time to seek safer alternatives to help patients improve their sleep. There are many promising candidates among medicinal plants (as outlined in Section 10.7).

Matthew Walker explains in his book why the insomnia drugs might result in premature death. First, we need to accept the premise that these drugs do not fully create a genuine state of sleep, with all the features of REM and NREM sleep. Instead, they create a state of sedation that mimics sleep. Hence a person who uses these drugs is, in fact, sleep-deprived. A feature of anyone who is sleep deprived is that they are more prone to infections and road accidents, both significant causes of death.

In contrast, there are preliminary data that herbs can actually support sleep architecture, meaning that they might represent the best and safest pharmacological option to treat insomnia and promote natural health-conferring sleep.

10.6 Insomnia and sleep hygiene

10.6.1 The four pillars of healthy sleep

According to Walker, these four pillars are:

1 **regularity:** same time to bed and rising
2 **continuity:** as few awakenings as possible

3 **quantity:** average 8 hours, and also adequate time for each stage of sleep (good sleep architecture)

4 **quality:** healthy electrical signature of sleep (good sleep architecture)

10.6.2 Classification of insomnia

The following basic differentiations are used to classify insomnia:

- difficulty falling asleep: sleep onset insomnia
- awakening during the night and difficulty falling asleep: sleep maintenance insomnia – often characteristic of adrenally depleted patients and those with fibromyalgia syndrome
- early morning awakening (sleep offset or terminal insomnia): can be linked to depression or poor sleep quality – often classified as one aspect of sleep maintenance insomnia
- a sense of not having enough sleep (non-restorative sleep): often characteristic of chronic fatigue syndrome

These different patterns of insomnia are treated in different ways when applying FHT.

10.6.3 Key aspects of sleep hygiene

The following tips will assist in promoting good sleep hygiene:

- The use of stimulants should be reduced, especially coffee, tea, guarana, and cola drinks.
- Just two glasses of wine with dinner is enough to reduce sleep quality by nearly 40%, and the effects are worse for young people.
- Unwinding at night can be important: a few drops of lavender oil added to an evening bath can help this process, or some other unwinding ritual.
- Other issues that might impact on sleep quality – such as pain, anxiety, or gastro-oesophageal reflux – need to be addressed.

- Avoid looking at screens – blue light, which turns off melatonin – especially in a poorly lit room, in the two hours before retiring and generally after 9 pm.
- Major causes of sleep-onset insomnia include anxiety, pain or discomfort, caffeine, and alcohol.
- Sleep maintenance insomnia can be linked to depression, sleep apnoea, hypoglycaemia, pain or discomfort, and alcohol.
- It is important to sleep in a darkened, cool, noise-free environment.
- Bed comfort is also relevant, and bed clothes should not be too warm.
- Be exposed to bright outdoor light for 30 minutes in the day.
- In healthy young women, sleep quality varies throughout the menstrual cycle (and is worse pre-menstrually).
- Exercise regularly and go to bed at a consistent time.

10.7 Key herbs for sleep: the evidence and clinical application

10.7.1 European valerian and sleep

In the 1980s Leathwood and Chauffard demonstrated that European valerian extract improved sleep latency and quality (versus placebo), but only for poor or irregular sleepers.[38] Results from subsequent trials have been mixed, but overall they do indicate a clear effect on subjective sleep quality.[39] Numerous earlier controlled clinical trials of valerian on its own or in combination with hops, passionflower, and/or lemon balm have demonstrated improvements in sleep parameters.

The Committee on Herbal Medicine Products of the European Medicines Agency concluded that

> aqueous ethanolic extracts of valerian root have a clinical effect in sleep disturbances as assessed by subjective ratings as well as by means of validated psychometric scales and EEG-recordings. . . . There is quite strong evidence from both clinical experience and sleep-EEG studies that the treatment effect increases during treatment over several weeks.[40]

10.7.2 Chaste tree and melatonin

Apparently according to Dioscorides (*De Materia Medica*, AD 40–80), when writing about chaste tree:

> A weight of 1 drachma in wine makes the menses come on earlier, detaches the embryo, attracts the milk, goes to your head and **brings sleep**.[41]

The circadian rhythm of melatonin secretion was measured in 20 healthy men aged 20–32 years following the intake for 14 days of a placebo or of various doses of an extract of chaste tree.[42] In an open, placebo-controlled study, the doses investigated were 120–480 mg / day of the extract (corresponding to approximately 0.6–2.4 g of the dried berries per day). These were taken as divided doses at 8.00, 14.00, and 20.00 hours. The concentration of melatonin in serum showed the typical nocturnal increase, beginning approximately one hour after the light had been turned off. Administration of chaste tree caused a dose-dependent increase of melatonin secretion when compared to the placebo treatment, especially during the night. Total melatonin output was approximately 60% higher in the group receiving chaste tree.

The authors observed that the feeling of fatigue or the promotion of sleepiness observed by some patients taking chaste tree during the trial might be a result of the stimulation of endogenous melatonin secretion. Indications for chaste tree should now include jet lag, sleep maintenance insomnia, and disturbed day–night rhythm (as with shift workers).

Based on that research, this has become one of my most important clinical uses of chaste tree for both men and women, and it is highly effective, provided an adequate dose is used. For jet lag, higher doses are needed: up to 5 g of DHE per day. It is also valuable in some cases of sleep onset insomnia.

10.7.3 Zizyphus seed and insomnia

The key Chinese herb for insomnia is Zizyphus seed (Suan Zao Ren) or the spiny jujube. A recent systematic review of RCTs of Chinese herbal medicine for insomnia found Zizyphus seed was the most used (in 190 of the 217 identified clinical trials).[43] Another systematic review of Zizyphus decoction on its own for primary insomnia found 12 clinical trials. The overall finding was that Zizyphus was more effective than benzodiazepines, but trial quality was noted to be poor.[44]

10.7.4 St John's wort and sleep

St John's wort (SJW) might also boost melatonin. In an uncontrolled trial involving 13 healthy volunteers, a significant increase in the nocturnal melatonin plasma concentration was observed after 3 weeks of administration of SJW.[45] Sleep disorders, as well as anxiety and depressive agitation, were reduced by SJW extract in 240 patients suffering from mild-to-moderate depression with anxiety in a 6-week RCT.[46]

10.7.5 Kava and sleep

Kava is not only the best herbal answer for anxiety, it also plays a very useful role in promoting healthy sleep, with very little "hangover" effect the next day from its use – although this can occur to a mild extent in some people. There is also clinical evidence to back this up.

In a pilot RCT involving 12 healthy volunteers over 4 days, a placebo was taken for the first 3 days, followed the next day by 3 divided doses totalling either 150 mg kava extract (containing 105 mg kavalactones) or 300 mg extract (containing 210 mg kavalactones).[47] With kava, the time to fall asleep and the light sleep phase were shortened, the deep sleep phase was lengthened, the duration of REM sleep was not influenced, and the length of wakeful phases in sleep EEG recordings was decreased.

A later double blind, multicentre RCT assessed a kava extract in sleep disturbances associated with anxiety disorders in 61 patients.[48] The dose of kava extract used was 200 mg / day (containing 140 mg kava lactones) over a period of 4 weeks. Statistically significant group differences were demonstrated in favour of the kava group, as measured by the sleep questionnaire SF-B subscores "Quality of sleep" and "Recuperative effect after sleep" ($p = 0.007$ and $p = 0.018$, respectively). Superior therapeutic efficacy was also demonstrated for kava extract over placebo by way of the Bf-S (Befindlichkeits-Skala) self-rating scale of well-being, the clinical global impression (CGI), and the Hamilton psychic anxiety sub-score ($p = 0.002$).

Insomnia was significantly relieved by the combination of kava and valerian ($p < 0.05$) and the individual treatments ($p < 0.01$).[49] On direct questioning, 16 patients (67%) reported no side effects while on kava, versus 10 (53%) for valerian and 10 (53%) for the combination.[50] The "commonest" such effects were vivid dreams with kava plus valerian (4 cases / 21%) and with valerian alone (3 cases / 16%).

10.7.6 Passionflower and sleep

In the first RCT (crossover design), 41 people found that a week of passionflower tea (2 g in one cup one hour before bed) was better than placebo (parsley tea) in terms of subjective sleep quality.[51] There was a significant improvement in sleep quality when taking the passionflower (5.2% mean increase relative to placebo; $p < 0.01$). No significant effects were found for the other parameters, although the participants had initially low levels of anxiety and only a small number had polysomnography recorded.

In a later RCT, in 110 patients diagnosed with insomnia according to the *DSM-5*, two weeks of passionflower treatment significantly improved total sleep time, compared to placebo.[52]

10.7.7 Mexican valerian and sleep

This herb is a highly underestimated option for treating insomnia and anxiety. Often the most positive feedback from patients suffering from these disorders is after they have taken Mexican valerian.

Valeriana edulis ssp. *procera*, commonly known as Mexican valerian, is widely used in Mexican traditional medicine for insomnia and anxiety. A crossover RCT ($n = 20$) compared Mexican with European valerian at equal doses (450 mg of dry extract) administered one hour before lights out in a sleep laboratory.[53] Mexican valerian reduced the number of awaking episodes, while both herbal treatments increased REM sleep; this last parameter showed greater improvement with European valerian. Both herbs diminished the time of N1 and N2 in NREM sleep, and they increased delta sleep (N3). Validated clinical tests showed that both species reduced morning sleepiness and did not affect anterograde memory (loss of short-term memory).

Chemical analysis of the hydroalcoholic extract of Mexican valerian indicated that the extract contained 0.26% of dihydroisovaltrate as the main valepotriate, and that it did not contain valerenic acid, which is a key active in European valerian. Hence, the two herbs are both phytochemically and therapeutically distinct, with Mexican valerian containing much higher levels of valepotriates.

10.8 FHT for insomnia: goals, actions, and herbs

Anxiolytic and hypnotic herbs are the mainstay of support. These can be taken throughout the day to prevent a build-up of tension or mental excitability that might result in insomnia (especially sleep onset insomnia). An additional dose is then recommended around one hour before bed. (See **Tables 10.1**, **10.2**, and **10.3**.)

Key aspects of FHT treatment are:

- For insomnia that is not severe, the herbs can be taken as a single dose before bed. Key herbs include valerian, Mexican valerian, Zizyphus, hops, passionflower, magnolia, lavender, kava, Californian poppy, and chamomile.
- Best results with valerian come from continuous use for at least 2 weeks (unless in a synergistic formulation with other herbs).

Table 10.1 Herbs and insomnia classification summary

Sleep problem	Herb
Sleep onset problems	▷ valerian, kava, Mexican valerian, passionflower, Zizyphus, Corydalis, chaste tree, Californian poppy, chamomile, magnolia, lavender, hops
Sleep maintenance problems	▷ St John's wort, chaste tree, valerian, kava, licorice and/or Rehmannia, magnolia
Restorative sleep problems	▷ Withania, Rhodiola, Korean ginseng, licorice, Rehmannia

Table 10.2 Example liquid herbal blends for anxiety

Anxiety			Anxiety with adrenal support		
Herb	Ratio	Amount	Herb	Ratio	Amount
▹ St John's wort	1:2	25 mL	▹ chamomile	1:2	30 mL
▹ passionflower	1:2	25 mL	▹ passionflower	1:2	20 mL
▹ skullcap	1:2	15 mL	▹ licorice	1:1	15 mL
▹ valerian	1:2	20 mL	▹ valerian	1:2	20 mL
▹ cramp bark	1:2	25 mL	▹ Rehmannia	1:2	20 mL
	Total	110 mL		Total	105 mL

Dose: 5 mL with water 3 times a day or 8 mL twice a day. Also consider additional kava tablets.

Dose: 5 mL with water 3 times a day or 8 mL twice a day. With additional chamomile tea.

▹ Antidepressant and nervine tonic herbs are indicated, especially if the insomnia is associated with fibromyalgia or is sleep maintenance insomnia. These include St John's wort, skullcap and saffron.
▹ If the patient is adrenally depleted and suffers from sleep maintenance insomnia, then adrenal tonics such as licorice or Rehmannia are indi-

Table 10.3 Example liquid herbal blends for insomnia

Sleep formula with kava liquid			Sleep onset insomnia			Sleep maintenance insomnia		
Herb	Ratio	Amount	Herb	Ratio	Amount	Herb	Ratio	Amount
▹ kava	1:1	45 mL	▹ valerian	1:2	30 mL	▹ valerian	1:2	25 mL
▹ passionflower	1:2	20 mL	▹ passionflower	1:2	30 mL	▹ St John's wort	1:2	25 mL
▹ Zizyphus	1:2	20 mL	▹ Zizyphus	1:2	30 mL	▹ chaste tree	1:2	30 mL
▹ Corydalis	1:2	20 mL	▹ Withania	2:1	15 mL	▹ skullcap	1:2	25 mL
	Total	105 mL		Total	105 mL		Total	105 mL

Dose: 10 mL with water one hour before bed.

Dose: 5 mL with water 3 times daily or 8 mL twice daily. Take the last dose one hour before bed. Also consider kava tablets before bed.

Dose: 5 mL with water 3 times daily or 8 mL twice daily. Take the last dose one hour before bed. Also consider kava tablets before bed and on awakening.

cated. These herbs will also help maintain blood sugar levels during the night.
- Tonic and adaptogenic herbs used throughout the day or before bed can help to break the vicious cycle of non-restorative sleep in stressed patients. Ashwagandha (Withania) can be a key herb for this.
- If pain interferes with sleep then analgesic herbs for pain management are indicated. For example, willow bark is useful for pain associated with inflammation, whereas Corydalis, cramp bark, kava and wild yam will help to alleviate pain associated with smooth muscle cramping.
- Research on chaste tree and melatonin represents a key development in the treatment of both onset and maintenance insomnia, but especially the latter.

10.8.1 Case history: protracted insomnia

A female patient aged 56 years, who worked as a medical receptionist, presented with a 5-year history of sleep maintenance insomnia. It began with her menopause and learning that her husband had cancer. Conventional treatments were of no benefit. Pattern was variable, she woke up between 1:00 and 4:30 am most nights and could not return to sleep, so was averaging about 5 hours' sleep a night.

Didn't like the liquid formula given, so eventually settled on tablets:

- chaste tree (3 g/day as tablets) and the combination: lemon balm, Zizyphus seed, magnolia, lavender oil; 3 of each throughout the day, delivering doses of 2 g (DHE), 2 g (DHE), 30 mg and 1.8 g (DHE), respectively
- kava (3.2 g DHE) and Mexican valerian (1 g DHE) tablets: 2–3 of each before bed, and then the same again if she wakes up

After 4 months: "going well". Sleeps through "99%" of the time, with no need for the extra kava or Mexican valerian tablets.

Benefit maintained for 5 years as long as the patient used herbs, albeit not every night and usually at lower doses than above.

References

1. American Psychiatric Association. (2013). *Diagnostic and Statistical Manual of Mental Disorders* (5th ed). Arlington, VA: American Psychiatric Publishing.
2. https://adaa.org/sites/default/files/GAD-7_Anxiety-updated_0.pdf
3. Slee A, Nazareth I, Bondaronek P, et al. Pharmacological treatments for generalised anxiety disorder: a systematic review and network meta-analysis. *Lancet*. 2019; **393**(10173): 768–777. doi:10.1016/S0140-6736(18)31793-8. PMID: 30712879.
4. Pakseresht S, Boostani H, Sayyah M. Extract of valerian root (*Valeriana officinalis* L.) vs. placebo in treatment of obsessive-compulsive disorder: a randomized double-blind study. *J Complement Integr Med*. 2011; **8**(1): Article 32. doi:10.2202/1553-3840.1465. PMID: 22718671.
5. Bone KM, Mills SY. *Principles and Practice of Phytotherapy: Modern Herbal Medicine*, 2nd ed. Elsevier, UK, 2013.
6. Pinheiro ML, Alcântara CE, de Moraes M, de Andrade ED. *Valeriana officinalis* L. for conscious sedation of patients submitted to impacted lower third molar surgery: a randomized, double-blind, placebo-controlled split-mouth study. *J Pharm Bioallied Sci*. 2014; **6**(2): 109–114. doi:10.4103/0975-7406.129176. PMID 24741279.
7. Roh D, Jung JH, Yoon KH, et al. Valerian extract alters functional brain connectivity: a randomized double-blind placebo-controlled trial. *Phytotherapy Research*. 2019 Apr; **33**(4): 939–948. doi:10.1002/ptr.6286. PMID: 30632220.
8. Movafegh A, Alizadeh R, Hajimohamadi F, et al. Preoperative oral *Passiflora incarnata* reduces anxiety in ambulatory surgery patients: a double-blind, placebo-controlled study. *Anesth Analg*. 2008; **106**(6): 1728–1732. doi:10.1213/ane.0b013e318172c3f9. PMID: 18499602.
9. Aslanargun P, Cuvas O, Dikmen B, et al. *Passiflora incarnata* Linneaus as an anxiolytic before spinal anesthesia. *J Anesth*. 2012; **26**(1): 3944. doi:10.1007/s00540-011-12656. PMID: 22048283.
10. Dantas LP, de Oliveira-Ribeiro A, de Almeida-Souza LM, et al. Effects of *Passiflora incarnata* and midazolam for control of anxiety in patients undergoing dental extraction. *Med Oral Patol Oral Cir Bucal*. 2017; **22**(1): e95–e101. PMID: 27918731.
11. Akhondzadeh S, Naghavi HR, Vazirian M, et al. Passionflower in the treatment of generalized anxiety: a pilot double-blind randomized controlled trial with oxazepam. *J Clin Pharm Ther*. 2001; **26**(5): 363–367. PMID: 11679026.
12. Schulz H, Jobert M, Hübner WD. The quantitative EEG as a screening instrument to identify sedative effects of single doses of plant extracts in comparison with diazepam. *Phytomedicine*. 1998; **5**(6): 449–458. doi:10.1016/S0944-7113(98)80041-X. PMID: 23196028.
13. Akhondzadeh S, Kashani L, Mobaseri M, et al. Passionflower in the treatment of opiates withdrawal: a double-blind randomized controlled trial. *J Clin Pharm Ther*. 2001; **26**(5): 369–373. PMID: 11679027.
14. Pratte MA, Nanavati KB, Young V, et al. An alternative treatment for anxiety: a systematic review of human trial results reported for the Ayurvedic herb ashwagandha (*Withania somnifera*). *J Altern Complement Med*. 2014; **20**(12): 901–908. doi:10.1089/acm.2014.0177. PMID: 25405876.
15. Chen HC, Hsieh MT, Shibuya TK. Suanzaorentang versus diazepam: a controlled double-blind study in anxiety. *Int J Clin Pharmacol Ther Toxicol*. 1986 Dec; **24**(12): 646–650. PMID: 2880811.

16. Hsieh MT, Chen HC. Suanzaorentang in cardiac patients with anxiety. *Eur J Clin Pharmacol.* 1986; **30**(4): 481–484. PMID: 2874989.
17. Haybar H, Javid AZ, Haghighizadeh MH, et al. The effects of *Melissa officinalis* supplementation on depression, anxiety, stress, and sleep disorder in patients with chronic stable angina. *Clin Nutr ESPEN.* 2018; **26**: 47–52. doi:10.1016/j.clnesp.2018.04.015.
18. Generoso MB, Soares A, Taiar IT, Cordeiro Q, Shiozawa P. Lavender oil preparation (Silexan) for treating anxiety: an updated meta-analysis. *J Clin Psychopharmacol.* 2017; **37**(1): 115–117. doi:10.1097/JCP.0000000000000615.
19. Mao JJ, Xie SX, Keefe JR, et al. Long-term chamomile (*Matricaria chamomilla* L.) treatment for generalized anxiety disorder: a randomized clinical trial. *Phytomedicine.* 2016; **23**(14): 1735–1742. doi:10.1016/j.phymed.2016.10.012. PMID: 27912875.
20. Milajerdi A, Jazayeri S, Shirzadi E, et al. The effects of alcoholic extract of saffron (*Crocus sativus* L.) on mild to moderate comorbid depression-anxiety, sleep quality, and life satisfaction in type 2 diabetes mellitus: a double-blind, randomized and placebo-controlled clinical trial. *Complement Ther Med.* 2018; **41**: 196–202. doi:10.1016/j.ctim.2018.09.023. PMID: 30477839.
21. Mazidi M, Shemshian M, Mousavi SH, et al. A double-blind, randomized and placebo controlled trial of saffron (*Crocus sativus* L.) in the treatment of anxiety and depression. *J Complement Integr Med.* 2016; **13**(2): 195–199. doi:10.1515/jcim-2015-0043. PMID: 27101556.
22. Ghajar A, Neishabouri SM, Velayati N, et al. *Crocus sativus* L. versus citalopram in the treatment of major depressive disorder with anxious distress: a double-blind, controlled clinical trial. *Pharmacopsychiatry.* 2017; **50**(4): 152–160. doi:10.1055/s-0042-116159. PMID: 27701683.
23. Lopresti AL, Drummond PD, Inarejos-García AM, Prodanov M. affron®, a standardised extract from saffron (*Crocus sativus* L.) for the treatment of youth anxiety and depressive symptoms: a randomised, double-blind, placebo-controlled study. *J Affect Disord.* 2018; **232**: 349–357. doi:10.1016/j.jad.2018.02.070.
24. Mills S, Bone K (Eds). *The Essential Guide to Herbal Safety.* Elsevier, St Louis, MI, 2005, pp 155–219.
25. Kuchta K, Schmidt M, Nahrstedt A. German kava ban lifted by court: the alleged hepatotoxicity of kava (*Piper methysticum*) as a case of ill-defined herbal drug identity, lacking quality control, and misguided regulatory politics. *Planta Med.* 2015; **81**(18): 1647–1653. doi:10.1055/s-0035-1558295. PMID: 26695707.
26. Boerner RJ, Sommer H, Berger W, et al. Kava-Kava extract LI 150 is as effective as Opipramol and Buspirone in generalised anxiety disorder: an 8-week randomized, double blind multi-centre clinical trial in 129 out-patients. *Phytomedicine.* 2003; **10**(Suppl 4): 38–49. PMID: 12807341.
27. Gastpar M, Klimm HD. Treatment of anxiety, tension and restlessness states with Kava special extract WS 1490 in general practice: a randomized placebo-controlled double-blind multicenter trial. *Phytomedicine.* 2003; **10**(8): 631–639. PMID: 14692723.
28. Sarris J, Stough C, Bousman CA, et al. Kava in the treatment of generalized anxiety disorder: a double-blind, randomized, placebo-controlled study. *J Clin Psychopharmacol.* 2013; **33**(5): 643–648. doi:10.1097/JCP.0b013e318291be67.
29. http://sleepdisorders.sleepfoundation.org/chapter-1-normal-sleep/stages-of-human-sleep
30. https://lucid.me/blog/5-brainwaves-delta-theta-alpha-beta-gamma
31. Walker, M. *Why We Sleep: Unlocking the Power of Sleep and Dreams.* Scribner, New York, 2017. [p 107]
32. *Ibid.* [p 4]

33. *Ibid.* [p 334]
34. https://www.dreams.co.uk/sleep-matters-club/data-shows-a-shocking-worldwide-lack-of-sleep
35. Walker, M. *Why We Sleep: Unlocking the Power of Sleep and Dreams.* Scribner, New York, 2017.
36. Kripke DF, Langer RD, Kline LE. Hypnotics' association with mortality or cancer: a matched cohort study. *BMJ Open.* 2012 Feb 27; **2**(1): e000850. doi:10.1136/bmjopen-2012-000850. PMID: 22371848.
37. Kripke DF. Hypnotic drug risks of mortality, infection, depression, and cancer: but lack of benefit. Version 3. *F1000Res.* 2016 May 19 [revised 2018 Jan 1]; **5**: 918. doi:10.12688/f1000research.8729.3. PMID: 27303633.
38. Leathwood PD, Chauffard F, Heck E, et al. Aqueous extract of valerian root (*Valeriana officinalis* L.) improves sleep quality in man. *Pharmacol Biochem Behav.* 1982; **17**(1): 65–71. PMID: 7122669.
39. Bone KM, Mills SY. *Principles and Practice of Phytotherapy: Modern Herbal Medicine*, 2nd ed. Elsevier, UK 2013, pp 923–934.
40. European Medicines Agency. *Assessment Report on* Valeriana Officinalis *L., Radix.* London, 29 November 2007.
41. Upton R, Petrone C, Graff A (Eds). *American Herbal Pharmacopoeia*, Santa Cruz, CA, American Herbal Pharmacopoeia, 2001.
42. Dericks-Tan JS, Schwinn P, Hildt C. Dose-dependent stimulation of melatonin secretion after administration of Agnus castus. *Exp Clin Endocrinol Diabetes.* 2003; **111**(1): 44–46. PMID: 12605350.
43. Yeung WF, Chung KF, Poon MM, et al. Chinese herbal medicine for insomnia: a systematic review of randomized controlled trials. *Sleep Med Rev.* 2012; **16**(6): 497–507. doi:10.1016/j.smrv.2011.12.005. PMID: 22440393.
44. Xie CL, Gu Y, Wang WW, et al. Efficacy and safety of Suanzaoren decoction for primary insomnia: a systematic review of randomized controlled trials. *BMC Complement Altern Med.* 2013; **13**: 18. doi:10.1186/1472-6882-13-18. PMID: 23336848.
45. Demisch L, et al. *AGNP-Symposium, 1991.* Cited in Scientific Committee of ESCOP. *ESCOP Monographs: Hyperici herba.* European Scientific Cooperative on Phytotherapy, Exeter, 1996.
46. Friede M, Henneicke von Zepelin HH, Freudenstein J. Differential therapy of mild to moderate depressive episodes (ICD–10 F 32.0; F 32.1) with St. John's wort. *Pharmacopsychiatry.* 2001; **34**(Suppl 1): S38–S41. PMID: 11518073.
47. Emser W, Bartylla K. Improvement of sleep quality. Effect of kava extract WS 1490 on the sleep pattern in healthy subjects. *TW Neurologie/Psychiatrie* 1991; **5**(11): 636–642.
48. Lehrl S. Clinical efficacy of kava extract WS 1490 in sleep disturbances associated with anxiety disorders. Results of a multicenter, randomized, placebo-controlled, double-blind clinical trial. *J Affect Disord.* 2004; **78**(2): 101–110. PMID: 14706720.
49. Wheatley D. Stress-induced insomnia treated with kava and valerian: singly and in combination. *Hum Psychopharmacol.* 2001; **16**(4): 353–356. PMID: 12404572.
50. Wheatley D. Kava and valerian in the treatment of stress-induced insomnia. *Phytother Res.* 2001; **15**(6): 549–551. PMID: 11536390.
51. Ngan A, Conduit R. A double-blind, placebo-controlled investigation of the effects of *Passiflora incarnata* (passionflower) herbal tea on subjective sleep quality. *Phytother Res.* 2011 Aug; **25**(8): 1153–1159. doi:10.1002/ptr.3400. PMID: 21294203.
52. Lee J, Jung HY, Lee SI, Choi JH, Kim SG. Effects of *Passiflora incarnata* Linnaeus on polysomnographic sleep parameters in subjects with insomnia disorder: a double-blind randomized placebo-controlled study. *Int Clin Psychopharmacol.* 2020; **35**(1): 29–35. doi:10.1097/YIC.0000000000000291.
53. Herrera-Arellano A, Luna-Villegas G, Cuevas-Uriostegui ML, et al. Polysomnographic evaluation of the hypnotic effect of *Valeriana edulis* standardized extract in patients suffering from insomnia. *Planta Med.* 2001; **67**(8): 695–699. PMID: 11731907.

APPLYING FUNCTIONAL HERBAL THERAPY

11

FHT for metabolic syndrome

This chapter provides a detailed examination of the role of FHT in correcting metabolic syndrome (MetS). It begins with a detailed definition of metabolic syndrome and its comorbidities. Next, the potential causes of insulin resistance (IR) are investigated, followed by an exploration of the key cellular and systemic targets for MetS. Finally, MetS management through lifestyle, diet, and FHT strategies is outlined.

Metabolism is the set of life-sustaining chemical reactions in organisms. The three main purposes of the metabolism are: the conversion of food to energy to run cellular processes; the conversion of food/fuel to building blocks for proteins, lipids, nucleic acids, and some carbohydrates; and the elimination of waste.[1]

One of the 12 core strategies of FHT (discussed in Chapter 2) is: "Address/correct metabolic imbalance". Hence, the information provided in this chapter also informs the implementation of this objective, even in people who do not meet the strict definition of MetS. One example is benign prostatic hyperplasia (BPH), which has been linked to metabolic imbalance and IR. Consequently, the management of a patient with BPH will involve the examination of whether metabolic correction, harnessing the protocols outlined in this chapter, is required.

Metabolic syndrome is the lifestyle challenge of our modern age. It truly represents a failure of the modern lifestyle. There is no other disorder that so comprehensively reflects the weaknesses in our present-day way of living: our eating habits, the quality and amount of our exercise, the degree of stress that we are under, all our many current immune challenges, and, indeed, the polluted environment in which we live. These factors all coalesce to manifest the potentially lethal problem we call metabolic syndrome. Even children are now suffering from this condition.

Scott Gottlieb, former Director General of the US FDA (Food and Drug Administration), said in 2018:

> Improving the nutrition and diet of Americans would be another transformative effort toward reducing the burden of many chronic diseases, ranging from diabetes to cancer to heart disease. The public health gains of such efforts would almost certainly dwarf any single medical innovation or intervention we could discover.[2]

Metabolic syndrome can definitely be included as part of the disease spectrum mentioned by Gottlieb. Hence, we can cheekily assert that, since in the United States supplements (including herbs) come under the category of dietary/nutritional intervention, we have the endorsement of the FDA in our objective to better understand and implement herbs for the management of MetS.

11.1 What is metabolic syndrome?

MetS has been given many names over the years as the understanding of the disorder slowly evolved. Some of these alternative terms for MetS are:

- syndrome X
- dysmetabolic syndrome X
- insulin resistance (IR) syndrome
- cardiometabolic syndrome
- cardiorenal syndrome
- prediabetes (rather vaguely applied)

Multiple labels have been used in the past, but the term mainly used today is metabolic syndrome, together with "cardiometabolic syndrome", which is sometimes referred to as a subcategory of MetS.

MetS is commonly characterised by four key clinical features:

1. obesity, especially abdominal obesity, as an indicator of visceral organ fat
2. impaired glucose metabolism; IR

3   hypertension

4   an atherogenic dyslipidaemia (but not necessarily an elevated LDL cholesterol)

The exact meaning of MetS has been the subject of much debate, with several groups arriving at slightly different definitions. In 2009, five key groups finally arrived at a harmonised definition, which is three or more of the following:[3]

1   **abdominal obesity:** waist ≥102 cm M (male); ≥88 cm F (female) for the United States/Canada, but varying with ethnicity

2   **dyslipidaemia:** high-density lipoprotein cholesterol (HDL-C) (<40 mg/dL M; <50 mg/dL F; <1.0 mmol/L M; <1.3 mmol/L F); triglycerides (≥150 mg/dL; ≥1.7 mmol/L) or treated

3   **hyperglycaemia:** fasting plasma glucose ≥100 mg/dL (≥5.6 mmol/L) or treated

4   **hypertension:** systolic blood pressure (BP) ≥130 mm Hg; diastolic BP ≥85 mm Hg or treated

Figure 11.1 illustrates the core characteristics of MetS and suggests the pathways of metabolic imbalance.[4] Components used to define MetS are indicated in blue. The underlying metabolic derangements are indicated in green. The authors of this review suggest that interventions can be targeted at one or multiple individual components (indicated by 1) or – better – at the potential underlying causes (indicated by 2). The approach of conventional medicine is to focus on the former, whereas the FHT approach is to address both factors 1 and 2. Microvascular dysfunction is noted as an early functional pathway connecting adipose tissue dysfunction to IR and the resulting metabolic derangements. Note that a low-grade inflammation is also considered to be a characteristic feature.

11.1.1 Comorbidities of metabolic syndrome

The following comorbidities are associated with MetS, highlighting the importance of the prevention and treatment of this syndrome:

1   twice the risk of large artery/cardiovascular disease (CVD)
2   five times the risk of type 2 diabetes (T2D)[5]

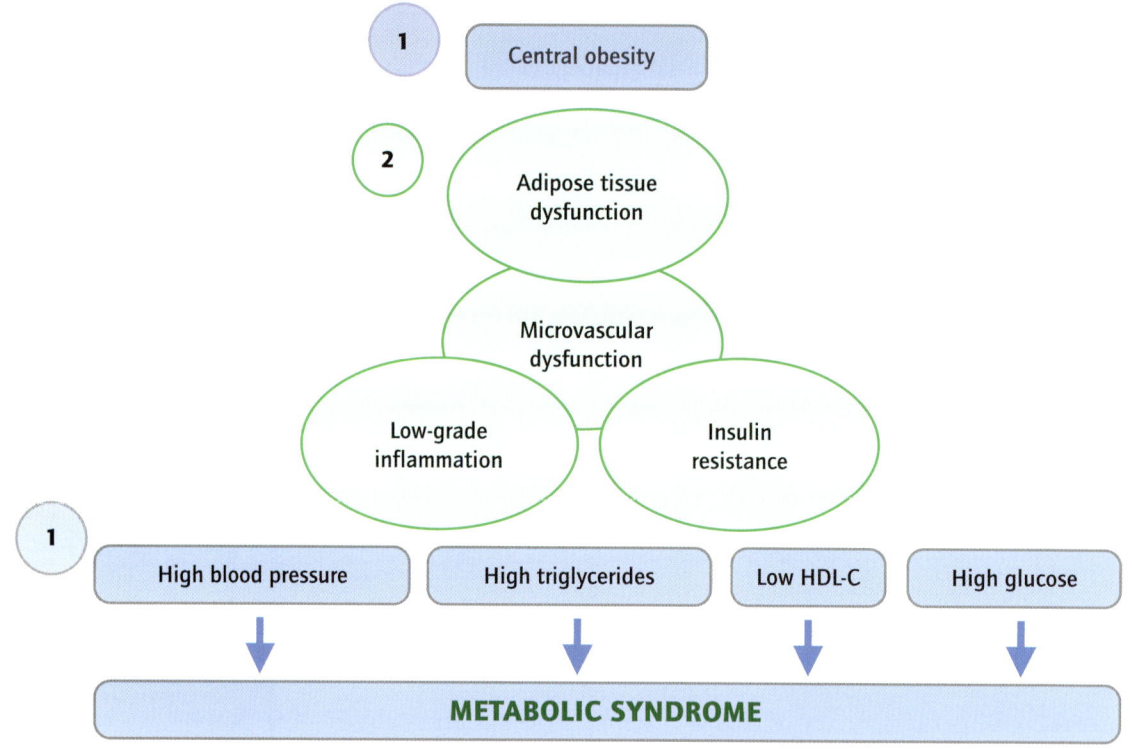

Figure 11.1 Characteristics of metabolic syndrome. [HDL-C = high-density lipoprotein cholesterol.]

3. non-alcoholic fatty liver disease (NAFLD)[6] – experts recently reached the consensus that the term NAFLD does not reflect current knowledge; "metabolic (dysfunction) associated fatty liver disease" (MAFLD) was suggested instead as a more appropriate overarching term[7]
4. gout[8]
5. polycystic ovary syndrome (PCOS)[9]
6. microalbuminuria and chronic kidney disease[10]
7. cancer[11]
8. dementia[12]
9. ageing male disorders, including BPH[13]

These comorbidities highlight the contribution of metabolic imbalance/dysfunction to the progression of a range of chronic diseases and provide a clear justification for including "correcting metabolic imbalance" as one of the 12 core strategies of FHT.

11.2 Causes of insulin resistance

Some of the key theories of contributing factors to IR include the following:

- intermittent hypoxia – obstructive sleep apnoea[14]
- the portal theory – visceral fat acting as an endocrine gland (see Section 11.2.1)[15]
- microcirculatory dysfunction (see Chapter 5)
- unregulated nutrient flux, especially fructose (see Section 11.2.2)
- toxins: dietary, environmental – endocrine disruptors – and internal (see Section 11.2.3)
- dysbiosis or lack of "old friends" (see Section 12.1.4)

Figure 11.2 illustrates several potential risk factors for IR and its physiological consequences.[16]

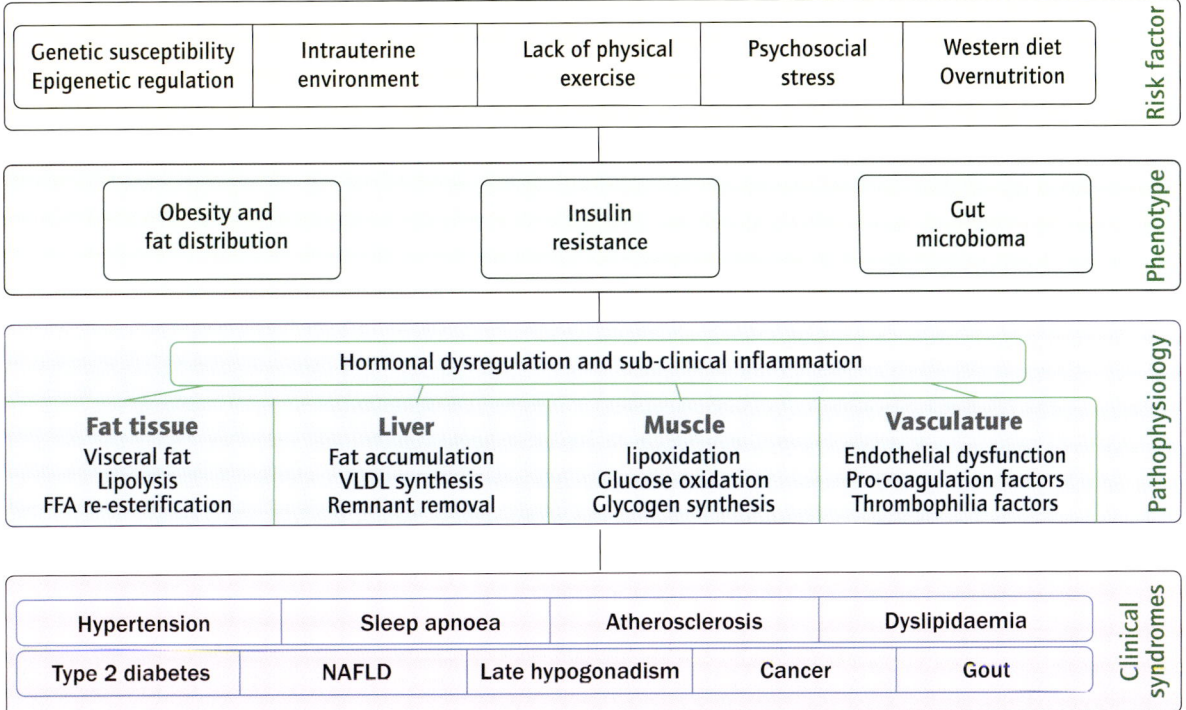

Figure 11.2 Possible risk factors for insulin resistance and its consequences. [FFA = free fatty acids; NAFLD = non-alcoholic fatty liver disease; VLDL = very low-density lipoprotein.]

11.2.1 The portal theory: visceral fat acting as an endocrine gland

Adipokines are adipose tissue hormones.[17] They include leptin and adiponectin, which promote insulin sensitivity. The adiponectin level in any individual is stable throughout the day, so it is often used as an indicator of adipose tissue endocrine function. The healthier a person is, the higher their adiponectin. Tumour necrosis factor α (TNF-α), resistin, and interleukin-6 (IL-6) are examples of adipokines that promote IR. In central obesity, leptin levels rise and adiponectin levels fall, but leptin resistance also develops. Hence, the appetite-suppressing effect of leptin fails.

The portal theory basically proposes that the liver is directly exposed to increased amounts of free fatty acids and pro-inflammatory adipokines released from visceral fat into the portal vein.[18] This then promotes the development of hepatic IR and liver steatosis, which explains how visceral obesity feeds the pathogenesis of IR.

11.2.2 Unregulated nutrient flux

The liver is the primary metabolic clearinghouse for four specific nutrients that are not insulin-regulated and lack an appropriate turn off mechanism for excessive substrate.[19] This results in enhanced lipogenesis and ectopic adipose storage in the liver.

The four nutrients are:

- trans-unsaturated fatty acids (trans-fats)
- branched-chain amino acids (BCAAs: valine, leucine, and isoleucine)
- ethanol
- fructose

In other words, these are nutrients that the body is not actually well adapted to deal with. We rely on the liver as a metabolic clearing house after nutrients are absorbed into the portal vein. Being neither essential nor regulated, the liver is obliged to process them, no matter how much is consumed. If they are consumed in excess, the high level of underutilised nutrient metabolites that result drives the creation and storage of fat in the liver, where it is not really needed. This then lowers hepatic insulin sensitivity. The problem is exacerbated by consuming these four substrates in nutrient-dense and/or liquid form, which rapidly floods the liver, overloading its limited capacity to metabolise them in a healthy way.

In a study involving three experimental groups: (1) participants with normal fasting glucose ($n = 30$), (2) participants with impaired fasting glucose ($n = 25$), and (3) participants with type 2 diabetes ($n = 15$), plasma BCAA levels were correlated with IR and inversely with adiponectin. The association remained after adjusting for age, sex, T2D, body mass index (BMI), as well as leptin and adiponectin.[20] Another study of 898 patients with hypertension found plasma levels of BCAAs and aromatic amino acids to be correlated with metabolic syndrome and IR.[21]

11.2.2.1 Fructose: uric acid and methylglyoxal

Another consequence of fructose acting as an unregulated nutrient is its capacity to generate a toxic by-product (methylglyoxal; MGO) and increase plasma uric acid levels, as shown in **Figure 11.3**.[22] As shown in the figure, fructose increases uric acid production by the liver. Fructose is metabolised there by several key enzymes. First, it is phosphorylated to fructose-1-P (fructose 1 phosphate) by the enzyme FRK C (fructokinase C). Fructose-1-P is then converted into glyceraldehyde-3-phosphate (G-3-P) via thiokinase (TKFC). Excessive fructose consumption can decrease the levels of intracellular ATP due to the quick process of phosphorylation by FRK C, forming ADP. Conversion of this ADP back to ATP increases AMP production. The excess AMP is then "dumped" by the liver, leading to its catabolism into uric acid, as shown.

The formation and accumulation of MGO, a highly reactive dicarbonyl compound, has been implicated in the pathogenesis of T2D, vascular complications of diabetes, and several other age-related chronic inflammatory diseases such as cardiovascular disease, cancer, and disorders of the central nervous system.[23] MGO is mainly formed as a by-product of glycolysis and is, under normal physiological circumstances, detoxified by the glyoxalase system. It is the major precursor of the nonenzymatic glycation of proteins

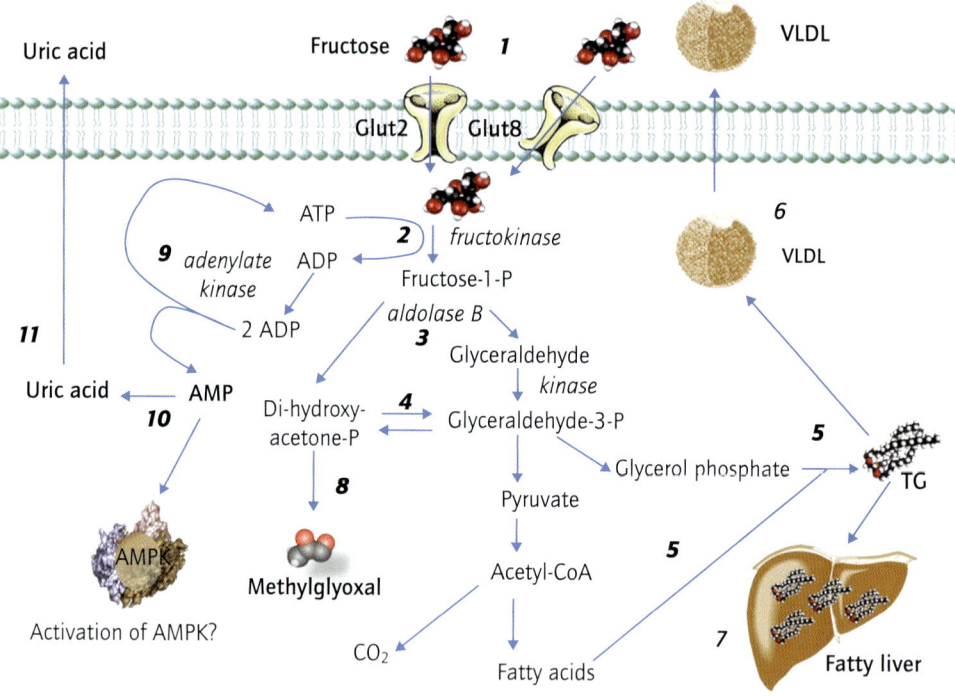

Figure 11.3 The hepatic metabolic impact of fructose. [Acetyl-CoA = acetyl coenzyme A; ADP = adenosine diphosphate; AMP = adenosine monophosphate; AMPK = adenosine monophosphate-activated protein kinase; TG = triglyceride; VLDL = very low density lipoprotein.]

and DNA, subsequently leading to the formation of advanced glycation end products (AGEs). MGO and MGO-derived AGEs can impact organs and tissues, affecting their functions and structure. As shown in Figure 11.3, the unregulated metabolism of fructose increases MGO production in the liver, either directly or via G-3-P.

Recent research published in *Cell Metabolism* suggests that MGO may cause many of the defects associated with T2D,[24] leading some to speculate that it might be the missing link in this disorder.[25] Using genetic engineering, the researchers turned off the enzyme that breaks down MGO in flies. MGO then accumulated in their bodies, and the flies developed IR. Later they became obese, and, as time went on, their glucose levels subsequently also became disrupted.

11.2.3 Toxins and metabolic syndrome

11.2.3.1 Endocrine disruptors

Various environmental chemicals have been shown to act as endocrine disruptors and obesogens.[26] A meta-analysis of nine studies compared highest versus lowest GGT (gamma-glutamyltransferase) levels and found a 63% increased risk of metabolic syndrome (independent of alcohol intake).[27] In this context GGT levels can be taken as a surrogate of environmental toxin exposure.

Epidemiological and experimental studies provide compelling evidence indicating that exposure to POPs (persistent organic pollutants) increases the risk of developing IR and metabolic disorders.[28] Body levels of POPs are linked to an increased risk of T2D, IR, and NAFLD, and it appears to be causal.[29] PCBs were positively associated with diabetes and prediabetes.[30] Organochlorines are also implicated in T2D; and, in one study, obesity was not linked to T2D provided that serum POPs were low.[31] PCBs, DDT metabolites, and dioxin were all associated with abdominal obesity.[32] The incidence of MetS was found to be higher in more POP-polluted regions of the United States.[33]

11.2.3.2 Dietary toxins

Dietary AGEs are mainly formed as a result of frying, grilling, or roasting foods rich in protein and fat. Human studies show consistently that dietary AGEs increase inflammation, oxidative stress, and endothelial dysfunction. Trials in people with early MetS have shown decreased IR, inflammation, and blood lipids after implementing low-AGE diets.[34] Dietary AGEs probably add to the total AGE load, accumulate in tissues, and interact with the AGE receptor (RAGE), driving inflammation. Hence, they may indirectly increase oxidation and inflammation, affect endothelial function, and promote IR.

11.2.4 Gut flora and metabolic syndrome

Recent studies suggest that an aberrant gut microbiota and an alteration of gut microbial metabolic activities in people with MetS have an important influence on several physiological functions. Some of these observations are illustrated in **Figure 11.4**.[35]

Ways in which gut microbiome changes can influence metabolism and body weight include:

- nutrient extraction: some gut bacteria might improve nutrient extraction from the diet, leading to a higher effective energy intake than might be expected[36,37]
- inflammatory overdrive via local – cross talk – and systemic (endotoxin, LPS) influences[38]
- metabolite-mediated mechanisms[39]
- endocannabinoid release – our understanding of the influence of this system on metabolism is growing at a rapid rate
- incretin production (see Section 11.3)
- GPR regulation: GPR41 and 43 receptors on submucosal immune cells in the intestine bind butyrate – an important SCFA produced by gut flora – and downregulate inflammation

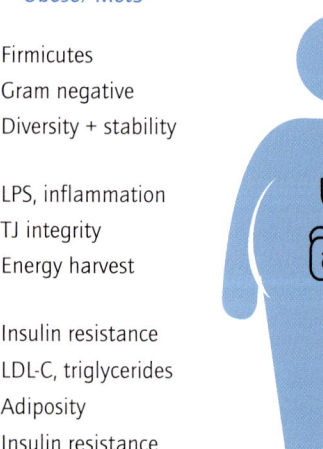
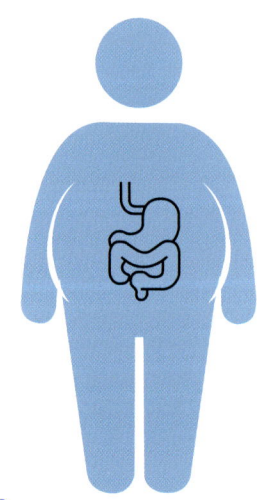

Normal/non-obese

Gut microbiome
↑ Bacteroidetes
↑ Proteobacteria
↑ Diversity + stability

Gut epithelium
↑ TJ integrity
↑ IEC differentiation
↑ SFCA production

Metabolic outcomes
↑ Insulin sensitivity
↑ Adaptive immunity
↓ Inflammation
↓ CVD risk

Balanced microbiome

Obese/MetS

↑ Firmicutes
↑ Gram negative
↓ Diversity + stability

↑ LPS, inflammation
↓ TJ integrity
↓ Energy harvest

↑ Insulin resistance
↑ LDL-C, triglycerides
↑ Adiposity
↑ Insulin resistance

Dysbiotic microbiome

Figure 11.4 An overview of the microbiome role in the development of obesity and metabolic syndrome. [CVD = cardiovascular disease; IEC = intestinal epithelial cells; LDL-C = low density lipoprotein cholesterol; LPS = lipopolysaccharide; MetS = metabolic syndrome; SCFA = short chain fatty acid; TJ = tight junction.]

11.3 Important cellular targets for MetS

These can be listed as follows:

- SIRT1 (sirtuin 1) and Nrf2 (detoxification, mitochondria)
- AMPK
- NFκB (nuclear factor kappa B): MetS is an inflammatory condition
- GPRs (G protein coupled receptors) (see Section 11.2) – and incretins
- 11β-HSD-1 (11-β-hydroxysteroid dehydrogenase type 1)
- mitochondria

SIRT1 is a key regulator of energy homeostasis and metabolism via PGC-1α (peroxisome proliferator-activated receptor-gamma coactivator 1alpha) and HIF-1α (hypoxia inducible factor 1-alpha) generation.[40] Studies have shown that SIRT1 controls both glucose and lipid metabolism in the liver, promotes fat mobilisation and stimulates brown remodelling of white fat in white adipose tissue, controls insulin secretion by the pancreas, senses nutrient availability in the hypothalamus, influences obesity-induced inflammation in macrophages, and modulates the activity of the circadian clock in metabolic tissues.

The key roles of Nrf2 are discussed in Chapter 6.

AMPK acts as the central energy switch (a cellular energy sensor), regulating how energy is produced and used in the body. The AMPK system senses and responds to changes in energy metabolism, both in the cell and in the whole body, via the AMP:ATP ratio. On activation of AMPK, catabolism is increased and anabolism decreased. AMPK regulates a diverse range of metabolic and physiological processes and is dysregulated in major chronic diseases, such as obesity, inflammation, diabetes, and cancer.[41]

Incretins are gut-derived peptides that increase glucose-stimulated insulin secretion. Though they are more relevant to our understanding of FHT for T2D, they are discussed briefly here. Incretins are produced by the enteroendocrine cells in the gastrointestinal tract in response to incoming nutrients. The main incretin hormones are GLP-1 (glucagon-like peptide 1) and GIP (gastric inhibitory polypeptide). As well as their role in managing blood glucose homeostasis, they also decrease appetite.[42] Some modern drugs for T2D treatment either mimic or modulate incretins.

The enzyme 11β-HSD-1 is an intracellular enzyme that catalyses the conversion of cortisone into cortisol.[43] It is well known that intracellular cortisol concentrations are determined not only by plasma levels, but also by the activity of 11β-HSD-1. Growing evidence suggests that MetS and central obesity may result from an increased bioavailability of cortisol at the tissue level (especially in liver and adipose tissue that overexpress this enzyme).[44]

Evidence increasingly supports the role of mitochondrial functional parameters in the genesis of various metabolism-related disorders. Biochemical pathways that modulate various mitochondrial functional indicators have been recognised in the diagnosis and prognosis of various disorders associated with energy metabolism, including MetS.[45] These include mitochondrial biogenesis, mitochondrial membrane potential, electron transport chain and ATP synthesis, intramitochondrial oxidative stress, and mitochondria-mediated cell death. Among other things, mitochondrial dysfunction contributes to the oxidative stress and systemic inflammation seen in MetS.[46]

11.4 Important systemic targets for MetS

Systemic targets in MetS can be listed as follows:

- gut flora
- environmental obesogens/endocrine disruptors/toxins
- microcirculation
- brown fat
- visceral adiposity
- stress responses/coping

The question of whether adults had brown adipose tissue and whether it could conceivably contribute to whole body energy usage in a meaningful way was a matter of vigorous debate until 2009. Three papers published in that year demonstrated that adult humans do, indeed, have brown adipose tissue, that it can be activated, and that this activation appears to be defective in obesity, completely reframing the debate.[47]

Compared with healthy lean controls, obese people display reduced brown adipose tissue (BAT) content. This reduction in active BAT mass appears to be more prevalent in visceral obesity. Concurrently, people with detectable BAT activity display lower blood glucose, triglyceride, and FFA levels, lower glycated haemoglobin (HbA1c) levels, and higher HDL cholesterol levels than people with no detectable BAT. BAT acts as an important "sink" for excess blood glucose and free fatty acid disposal. Thus, loss of BAT function in association with visceral obesity could contribute to the development of IR and hyperlipidaemia.[48]

In terms of stress response, a multicohort study used data from seven studies in Finland, France, Sweden, and the United Kingdom to examine the association between work stress and mortality.[49] In men with cardiometabolic disease, the contribution of job strain to risk of death was clinically significant and independent from conventional risk factors and their treatment and from measured lifestyle factors. It was concluded that standard care targeting conventional risk factors is therefore unlikely to mitigate the mortality risk associated with job strain in this population.

11.5 Overview of FHT objectives for the management of MetS

FHT objectives for the management and amelioration of MetS and IR are as follows:

1. reducing waist measurement – abdominal/visceral fat loss
2. stress reduction with adequate sleep quality/quantity (see Chapter 10)
3. adequate and appropriate exercise
4. appropriate dietary changes
5. carefully selected herbs to address the underlying causes and cellular and systemic targets

11.5.1 Exercise and MetS

High-intensity interval training (HIIT) is an effective strategy to boost levels of clinically relevant exercise in time-poor patients with MetS. Low-volume HIIT (51 minutes/week) was found to be at least as effective in ameliorating MetS as high-volume HIIT (114 min/week) or continuous training (150 min/week).[50] Participants in the HIIT groups trained three times a week (with at least a day between sessions). Low-volume-HIIT sessions were preceded by a 10-min warm-up and followed by a 3-min cool-down, both at 60–70% peak heart rate. The low-volume HIIT protocol consisted of only one bout of 4-min interval at 85–95% peak heart rate.

11.5.2 Diet and MetS

Although the following review looked specifically at T2D, it is also relevant to MetS. The review identified 20 RCTs lasting more than 6 months in people with T2D ($n = 3073$).[51] The four dietary patterns that showed the most benefit were the low-carbohydrate, low glycaemic index (GI), Mediterranean, and high-protein diets. All led to improved glycaemic control, but the strongest effect was found to be for the Mediterranean diet. The low-carb and Mediterranean diets led to the greatest weight loss (which was relatively small), and both increased HDL-cholesterol, but the high-protein diet did not.

Other dietary considerations based on the issues highlighted in this chapter include:

- fibre from multiple plant sources
- principally a plant-based diet
- minimal added sugar
- no consumption of sugary drinks (including juices), low-fructose fruits, organic animal fat (dairy, meat), and low BCAA proteins
- reduced haem iron intake via meat, fish, and poultry (MetS is linked to high ferritin)
- no consumption of synthetic trans-fats
- minimal alcohol
- the 5-point microcirculation phytonutrient plan – low-fructose version, with low-sugar strawberries and blackberries (see Chapter 5.1.3)

11.5.3 FHT prescribing for MetS

According to the principles of FHT, prescribing herbs for MetS should have the following objectives:

1. reducing nutrient flux and lowering the glycaemic index of meals
2. hitting the cellular targets
3. hitting the systemic targets
4. improving glycaemic control – more important for T2D, but also relevant for MetS
5. correcting the standout disturbances, especially lipids, hypertension
6. addressing any associated diseases/dysfunctions/comorbidities, such as gout, NAFLD, and BPH

11.5.3.1 Reducing nutrient flux

One of the reasons for the variation in the GI of different foods is the presence of phytochemicals that modify carbohydrate digestion and absorption. The GI of each meal can be lowered by including the following with the meal:

- mucilage herbs: slippery elm, linseed (flaxseed), psyllium
- tannins and other polyphenols that inhibit digestive enzymes – for example, grape seed, green tea
- Gymnema, which disrupts glucose uptake

Any meal can be turned into a low-GI meal with the help of these herbs.

Mucilages and tannins will also reduce nutrient flux by slowing the absorption of BCAAs and other macronutrients. This will enable the liver to metabolise unregulated nutrients more effectively.

11.5.3.2 Key herbs for the management of MetS

Nigella. In an open trial ($n = 159$), Nigella seed (0.5 g/day) plus standard drug treatment for 6 weeks led to a greater improvement in fasting blood glucose than standard drug treatment alone (decrease from baseline of 28.7% vs. 14.8%, respectively; $p = 0.01$).[52]

In one RCT, the effect of Nigella seed (3 g/day) was assessed over 12 weeks in people at risk of MetS. Lipid levels improved significantly from baseline ($p \leq 0.001$), with favourable changes in HDL-cholesterol (+0.24 mmol/L), LDL-cholesterol (−0.22 mmol/L), and triglycerides (−0.1 mmol/L).[53]

In another RCT ($n = 30$), Nigella seed (1 g/day for 2 months) taken by menopausal women with MetS resulted in metabolic improvements: total cholesterol, LDL cholesterol, and triglycerides were all significantly reduced compared to baseline (by 16.1, 27.2 and 22.2%, respectively) and compared with placebo (both $p < 0.05$).[54]

Meta-analysis of 11 RCTs ($n = 860$) found that short-term treatment with Nigella significantly reduced SBP (systolic blood pressure) and DBP (diastolic blood pressure) levels.[55] Preparations of Nigella either in seed powder or in oil demonstrated different lowering effects (in favour of the former) on both SBP and DBP. Meta-analysis of 11 RCTs ($n = 783$) showed that Nigella exerted a moderate effect on reducing body weight, BMI, and waist circumference.[56]

Bitter melon. Bitter melon is the fruit of *Momordica charantia*, a tropical vegetable and Ayurvedic herb. In a small crossover acute study ($n = 10$) a single dose of bitter melon extract reduced postprandial glucose in half of the prediabetic participants.[57] In a crossover RCT ($n = 52$ with prediabetes), bitter melon (2.5 g/day of dried fruit) for 8 weeks led to decreased fasting blood glucose compared to placebo (0.31 mmol/L; $p \leq 0.031$).[58]

Cinnamon and fenugreek. Oral administration of cinnamon extract significantly increased UCP1 (uncoupling protein 1) expression in subcutaneous adipose tissue *in vivo*.[59] This suggests that it might help with conversion of adipose tissue to brown fat.

In an RCT ($n = 116$, MetS), cinnamon (3 g/day for 16 weeks) significantly reduced fasting blood glucose ($p = 0.001$), HbA1c (2.6 units, $p = 0.023$), waist circumference (4.8 cm, $p = 0.002$), and BMI (1.3, $p = 0.001$) as compared to placebo.[60] The prevalence of MetS was reduced significantly: (34.5%) versus placebo (5.2%).

While there are no clinical trials of the use of fenugreek in MetS, the many clinical trials of its use for T2D suggest its value also for the former. One review suggested:

Based on the beneficial metabolic properties that have been demonstrated, 4-hydroxyisoleucine, a simple, plant-derived amino acid (from fenugreek), may represent an attractive new candidate for the treatment of all key components of metabolic syndrome.[61]

Berberine. In a small RCT with patients with MetS (n = 24), berberine at 1,500 mg/day resulted in a significant remission rate of 36%. It also lowered SBP, triglycerides and IR.[62] However, there is also high-level evidence from meta-analysis that berberine lowers chronic inflammation,[63] blood lipids,[64] and blood glucose in T2D.[65]

Curcumin. One RCT (n = 117, MetS) demonstrated that 8 weeks of supplementation with curcumin at 1,000 mg/day curcuminoids plus 5 mg piperine was associated with a significant increase in serum adiponectin levels ($p < 0.001$) and a reduction in serum leptin ($p < 0.001$). The serum leptin:adiponectin ratio was also improved by the curcumin ($p < 0.001$). These beneficial effects remained significant after adjustment for changes in serum lipids and glucose concentrations, and for baseline differences in BMI, serum glucose, and glycated haemoglobin (as potential confounders of the treatment response).[66]

In another long-term RCT (n = 213, T2D, 1,500 mg/day of curcuminoids for 6 months), curcumin intervention significantly reduced pulse wave velocity, increased serum adiponectin, and decreased leptin. These results were associated with reduced levels of IR, triglycerides, uric acid, visceral fat, and total body fat.[67]

Bitter herbs and incretins. Several bitter herbs have been shown to increase GLP-1 release *in vitro* via stimulating the bitter taste receptors expressed on enteroendocrine cells.[68,69] While these are *in vitro* results, the model does have some relevance to the clinical situation, because these receptors are on the surface of the gut lumen and will be in direct contact with ingested herbs.

This suggests a role for bitter herbs in improving glucose homeostasis and IR, especially in the case of MetS, and there are some clinical data to support this. In one study, bitter hops extract resulted in improvements in BMI, glycaemic control, and body fat. Patients were given just 16–48 mg/day of isohumulones (hop bitter acids) in capsule form in this double-blind RCT

(n = 94 patients, prediabetes).[70] In a later RCT, a liquid hop extract (matured bitter acids 35 mg/day from about 1 g hops) for 12 weeks caused a significant reduction in visceral fat in healthy overweight people.[71]

Green tea. Meta-analysis of 20 RCTs found that green tea decreased systolic BP and LDL-cholesterol.[72] In a pilot trial (n = 15, healthy participants), green tea catechin with caffeine acutely increased energy expenditure, associated with an increase in BAT activity, and chronically increased non-shivering cold-induced thermogenesis.[73] In an RCT (n = 35, MetS), green tea for 8 weeks increased whole blood glutathione (Nrf2 effect) and reduced plasma iron.[74] In another meta-analysis of 5 RCTs in MetS, green tea lowered BMI.[75]

Gymnema. Until recently, Gymnema trials were all conducted on people with T2D. However, a small RCT (n = 24) over 12 weeks on people with MetS compared Gymnema (at 600 mg/day) with a placebo. Use of the herb decreased body weight, BMI, and VLDL levels (from baseline), but without changes in insulin secretion and insulin sensitivity. No change was observed in the placebo group. The low dose used might explain why the Gymnema did not reduce IR.

Resveratrol. In a small RCT (n = 11, men with obesity but no other metabolic alteration), resveratrol (150 mg/day for 30 days) activated AMPK in muscle and increased SIRT1 and PGC-1α, with higher lipolysis in adipose tissue. Treatment also led to a decrease in glucose, insulin, and IR.[76]

A meta-analysis of 21 trials in overweight and obese people found that resveratrol significantly lowered total cholesterol, BP, and fasting glucose.[77]

But more is not necessarily better: in an RCT (n = 74), resveratrol (1,000mg/day for 16 weeks) increased LDL-cholesterol and fructosamine.[78]

Other herbs. In a pilot study (n = 11, MetS patients), taking Ginkgo for 2 months decreased hs-CRP from 8.9 to 4.9 mg/L (-44.4%, $p < 0.044$) and IR from 3.1 to 2.60 (-15.3%, $p < 0.012$), as well as inducing beneficial changes in inflammatory and oxidative stress biomarkers.[79]

In an RCT (n = 30 overweight and obese subjects), Coleus extract (with 25 mg forskolin) for 12 weeks lowered insulin levels and IR ($p = 0.001$ and 0.01, respectively) compared to placebo.[80]

In another RCT (*n* = 44, MetS), saffron (100 mg/day for 12 weeks) reduced inflammatory cytokines, hs-CRP, fasting blood glucose, cholesterol, and triglycerides and increased HDL-cholesterol.[81]

Licorice is well documented to inhibit the activity of 11β-HSD-2 (11-β-hydroxysteroid dehydrogenase type 2). This is responsible for its aldosterone-like side effects. A group of Italian scientists found that licorice taken for 2 months reduced body fat mass in 15 healthy volunteers without any change in calorie intake. BMI did not change. The authors attributed this effect to inhibition of 11β-HSD-1 at adipocytes.[82] Similar results have been observed clinically for the glycyrrhizin analogue carbenoxolone.[83]

11.5.3.3 Key herbs for cellular and systemic targets

Table 11.1 lists the key herbs for correcting metabolic dysfunction and the principal reason for their use, mainly in terms of cellular and systemic targets.

Table 11.2 lists the key herbs for correcting metabolic dysfunction, classified according to their cellular or systemic targets.

Table 11.1 Key herbs and their uses

Effective herbs	Principal use
▸ Nigella (black seed)	↓ BG, corrects lipids, ↓ BP, ↓ body weight
▸ Ginkgo	Nrf2, mitochondria, ↓ inflammation, MC
▸ curcumin/turmeric	↑ adiponectin, ↓ leptin, ↓ inflammation Nrf2, MC, corrects lipids, ↓ IR, ↑ AMPK
▸ bitter melon	incretin effect, ↓ BG, ↓ IR
▸ green tea	↑ brown fat, ↓ visceral fat, ↓ BP, Nrf2
▸ Reynoutria/Polygonum (resveratrol)	↑ AMPK, Nrf2, ↑ SIRT1
▸ cinnamon	↓ BG and see above
▸ Phellodendron (berberine)	↑ AMPK, ↓ BG, corrects lipids, ↓ BP, ↓ inflammation

Note. AMPK = adenosine monophosphate-activated protein kinase; BG = blood glucose; BP = blood pressure; IR = insulin resistance; MC = microcirculation.

Table 11.2 Effective herbs and their cellular or systemic metabolic targets

Effective herbs	Cellular or systemic target
▹ Nrf2 herbs	detoxification and intracellular antioxidant effects
▹ Rhodiola, ginseng, Ginkgo; Nrf2 herbs, SIRT1 herbs, and AMPK herbs	mitochondrial function
▹ curcumin/turmeric	↑ adiponectin, ↓ leptin
▹ Ginkgo, gotu kola, grape seed, bilberry, and garlic	microcirculatory and general cardiovascular health (such as ↓BP)
▹ curcumin/turmeric, Ginkgo, saffron, Phellodendron (berberine)	↓ NFκB and inflammatory cytokines and markers
▹ green tea, ginger, cinnamon?	↑ brown fat and ↓ visceral fat
▹ Nigella, curcumin/turmeric, garlic	abnormal lipids
▹ Polygonum/Reynoutria (resveratrol), milk thistle	SIRT1
▹ curcumin/turmeric, Phellodendron (berberine), Polygonum/Reynoutria (resveratrol)	AMPK
▹ licorice (but watch for ↑ BP due to ↓ 11β-HSD-2 at kidneys)	↓ 11βHSD-1 at muscle and adipose tissue
▹ bitter herbs (such as feverfew, gentian, wormwood)	↑ incretins
▹ garlic, ginger, Coleus, bioavailable curcumin	prothrombotic state
▹ Bowel flora protocol with extra fibre	fibre, SCFAs, and GPRs

Note. 11β-HSD-2 = 11-β-hydroxysteroid dehydrogenase type 2; AMPK = adenosine monophosphate-activated protein kinase; BP = blood pressure; GPR = G protein-coupled receptor; NFκB = nuclear factor kappa B; SCFAs = short chain fatty acids.

11.5.3.4 Key herbs for improving glycaemic control

The major herbs useful for improving glycaemic control are listed in **Table 11.3**.

The use of these key and supporting herbs is supported by clinical trial data.

Table 11.3 Key and supporting herbs for better glycaemic control

Key herbs	Supporting herbs
▸ Nigella (black seed)	▸ bitters (boost incretin effect)
▸ Gymnema (long term)	▸ milk thistle
▸ fenugreek	▸ Ginkgo
▸ Polygonum/Reynoutria (resveratrol)	▸ sage
▸ bitter melon	▸ curcumin/turmeric
▸ green tea	▸ Korean ginseng
▸ cinnamon	▸ Coleus
▸ Phellodendron (berberine)	▸ ginger

11.5.4 How to approach the individual MetS patient with FHT

The FHT therapeutic pyramid for MetS is outlined in **Figure 11.5**. The clinical features of the case, together with diet, exercise, and stress management, comprise the core baseline. Next, always keep in mind that this is a

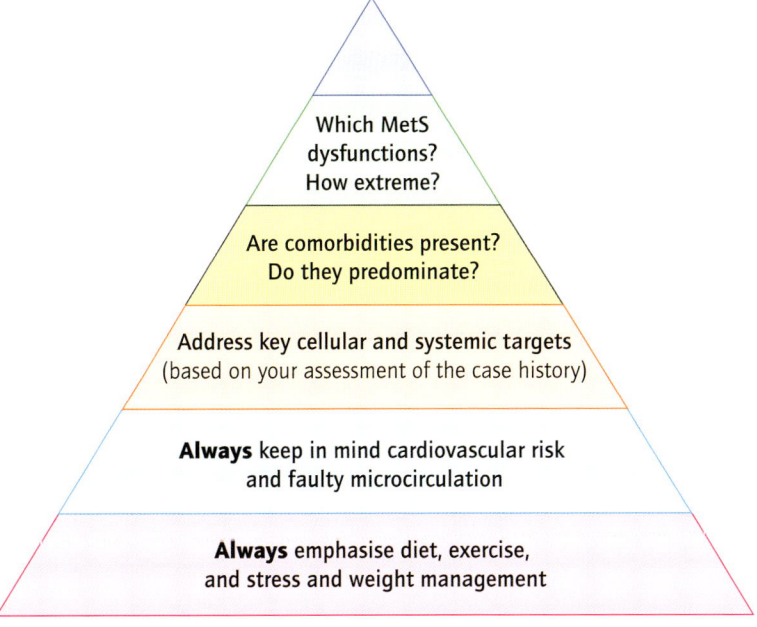

Figure 11.5 The FHT therapeutic pyramid for MetS.

condition of enhanced cardiovascular risk, and compromised microcirculation contributes to this. Then address relevant cellular and systemic targets based on an assessment of the case history. Some of these might be targeted specifically, but others will be targeted coincidentally, according to the herb that is selected. Next, identify any co-morbidities present and whether they predominate. Finally, determine which of the metabolic syndrome dysfunctions are being expressed, and how extreme.

To reiterate: above all, be guided by the clinical features of the case. This is illustrated by the sample protocols in Section 11.6.

11.5.4.1   The 8-point dietary BP plan

The key elements of this are as follows:

- the DASH dietary guidelines: diet high in fruit, vegetables, whole grains, low-fat dairy products, fish, chicken, and lean meats

And as a major part of this:

- berries, especially low sugar strawberries and blackberries
- cocoa (90% chocolate, 20 g/day), or cocoa with a natural sweetener
- green tea and hibiscus tea – several cups per day of each
- garlic as 1–2 fresh, crushed raw cloves/day
- boost dietary nitrate: beetroot as juice or supplement – plus sunlight to increase its conversion to NO; spinach is a lower-sugar alternative
- fibre, especially 30 g/day of freshly milled linseed (flaxseed)
- reduce salt to 3 g/day, increase potassium

11.5.4.2   What about high cholesterol?

High plasma LDL-cholesterol is not a necessary feature of MetS, but it can occur in conjunction with it. It is best addressed by selecting herbs that will not only lower cholesterol, but also provide other health benefits in terms of improving symptoms, hitting targets, and correcting metabolic dysfunction. The best examples of such herbs are Nigella, garlic, Phellodendron (berberine), and turmeric/curcumin.

11.6 Protocol examples

11.6.1 MetS with hypertension predominating

- Nigella, bitter melon, cinnamon, and fenugreek
  AND/OR
  Phellodendron (berberine)
- garlic, Coleus
- 8-point dietary BP Plan (see Section 11.5.4.1)

11.6.2 MetS with high triglycerides and LDL-cholesterol predominating

- Nigella, bitter melon, cinnamon, and fenugreek
  AND/OR
  Phellodendron (berberine)
- garlic
- bioavailable curcumin

11.6.3 MetS with lipids and hypertension predominating

- Nigella, bitter melon, cinnamon, and fenugreek
  AND/OR
  Phellodendron (berberine)
- garlic, Coleus
- 8 Point Dietary BP Plan (see Section 11.5.4.1)

11.6.4 MetS with poor appetite control

- Nigella, bitter melon, cinnamon, and fenugreek
  AND
  gentian, wormwood, feverfew, ginger, and tangerine peel
  AND
  Gymnema

11.6.5 MetS with high blood glucose predominating

- Nigella, bitter melon, cinnamon, and fenugreek
  AND/OR
  gentian, wormwood, feverfew, ginger, and tangerine peel
  AND/OR
  Polygonum/Reynoutria, Ginkgo, milk thistle, Korean ginseng, and grape seed
- Phellodendron (berberine)
- Gymnema

11.6.6 MetS with previous heart attack

- Nigella, bitter melon, cinnamon, and fenugreek
  AND/OR
  Phellodendron (berberine)
- bioavailable curcumin
  AND
  garlic
- gotu kola, Ginkgo, grape seed

11.6.7 MetS with previous heart attack & under work/life stress

- Nigella, bitter melon, cinnamon, and fenugreek
  AND/OR
  Phellodendron (berberine)
- bioavailable curcumin

- gotu kola, Ginkgo, and grape seed
  AND
  kava, valerian
- Rehmannia, Withania (ashwagandha), etc.

11.6.8 MetS with gout predominating

- Nigella, bitter melon, cinnamon, and fenugreek
  AND/OR
  Phellodendron (berberine)
- bioavailable curcumin
  AND
  dandelion leaf and celery

11.6.9 MetS but too tired to exercise

- Nigella, bitter melon, cinnamon, and fenugreek
  AND/OR
  Phellodendron (berberine)
- bioavailable curcumin
  AND
  Rhodiola and Korean ginseng

11.6.10 MetS with recurrent cellulitis

- Nigella, bitter melon, cinnamon, and fenugreek
- bioavailable curcumin
- gotu kola, Ginkgo and grape seed
- Echinacea root

AND

- 5-point microcirculation dietary plan (low-sugar version):
  - boost dietary nitrate: green leafy vegetables, especially spinach
  - increase cocoa intake: 20 g/day with a natural sweetener
  - increase berry anthocyanin intake: one cup a day of strawberries and blackberries
  - fresh raw crushed garlic: ½–1 clove/day
  - increase herbs and spices: especially green tea (3–4 cups/day with meals), turmeric, and ginger

11.6.11 Older male with MetS and low testosterone

- Nigella, bitter melon, cinnamon, and fenugreek
  AND/OR
  Phellodendron (berberine)
- bioavailable curcumin
- Rhodiola and Korean ginseng
  AND/OR
  Tribulus leaf

11.6.12 MetS with clear history of toxin exposure

- Nigella, bitter melon, cinnamon, and fenugreek
  AND/OR
  Phellodendron (berberine)
- bioavailable curcumin
- rosemary, green tea, turmeric, and grape seed
- garlic
- Schisandra

11.6.13 MetS with chronic kidney disease

- Nigella, bitter melon, cinnamon, and fenugreek
  AND/OR
  Phellodendron (berberine)
- bioavailable curcumin
- gotu kola, Ginkgo and grape seed
  AND
  5-point microcirculation dietary plan (low-sugar version)
  ALSO CONSIDER
- Polygonum/Reynoutria, Ginkgo, milk thistle, Korean ginseng and grape seed
  AND
  Astragalus, Bupleurum, and Rehmannia

References

1. https://en.wikipedia.org/wiki/Metabolism
2. https://www.fda.gov/news-events/speeches-fda-officials/reducing-burden-chronic-disease-03292018
3. Samson SL, Garber AJ. Metabolic syndrome. *Endocrinol Metab Clin North Am.* 2014; **43**(1): 1–23. doi:10.1016/j.ecl.2013.09.009.
4. van Greevenbroek MM, Schalkwijk CG, Stehouwer CD. Dysfunctional adipose tissue and low-grade inflammation in the management of the metabolic syndrome: current practices and future advances. *F1000Res.* 2016 Oct 13; **5**: 2515. doi:10.12688/f1000research.8971.1.
5. Samson SL, Garber AJ. Metabolic syndrome. *Endocrinol Metab Clin North Am.* 2014; **43**(1): 1–23. doi:10.1016/j.ecl.2013.09.009.
6. Tarantino G, Finelli C. What about non-alcoholic fatty liver disease as a new criterion to define metabolic syndrome? *World J Gastroenterol.* 2013; **19**(22): 3375–3384. PMID: 23801829.
7. Eslam M, Sanyal AJ, George J; International Consensus Panel. MAFLD: a consensus-driven proposed nomenclature for metabolic associated fatty liver disease. *Gastroenterology.* 2020; **158**(7): 1999–2014. doi:10.1053/j.gastro.2019.11.312.
8. Thottam GE, Krasnokutsky S, Pillinger MH. Gout and metabolic syndrome: a tangled web. *Curr Rheumatol Rep.* 2017 Aug 26; **19**(10): 60. PMID: 28844079.
9. Sirmans SM, Pate KA. Epidemiology, diagnosis and management of polycystic ovary syndrome. *Clin Epidemiol* 2013; **6**: 1–13. PMID: 24379699.
10. Nistala R, Whaley-Connell A. Resistance to insulin and kidney disease in the cardiorenal metabolic syndrome; role for angiotensin II. *Mol Cell Endocrinol.* 2013; **378**(1–2): 53–58. PMID: 23416840.
11. Hursting SD. Obesity, energy balance and cancer: a mechanistic perspective. *Cancer Treat Res* 2014; **159**: 21–33. PMID: 24114472.
12. Misiak B, Leszek J, Kiejna A. Metabolic syndrome, mild cognitive impairment and Alzheimer's disease: the emerging role of systemic low grade inflammation and adiposity. *Brain Res Bull*; **89**(3–4): 144–149. PMID: 22921944.
13. Sebastianelli A, Gacci M. Current status of the relationship between metabolic syndrome and lower urinary tract symptoms. *Eur Urol Focus.* 2018 Mar 27; **4**(1): 25–27. doi:10.1016/j.euf.2018.03.007. PMID: 29602736.
14. Drager LF, Togeiro SM, Polotsky VY, et al. Obstructive sleep apnea: a cardiometabolic risk in obesity and the metabolic syndrome. *J Am Coll Cardiol.* 2013; **62**(7): 569–576.
15. Item F, Konrad D. Visceral fat and metabolic inflammation: the portal theory revisited. *Obes Rev.* 2012; **13**(Suppl 2): 30–39. doi:10.1111/j.1467-789X.2012.01035.x.
16. Hanefeld M, Pistrosch F, Bornstein SR, Birkenfeld AL. The metabolic vascular syndrome: guide to an individualized treatment. *Rev Endocr Metab Disord.* 2016; **17**(1): 5–17. doi:10.1007/s11154-016-9345-4.
17. Beale EG. Insulin signalling and insulin resistance. *J Investig Med.* 2013 Jan; **61**(1): 11–14. PMID: 23111650.
18. Item F, Konrad D. Visceral fat and metabolic inflammation: the portal theory revisited. *Obes Rev.* 2012; **13**(Suppl 2): 30–39. doi:10.1111/j.1467-789X.2012.01035.x.
19. Bremer AA, Mietus-Snyder M, Lustig RH. Toward a unifying hypothesis of metabolic syndrome. *Pediatrics* 2012; **129**(3): 557–570. PMID: 22351884.
20. Connelly MA, Wolak-Dinsmore J, Dullaart RPF. Branched chain amino acids are associ-

ated with insuilin resistance independent of leptin and adiponectin in subjects with varying degrees of glucose tolerance. *Metab Syndr Relat Disord.* 2017 May; **15**(4): 183–186. PMID: 28437198.
21. Weng L, Quinlivan E, Gong Y, et al. Association of branched and aromatic amino acids levels with metabolic syndrome and impaired fasting glucose in hypertensive patients. *Metab Syndr Relat Disord.* 2015 Jun; **13**(5): 195–202. PMID: 25664967.
22. Gugliucci A. Fructose surges damage hepatic adenosyl-monophosphate-dependent kinase and lead to increased lipogenesis and hepatic insulin resistance. *Med Hypotheses.* 2016; **93**: 87–92. doi:10.1016/j.mehy.2016.05.026.
23. Schalkwijk CG, Stehouwer CDA. Methylglyoxal, a highly reactive dicarbonyl compound, in diabetes, its vascular complications, and other age-related diseases. *Physiol Rev.* 2020; **100**(1): 407–461. doi:10.1152/physrev.00001.2019.
24. Moraru A, Wiederstein J, Pfaff D, et al. Elevated levels of the reactive metabolite methylglyoxal recapitulate progression of type 2 diabetes. *Cell Metab.* 2018; **27**(4): 926–934. doi:10.1016/j.cmet.2018.02.003.
25. https://theconversation.com/have-we-got-the-causes-of-type-2-diabetes-wrong-93326
26. Janesick A, Blumberg B. Obesogens, stem cells and the developmental programming of obesity. *Int J Androl* 2012; **35**(3): 437–448. PMID: 22372658.
27. Liu CF, Zhou WN, Fang NY. Gamma-glutamyltransferase levels and risk of metabolic syndrome: a meta-analysis of prospective cohort studies. *Int J Clin Pract.* 2012; **66**(7): 692–698. PMID: 22698421.
28. Kim YA, Park JB, Woo MS, Lee SY, Kim HY, Yoo YH. Persistent organic pollutant-mediated insulin resistance. *Int J Environ Res Public Health.* 2019; **16**(3): 448. doi:10.3390/ijerph16030448.
29. Ruzzin J, Lee DH, Carpenter DO, et al. Reconsidering metabolic diseases: the impacts of persistent organic pollutants. *Atherosclerosis.* 2012; **224**(1): 1–3. PMID: 22472455.
30. Gasull M, Pumarega J, Teliaz-plaza, M, et al. Blood concentrations of persistent organic pollutants and prediabetes and diabetes in the general population of Catalonia. *Environ Sci Technol.* 2012 Jul 17; **46**(14): 7799–7810. PMID: 22681243.
31. Lee DH. Persistent organic pollutants and obesity-related metabolic dysfunction: focusing on type 2 diabetes. *Epidemiol Health* 2012; **34**: e2012002. doi:10.4178/epih/e2012002. PMID: 22323980.
32. Lee DH, Lind, L, Jacobs, DR Jr, et al. Associations of persistent organic pollutants with abdominal obesity in the elderly: The Prospective Investigation of the Vasculature in Uppsala Seniors (PIVUS) study. *Environ Int.* 2012; **40**: 170–178. PMID: 21835469.
33. Sergeev AV, Carpenter, DO. Increase in metabolic syndrome-related hospitalisations in reaction to environmental sources of persistent organic pollutants. *Int J Environ Res Public Health* 2011; **8**(3): 762–776. PMID: 21556177.
34. Luévano-Contreras C, Gómez-Ojeda A, Macías-Cervantes MH, et al. Dietary advanced glycation end products and cardiometabolic risk. *Curr Diab Rep.* 2017 Aug; **17**(8): 63. doi:10.1007/s11892-017-0891-2. PMID: 28695383.
35. Green M, Arora K, Prakash S. Microbial medicine: prebiotic and probiotic functional foods to target obesity and metabolic syndrome. *Int J Mol Sci.* 2020 Apr 21; **21**(8): e2890. doi:10.3390/ijms21082890.
36. D'Aversa F, Tortora A, Ianiro G, et al. Gut microbiota and metabolic syndrome. *Intern Emerg Med.* 2013; **8**(Suppl 1): S11–S5.
37. Kovatcheva-Datchary P, Arora T. Nutrition, the gut microbiome and the metabolic syndrome. *Best Pract Res Clin Gastroenterol.* 2013; **27**(1): 59–72.
38. Piya MK, Harte AL, McTernan PG. Metabolic endotoxaemia: is it more than just a gut feeling? *Curr Opin Lipidol.* 2013; **24**(1): 78–85.

39. Burcelin R, Garidou L, Pomié C. Immuno-microbiota cross and talk: the new paradigm of metabolic diseases. *Semin Immunol.* 2012; **24**(1): 67–74.
40. Li X. SIRT1 and energy metabolism. *Acta Biochim Biophys Sin (Shanghai).* 2013; **45**(1): 51–60. doi:10.1093/abbs/gms108.
41. Jeon SM. Regulation and function of AMPK in physiology and diseases. *Exp Mol Med.* 2016; **48**(7): e245. doi:10.1038/emm.2016.81.
42. Spreckley E, Murphy KG. The L-cell in nutritional sensing and the regulation of appetite. *Front Nutr.* 2015 Jul 20; **2**: 23. doi:10.3389/fnut.2015.00023.
43. Gregory S, Hill D, Grey B, et al. 11β-Hydroxysteroid dehydrogenase type 1 inhibitor use in human disease: a systematic review and narrative synthesis. *Metabolism.* 2020 Apr 23 [published online ahead of print]; **108**: 154246. doi:10.1016/j.metabol.2020.154246.
44. Anagnostis P, Katsiki N, Adamidou F, et al. 11beta-Hydroxysteroid dehydrogenase type 1 inhibitors: novel agents for the treatment of metabolic syndrome and obesity-related disorders?. *Metabolism.* 2013; **62**(1): 21–33. doi:10.1016/j.metabol.2012.05.002.
45. Anupama N, Sindhu G, Raghu KG. Significance of mitochondria on cardiometabolic syndromes. *Fundam Clin Pharmacol.* 2018; **32**(4): 346–356. doi:10.1111/fcp.12359.
46. Prasun P. Mitochondrial dysfunction in metabolic syndrome. *Biochim Biophys Acta Mol Basis Dis.* 2020 May 16 [published online ahead of print]; **1886**(1): 165838. doi:10.1016/j.bbadis.2020.165838.
47. Lockie SH, Stefanidis A, Oldfield BJ, Perez-Tilve D. Brown adipose tissue thermogenesis in the resistance and reversal of obesity: a potential new mechanism contributing to the metabolic benefits of proglucagon-derived peptides. *Adipocyte.* 2013; **2**(4): 196–200. PMID: 24052894.
48. Chait A, den Hartigh LJ. Adipose tissue distribution, inflammation and its metabolic consequences, including diabetes and cardiovascular disease. *Front Cardiovasc Med.* 2020 Feb 25; **7**: 22. doi:10.3389/fcvm.2020.00022.
49. Kivimäki M, Pentti J, Ferrie JE, et al. Work stress and risk of death in men and women with and without cardiometabolic disease: a multicohort study. *Lancet Diabetes Endocrinol.* 2018; **6**(9): 705–713. doi:10.1016/S2213-8587(18)30140-2.
50. Ramos JS, Dalleck LC, Borrani F, et al. Low-volume high-intensity interval training is sufficient to ameliarate the severity of metabolic syndrome. *Metab Syndr Relat Disord.* 2017 Sep; **15**(7): 319–328. PMID: 28846513.
51. Ajala O, English P, Pinkney J. Systemic review and meta-analysis of different dietary approaches to the management of type 2 diabetes. *Am J Clin Nutr.* 2013; **97**(3): 505–516. PMID: 23364002.
52. Shah AS, Khan GM, Badshah A, et al. *Nigella sativa* provides protection against metabolic syndrome. *Afr J Biotechnol.* 2012; **11**(48): 10919–10925.
53. Al Dhaheri A. The effect of black seed powder on blood glycaemia, blood lipidemia and body composition on adults at risk for cardiovascular diseases. Dubai Nutrition Conference. Dubai, 2016.
54. Ibrahim R, Hamdan N, Mahmud R, et al. A randomised controlled trial on hypolipidemic effects of *Nigella sativa* seeds powder in menopausal women. *J Transl Med.* 2014; **12**: 82. doi:10.1186/1479-5876-12-82. PMID: 24685020.
55. Sahebkar A, Soranna D, Liu X, et al. A systematic review and meta-analysis of randomized controlled trials investigating the effects of supplementation with *Nigella sativa* (black seed) on blood pressure. *J Hypertens.* 2016; **34**(11): 2127–2135. doi:10.1097/HJH.0000000000001049.
56. Namazi N, Larijani B, Ayati MH, Abdollahi M. The effects of *Nigella sativa* L. on obesity: a systematic review and meta-analysis. *J Ethnopharmacol.* 2018; **219**: 173–181. doi:10.1016/j.jep.2018.03.001.

57. Boone CH, Stout JR, Gordon JA, et al. Acute effects of a beverage containing bitter melon extract (CARELA) on postprandial glycemia among prediabetic adults. *Nutr Diabetes.* 2017 Jan 16; **7**(1): e241. doi:10.1038/nutd.2016.51. PMID: 28092345.
58. Krawinkel MB, Ludwig C, Swai ME, et al. Bitter gourd reduces elevated fasting plasma glucose levels in an intervention study among prediabetics in Tanzania. *J Ethnopharmacol.* 2018 Apr 24; **216**: 1–7. doi: 10.1016/j.jep.2018.01.016. PMID: 29339109.
59. Kwan HY, Wu J, Su T, et al. Cinnamon induces browning in subcutaneous adipocytes. *Sci Rep.* 2017 May 26; **7**(1): 2447. doi:10.1038/s41598-017-02263-5. PMID: 28550279.
60. Gupta Jain S, Puri S, Misra A, Gulati S, Mani K. Effect of oral cinnamon intervention on metabolic profile and body composition of Asian Indians with metabolic syndrome: a randomized double-blind control trial. *Lipids Health Dis.* 2017 Jun 12; **16**(1): 113. doi: 10.1186/s12944-017-0504-8. PMID: 28606084.
61. Jetté L, Harvey L, Eugeni K, et al. 4-Hydroxyisoleucine: a plant-derived treatment for metabolic syndrome. *Curr Opin Investig Drugs.* 2009 Apr; **10**(4): 353–358. PMID: 19337956.
62. Pérez-Rubio KG, González-Ortiz M, Martínez-Abundis E, Robles-Cervantes JA, Espinel-Bermúdez MC. Effect of berberine administration on metabolic syndrome, insulin sensitivity, and insulin secretion. *Metab Syndr Relat Disord.* 2013; **11**(5): 366–369. doi:10.1089/met.2012.0183.
63. Beba M, Djafarian K, Shab-Bidar S. Effect of berberine on C-reactive protein: a systematic review and meta-analysis of randomized controlled trials. *Complement Ther Med.* 2019; **46**: 81–86. doi:10.1016/j.ctim.2019.08.002.
64. Ju J, Li J, Lin Q, Xu H. Efficacy and safety of berberine for dyslipidaemias: a systematic review and meta-analysis of randomized clinical trials. *Phytomedicine.* 2018; **50**: 25–34. doi:10.1016/j.phymed.2018.09.212.
65. Liang Y, Xu X, Yin M, et al. Effects of berberine on blood glucose in patients with type 2 diabetes mellitus: a systematic literature review and a meta-analysis. *Endocr J.* 2019; **66**(1): 51–63. doi:10.1507/endocrj.EJ18-0109.
66. Panahi Y, Hosseini MS, Khalili N, et al. Effects of supplementation with curcumin on serum adipokine concentrations: a randomized controlled trial. *Nutrition.* 2016; **32**(10): 1116–1122. doi:10.1016/j.nut.2016.03.018.
67. Chuengsamarn S, Rattanamongkolgul S, Phonrat B, Tungtrongchitr R, Jirawatnotai S. Reduction of atherogenic risk in patients with type 2 diabetes by curcuminoid extract: a randomized controlled trial. *J Nutr Biochem.* 2014; **25**(2): 144–150. doi:10.1016/j.jnutbio.2013.09.013.
68. Yu Y, Hao G, Zhang Q, et al. Berberine induces GLP–1 secretion through activation of bitter taste receptor pathways. *Biochem Pharmacol.* 2015; **97**(2): 173–177. doi:10.1016/j.bcp.2015.07.012.
69. Li J, Xu J, Hou R, et al. Qing-Hua granule induces GLP–1 secretion via bitter taste receptor in db/db mice. *Biomed Pharmacother.* 2017; **89**: 10–17. doi:10.1016/j.biopha.2017.01.168.
70. Obara K, Mizutani M, Hitomi Y, Yajima H, Kondo K. Isohumulones, the bitter component of beer, improve hyperglycemia and decrease body fat in Japanese subjects with prediabetes. *Clin Nutr.* 2009; **28**(3): 278–284. doi:10.1016/j.clnu.2009.03.012.
71. Morimoto-Kobayashi Y, Ohara K, Ashigai H, et al. Matured hop extract reduces body fat in healthy overweight humans: a randomized, double-blind, placebo-controlled parallel group study. *Nutr J.* 2016 Mar 9; **15**: 25. doi:10.1186/s12937-016-0144-2.
72. Onakpoya I, Spencer E, Heneghan C. The effect of green tea on blood pressure and lipid profile: a systematic review and meta-analysis of randomized clinical trials. *Nutr Metab Cardiovasc Dis.* 2014 Aug; **24**(8): 823–836. PMID: 24675010.
73. Yoneshiro T, Matsushita M, Hibi M, et al. Tea catechin and caffeine activate brown adi-

pose tissue and increase cold-induced thermogenic capacity in humans. *Am J Clin Nutr.* 2017 Apr; **105**(4): 873–881. PMID: 28275131.
74. Basu A, Betts NM, Mulugeta A, et al. Green tea supplementation increases glutathione and plasma antioxidant capacity in adults with the metabolic syndrome. *Nutr Res.* 2013 Mar; **33**(3): 180–187. PMID: 23507223.
75. Zhong X, Zhang T, Liu Y, et al. Short-term weight-centric effects of tea or tea extract in patients with metabolic syndrome: a meta-analysis of randomized controlled trials. *Nutr Diabetes.* 2015 Jun 15; **5**: e160. doi:10.1038/nutd.2015.10. PMID: 26075637.
76. Timmers S, Konings E, Bilet L, et al. Calorie restriction-like effects of 30 days of resveratrol supplementation on energy metabolism and metabolic profile in obese humans. *Cell Metab.* 2011 Nov 2; **14**(5): 612–622. PMID: 22055504.
77. Huang H, Chen G, Liao D, et al. The effects of resveratrol intervention on risk markers of cardiovascular health in overweight and obese subjects: a pooled analysis of randomized controlled trials. *Obes Rev.* 2016 Dec; **17**(12): 1329–1340. PMID: 27456934.
78. Kjær TN, Ornstrup MJ, Poulsen MM, et al. No beneficial effects of resveratrol on the metabolic syndrome: a randomized placebo-controlled clinical trial. *J Clin Endocrinol Metab.* 2017 May 1; **102**(5): 1642–1651. PMID: 28182820.
79. Siegel G, Ermilov E, Knes O, et al. Combined lowering of low-grade systemic inflammation and insulin resistance in metabolic syndrome patients treated with Ginkgo biloba. *Atherosclerosis.* 2014 Dec; **237**(2): 584–588. PMID: 25463092.
80. Loftus HL, Astell KJ, Mathai ML, et al. Coleus forskohlii extract supplementation in conjunction with a hypocaloric diet reduces the risk factors of metabolic syndrome in overweight and obese subjects: a randomized controlled trial. *Nutrients.* 2015 Nov 17; **7**(11): 9508–9522. PMID: 2659394.
81. Kermani T, Zebarjadi M, Mehrad-Majd H, et al. Anti-inflammatory effect of *Crocus sativus* on serum cytokine levels in subjects with metabolic syndrome: a randomized, double-blind, placebo-controlled trial. *Curr Clin Pharmacol.* 2017; **12**(2): 122–126. PMID: 28637418.
82. Armanini D, De Palo CB, Mattarello MJ, et al. Effect of licorice on the reduction of body fat mass in healthy subjects. *J Endocrinol Invest.* 2003; **26**(7): 646–650. doi:10.1007/BF03347023.
83. Anagnostis P, Katsiki N, Adamidou F, et al. 11β-Hydroxysteroid dehydrogenase type 1 inhibitors: novel agents for the treatment of metabolic syndrome and obesity-related disorders? *Metabolism.* 2013; **62**(1): 21–33. doi:10.1016/j.metabol.2012.05.002.

12

FHT strategies for atopy, asthma, and allergic rhinitis

This chapter explores FHT strategies for the prevention and management of atopy, asthma, and allergic rhinitis (AR). It is a fascinating observation that until the late nineteenth century, these disorders were not so prevalent. Since then, there have been steep rises in asthma (especially in children) and, more recently, an epidemic of peanut and other types of anaphylactic food allergies. We are, in fact, experiencing a pandemic of allergy, to the point where some pundits are saying that in a few decades every child will have some form of atopy.

Our lifestyles are moving further and further from what is natural, and this seems to be feeding the process. But what is specifically behind this, and how do we credibly address it in clinical practice, both in a preventative and a curative context? Furthermore, how do we keep up to date with all the research and make sense of the many different factors and causes that are being identified for what are very complex health issues?

In the mid-1980s, as a new graduate, I saw my first patient with asthma. I did not have much of an understanding of what to do, other than using bronchodilating and expectorant herbs. These are still important in asthma therapy, but with the development of our biomedical understanding of atopic conditions, we now have much more information to work with.

You might be reflecting that asthma and allergies are too complex and that you are sceptical that herbal therapies can have any impact on them. Perhaps you are baffled by the complexity of the research and wondering what the key issues are that we should focus on. You might, on the other hand, feel that you already treat asthma and allergies very well and are wondering what the FHT prescribing system has to offer that is new.

By the end of this chapter you might agree that, while we have relatively few clinical trials that directly show the benefits of herbs in atopy, we can still arrive at a highly evidence-based approach by applying FHT principles. This involves having an accurate biomedical understanding of the underlying disease and then individualising that information to the person in front of us.

12.1   FHT and atopy

12.1.1   The rise of atopy

The term atopy refers to the tendency to develop allergic diseases such as AR (hay fever), asthma, and atopic dermatitis (eczema). Atopy is typically associated with a heightened immune reaction to common allergens, especially inhaled allergens – such as pollen and dust mite – and to food allergens. This particularly involves an inappropriate IgE (immunoglobulin E) immune pathway response. (It is thought that IgE originally evolved as a defence mechanism against parasitic infestation.)

Even in mainstream thinking, for example in published research and reviews, atopy is considered to be a mosaic disease, where many inciting factors are involved. These include our microbiome (skin, lung, and gut), the timing of our initial exposure to allergens, defective body barriers, our exposure to air pollution (especially in the case of asthma), and several other factors, such as diet, socioeconomic status, and stress.[1] The true picture is even larger than this short list, and it dictates that we cannot appropriately address allergies with a main strategy that involves a symptomatic or superficial approach.

We are living in an allergy pandemic. Hay fever was only first described in the nineteenth century, and its rise is thought to be due to the first improved levels of hygiene that began at the time.[2] In addition, higher levels of pollen caused by changes in agriculture may have played a role. The major changes in hygiene in the West had all taken place by 1920, yet childhood asthma only started to increase alarmingly in the 1960s. The major social change that occurred then was television, and it adjusted our way of life so that it became more an indoor than an outdoor one. There are some researchers who posit that this could be the key factor in the rise of the asthma epidemic. Since 1990, there has been an epidemic of food allergy, especially to peanuts.

Just recently, we are witnessing the rise of an alpha-gal allergy. Galactose-alpha-1,3-galactose (alpha-gal) is a sugar found in mammalian meat, and it is also present in glycoproteins from tick saliva. A person bitten by a tick can become sensitised to this sugar, and this develops into an allergy to mammalian meat.[3] The tick is the trigger – but why is it on the increase?

The recent rise of atopic disease is illustrated in **Figure 12.1**.[4] Note that the vertical axis is a logarithmic scale.

The allergy pandemic completely challenges the comfortable assumption that our modern way of life is healthy. Something is very wrong! The way we

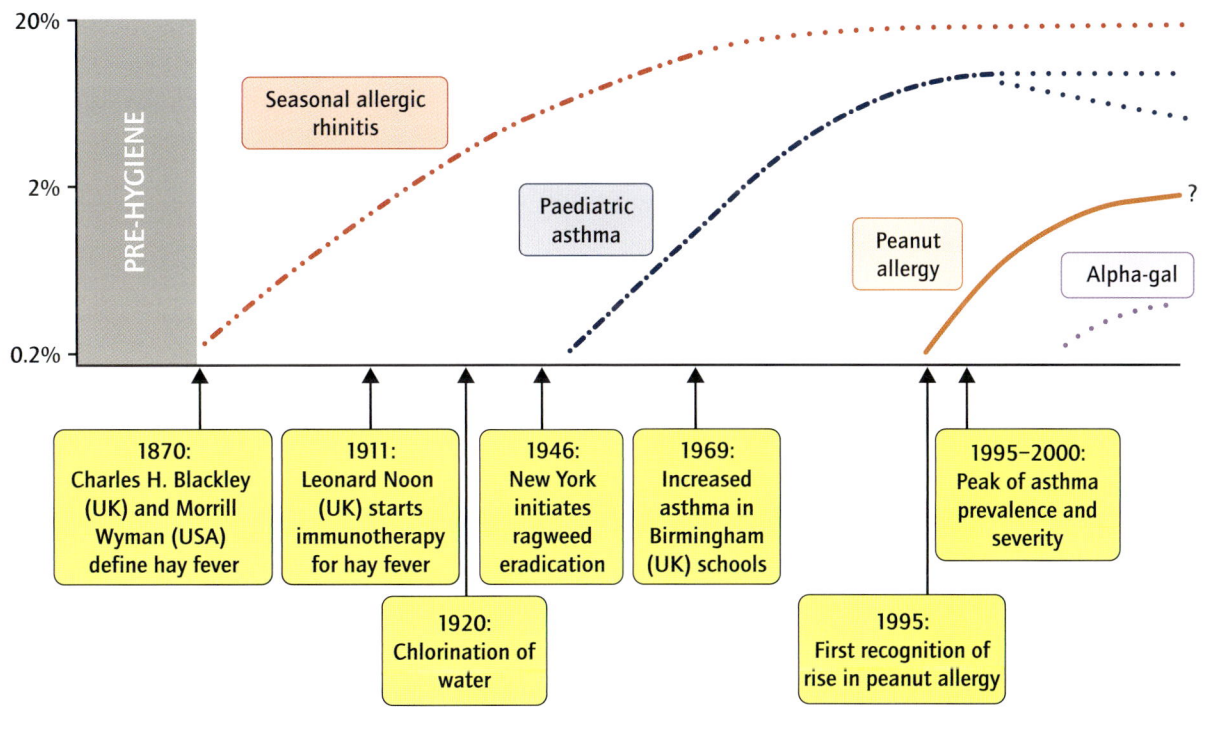

Figure 12.1 The rise of atopic diseases.

currently live our lives needs to change if we are to have any hope of reducing the relentless march towards a 100% incidence of atopy.

12.1.2 Toxins and allergy

Chapter 7 detailed the contribution of environmental toxin exposure to chronic disease, and allergy is no exception. As one might expect, one of the worst forms of toxin exposure in the world today is air pollution. Exposure to traffic-related air pollutants has been implicated in the development, persistence, and exacerbation of asthma.[5]

Environmental chemical exposure is a hidden factor that is often underestimated in allergy. Pesticide exposure – either environmental or occupational – and herbicide exposure have both been linked to a higher incidence of asthma.[6] Toxins can be deleterious each on their own, but what we face in modern lifestyle is a cocktail of toxins, often at quite low levels. One study demonstrated this by showing that exposure to endotoxin – a natural internal toxin, also known as LPS – enhances the respiratory toxicity of phthalates in adults, leading to wheezing and to asthma.[7] Maternal smoking during pregnancy contributes to asthma severity and poor lung function in offspring.[8] Obviously, parents should not smoke around their children. But this study found that even mothers' smoking during pregnancy had an effect, because the toxins absorbed into their bloodstream from the smoke impacted the unborn child.

12.1.3 Barrier function in atopy

Perhaps an even larger issue than toxin exposure is the concept of challenges to healthy barrier function and how they contribute to atopy. The gut barrier is certainly important in preventing the development of allergy. But even more relevant here than the gut barrier is the skin barrier. A malfunction or disruption of the skin barrier is possibly the cause of all forms of atopic allergy. This is the theory known as "atopic march".

> Epidermal barriers face harsh challenges in modern life. Features of current lifestyles, such as frequent bathing and regular use of soap, and living within

concrete jungles with air conditioning that dehumidifies the air, may accelerate sub-cutaneous barrier impairment.[9]

This quote lists some of the challenges to our skin barrier in modern life. These days we are all having one or two showers a day, often using harsh soaps or detergents. One UK dermatologist proposed that the biggest cause of allergy was the many things that are done to damage the skin in babies. This included the frequent washing, the detergents used on the clothes, the detergent used to wash the baby and the creams that were applied (often containing detergents). He was particularly critical of aqueous cream because it contains sodium lauryl sulfate, which strips the protective lipid barrier from the skin. This has been supported by research.[10]

When considering the relationship between barrier and atopy, and particularly the skin barrier, we have contributions from the outside going in damaging the barrier, but we also have contributions from the inside going out.[11] One of the key "inside" factors discovered is defects in a structural protein in the epidermis called filaggrin. Mutation in the filaggrin gene is the most significant risk factor for developing atopic dermatitis. But it also confers risk for food allergy, asthma, and AR. How can that be the case? As mentioned above, this is the theory of atopic march, which suggests that irrespective of the type of atopy, the initial sensitisation to the allergen occurs through the skin. In other words, the baby or child who develops a peanut allergy first gets sensitised by touching the peanuts. We first get sensitised to dust mites by crawling around (as babies do) and being exposed to the dust mite that way.

The atopic march theory really highlights the importance of having a healthy skin barrier and doing those things that support it from an early age. As well as filaggrin, the skin barrier contains lipids including ceramides. It also has tight junctions maintaining its integrity. These are the key components for a healthy skin barrier.

One of the analogies we can use when talking to patients about this is the oilskin jacket. The fabric is like the filaggrin and the tight junctions are the tightness of the weave of that fabric. The oil that makes the jacket impervious to water is the equivalent of the skin lipids, including the ceramides. These three components work together to make the barrier effective against moisture loss (or moisture ingress, if we are talking about a jacket). Hence, an important issue for maintaining skin health is to stop trans-epidermal water loss (TEWL). The skin can dry out and lose its protective nature. Also, skin pH needs to be acidic, so anything alkaline should not be applied to the skin. Skin microbiome alterations can also detrimentally affect the skin barrier.[12]

12.1.3.1 Atopic march

The concept of atopic march is illustrated in **Figure 12.2**.[13] We start with eczema, which peaks in childhood and then declines. This is followed by food allergy, then asthma, and, eventually, allergic rhinitis (AR).

Of the various observations that support the concept of atopic march, one key study will be mentioned here.[15] This investigated children up to one year of age in three monthly groupings and found that the more severe the atopic dermatitis, the greater the likelihood of food allergy.

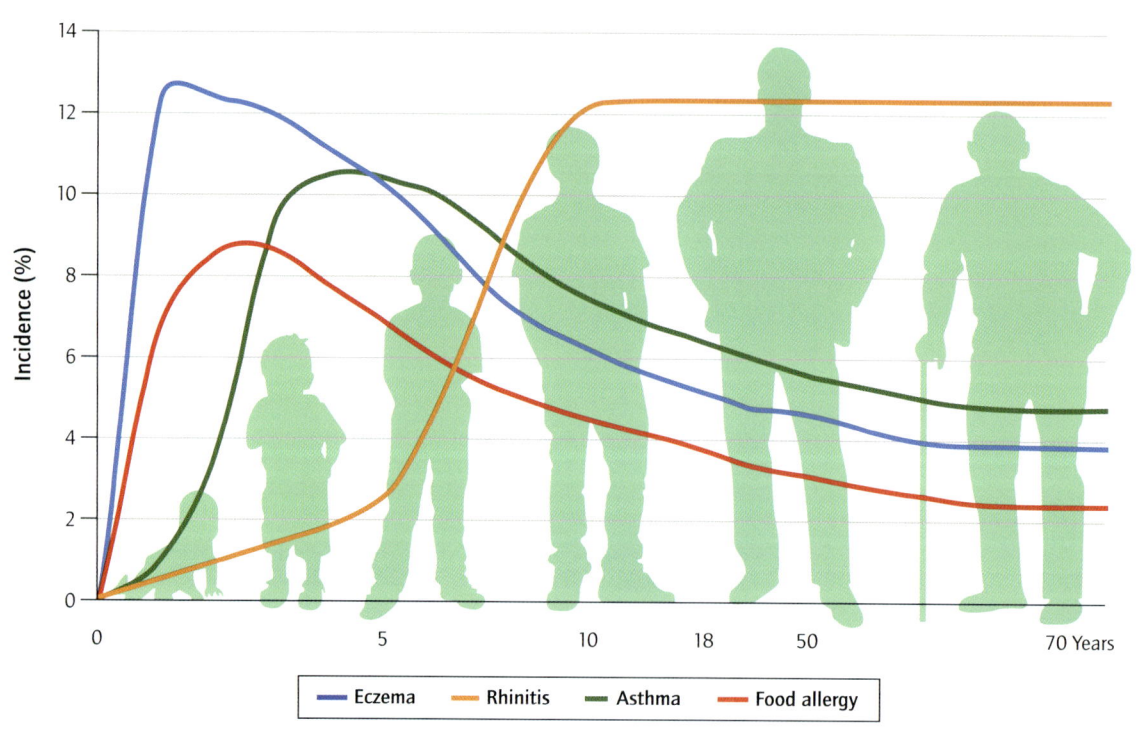

Figure 12.2 The atopic march timeline.[14]

12.1.3.2 Barrier function in AR and asthma

Barrier function is also important in AR and asthma. For example, a clinical trial in AR sufferers found that a drug-free nasal spray – one that forms a barrier on the nasal mucosa – reduced allergic reactions induced by dust mite allergen challenge.[16] This is an example of using an artificial barrier to supplement an impaired barrier.

The following quote from Matzinger concerning the lung barrier in asthma states, very eloquently:

> People have been trying to figure out what is wrong with the immune system in people that become allergic. I think that we have been asking the wrong question . . . rather than looking at the immune system in children who have asthma, we should be looking at their lungs.[17]

In other words, we should shift our focus to the lungs and, particularly, the lung barrier. Factors that can damage the lung barrier include cigarettes, air pollutants, oxidants, viruses, and bacteria.[18] Pseudomonas, which can occur as a chronic lung infection (especially in cystic fibrosis), damages the lung barrier and opens it up to allergen penetration.

The gut barrier is also important in managing allergy. One study found that aberrant (reduced) immunoglobulin A (IgA) responses to gut microbiota during infancy preceded the development of asthma and allergic disease in the first seven years of life.[19] The researchers suggested their findings possibly indicate an impaired gut mucosal barrier function in allergic children.

When aiming to improve any barrier in the body, we need to consider the three key aspects of effective barrier function: the physical barrier, the ecological barrier (microbiome), and the immune barrier.

12.1.4 The hygiene and old friends hypotheses

At this stage it is worth while briefly examining the hygiene hypothesis and how it has been modified into the "old friends" hypothesis. The hygiene hypothesis posited that, essentially due to our obsession with cleanliness and hygiene in modern life, we do not have enough exposure to beneficial microbes as children. As a result, our immune system does not mature in an appropriate manner and becomes more allergy-prone.[20] We now know that the hygiene hypothesis is not entirely correct, but it contains elements of truth.

The hygiene hypothesis was first proposed by Strachan in 1989 to explain some curious observations. Gerard and co-workers had observed, for example, a lower prevalence of allergy in indigenous populations in Northern Canada, compared to urban Caucasian populations. It was proposed that the indigenous people were living more naturally and had higher exposures to various bacterial infections, which helped mature the immune system.

It was not very long before flaws were seen in the hygiene hypothesis. Ultimately this led to the suggestion in 2003 by Graham Rook of a modified perspective, which became known as the "old friends" hypothesis.

Going into more detail about these issues, the early mechanistic understanding of the hygiene hypothesis evolved from an understanding of the functions of helper T cells – specifically, Th1 and Th2. The theory was that that we are born with Th2 responses predominating. Since that promotes antibody production, it potentially predisposes us to allergic responses by the immune system, with IgE production. As we become exposed to bacterial infections throughout early life, our immune response matures, bringing Th1 responses into dominance (as these are more important to fight bacterial infection). This shifts the immune system away from a tendency to allergic responses.

What are the flaws in the hygiene hypothesis? One key flaw is that the Th1/Th2 paradigm is now known to be overly simplistic. For example, Th17 cells are also involved in allergic disease. But, more specifically, the hygiene hypothesis has largely been modified by a recognition of the role of regulatory T cells. These cells prevent immune responses against harmless environmental proteins, which might otherwise be allergens, and also induce peripheral tolerance against self-antigens. Our microbiome plays a key role in their development, as they are particularly expressed in the gut. Their discovery led to the current view, or variant, of the hygiene hypothesis, which is the old friends hypothesis.[21] Acting above the helper T cells, and regulating their responses, are the regulatory T cells.

Hence, the old friends variant of the hygiene hypothesis emphasises the importance of adequate and responsive levels of regulatory T cells (Tregs) that are developed by our exposure to friendly, beneficial bacteria and even worms (the old friends). Old friends particularly comprise the ancient infections, commensal microbiota, and environmental organisms (from animals, soil, plants, and so on). This is elaborated in **Figure 12.3**.

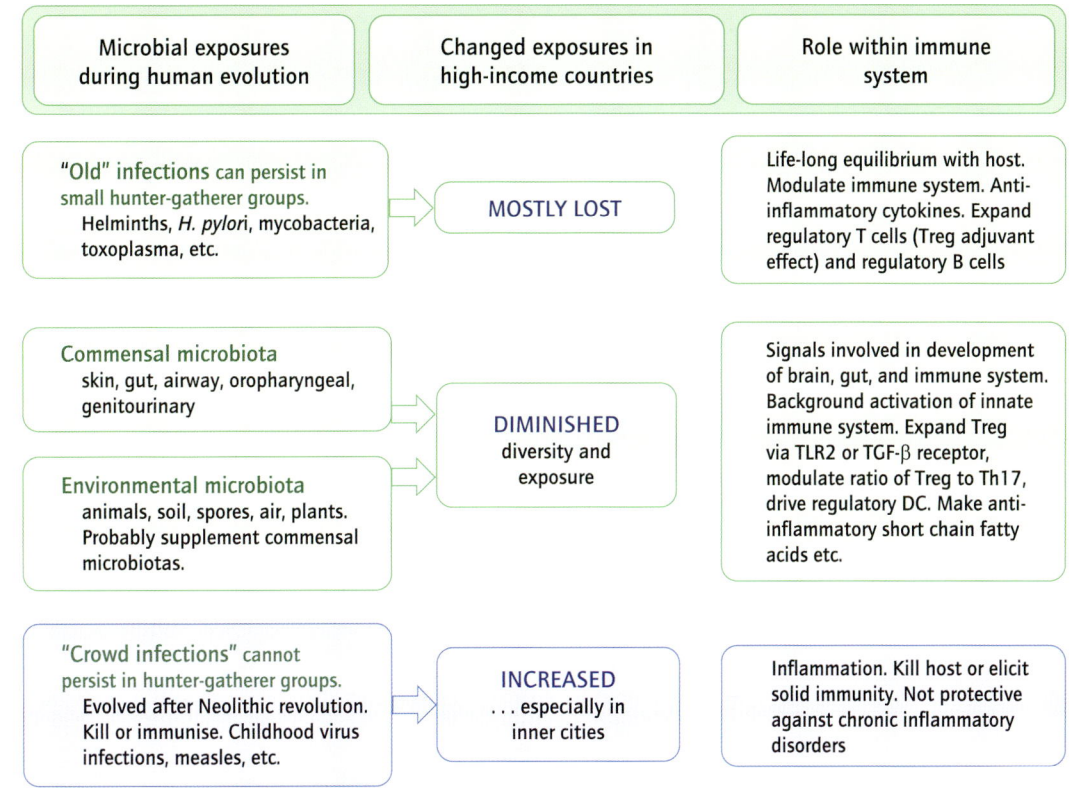

Figure 12.3 The "old friends" variant of the hygiene hypothesis.[22]

There are two critical implications of the old friends hypothesis:

- Adequate exposure to our old friends is needed to enhance Treg level and function.
- Adequate dietary fibre and a balanced gut microbiome is vital, because that also ensures healthy Tregs.

The old friends variant of the hygiene hypothesis also elevates the following to a new importance in allergy:

- digestive health, especially a healthy gut flora and diet
- appropriate processing of dietary proteins, since these are potential allergens

Thus, the bowel flora/barrier protocol (Chapter 8) now has a rational basis in the treatment of all allergic disorders in both children and adults.

12.1.4.1 The hygiene drivers of allergy

Examining now in more detail the principal drivers of the impact of hygiene on allergy incidence, these were clean water, less contaminated food, and helminth eradication. Other, secondary, elements included decreased exposure to farm animals and smaller family sizes.[23] However, the larger context here has been the movement of our way of life away from nature. Relevant lifestyle and medical changes included immunisation, broad-spectrum antibiotics (probably a very significant factor), toxin exposure, and the use of paracetamol (acetaminophen) to treat fever.[24]

But perhaps the most significant factor could be the advent of television, because it decreased outdoor play, decreased physical activity, increased body weight, and possibly even caused changes in breathing patterns while watching television, including a decline in sighs. Changes in the home to increase comfort also played a role, by increasing time indoors, with more exposure to indoor allergens. It is a whole package, a range of lifestyle changes, which the old friends and hygiene hypotheses reflect only in part.[25]

12.1.5 Atopy and our microbiome

Examining briefly the role the microbiome plays in atopy, it is not just a case of focusing on the gut microbiome: the lung microbiome, the nasopharyngeal microbiome, and the skin microbiome are also relevant.[26]

Figure 12.4 outlines some of the significant microbes and related factors and their impact on key immune cells in asthma.

As shown in the figure, the immune system is influenced by our microbiome in a myriad ways, many of which we are only beginning to understand. With respect to asthma, four key areas of microbiome-immune interactions are particularly relevant. Tregs have a critical role in regulating asthma pathogenesis and preventing asthma in healthy individuals, and the microbiome plays a large role in the generation and maintenance of Tregs. Microbial products, particularly short-chain fatty acids (SCFAs), microbe–microbe interactions, and microbial sensing by elements of the immune system all contribute to Treg formation and function. Dendritic cells (DCs) can also play key regulatory roles in the context of asthma. Multiple microbiome-

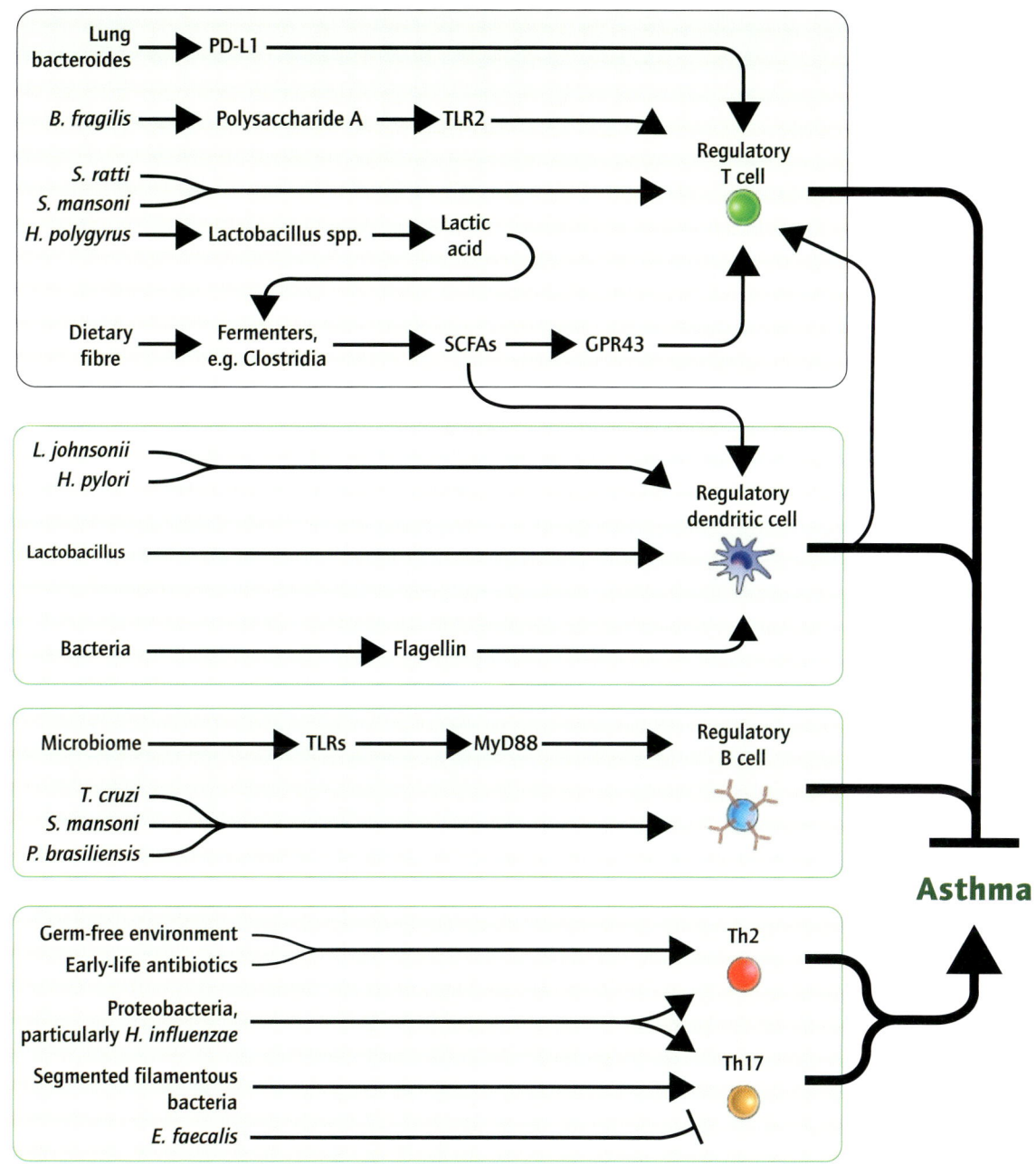

Figure 12.4 Immune microbiome interactions in asthma.[27] [GPR43 = G protein-coupled receptor 43; MyD88 = Myeloid differentiation primary response 88; PD-L1 = programmed death-ligand 1; SCFAs = short chain fatty acids; TLR = toll-like receptor.]

related mechanisms drive regulatory DC formation, including sensing of bacterial products such as flagellin and the production of SCFAs by certain microorganisms. Regulatory DCs may also promote the formation of Tregs. The role of the microbiome in generating regulatory B cells (Bregs) is less clear, but similar mechanisms seem to play a role in this process. Pathogenic Th2 and Th17 immune responses can also be driven by the microbiome. The absence of microorganisms, particularly early in life, can drive a Th2 response to allergen, as in the germ free (GF) mouse. Similarly, early-life antibiotic use can promote Th2 responses. Proteobacteria, particularly *Haemophilus influenzae*, can induce either a Th2 or a Th17 response, depending on the timing of infection. Other specific organisms can either inhibit or promote Th17 responses.

A study showed a strong association between the use of proton pump inhibitors and antibiotics during the first 6 months of life and the subsequent development of allergic disease.[28] The authors' recommendation, after reviewing a vast amount of evidence, was that acid-suppressive medications and antibiotics should be used during infancy only in situations of clear clinical benefit. These drugs probably alter the gut microbiome.

12.1.6 New herbs for atopy

In addition to herbs commonly used for atopy, such as Albizia and Baical skullcap, recent clinical trials have suggested some new options. As a key example, there are four clinical trials of the use of Nigella seed in AR.[29] While doses used varied from 250 to 2,000 mg DHE a day, at least 2,000 mg a day gives the best clinical outcomes. Trials have also shown similar benefits to antihistamine drugs and Montelukast, an immune-modulating drug. Results for the trial of Montelukast versus Nigella in AR are shown in **Table 12.1**.[30]

Referring to the table for the drug, daytime symptom scores improved, eye symptoms were also improved, and eosinophil count dropped. However, night symptoms did not change with the drug. Looking at Nigella, daytime symptom improvements were equal to that of the drug, as was the case for eye symptoms. Night symptom scores actually improved, a result that is better than that of the drug. The eosinophil count also dropped, providing an objective measure of the benefit of Nigella.

Table 12.1 Montelukast versus Nigella in allergic rhinitis[31]

	Study group 1 (Montelukast)			Study group 2 (*N. sativa*)		
	Day 0	Day 7	Day 14	Day 0	Day 7	Day 14
Daytime SS	25.00	19.20 $p < .001$	4.20 $p < .001$	23.86	13.12 $p < .001$	2.90 $p < .001$
Ophthalmic SS	13.6	10.31 $p < .001$	7.60 $p < .001$	13.90	9.63 $p < .001$	2.15 $p < .001$
Night time SS	12.2	12.13 $p < .639$	11.58 $p < .006$	12.98	11.41 $p < .001$	6.32 $p < .001$
EC	8.23	5.16 $p < .029$	4.30 $p < .003$	7.70	4.60 $p < .037$	3.10 $p < .007$

Note. SS = Symptom score; EC = Total eosinophil count (%/mm^3); *p*-values vs pre-treatment Day 0.

In terms of Nigella and asthma, the data from one clinical trial were promising.[32] Results were provided for 1 g and 2 g a day versus placebo. Over the course of the trial, the placebo did show an improvement, but there was a better and a similar improvement for Nigella at both doses, compared to the placebo. The conclusion that might be drawn from this is that either dose was equally effective. However, in terms of the objective measure of forced expiratory volume in one second, this only increased significantly in the higher dose group.

Sulforaphane from broccoli sprouts is providing interesting outcomes in the context of Nrf2 (see Chapter 6) and atopy. A few pharmacological studies have established the proof of principle of Nrf2 herbs acting as barrier-enhancing treatments. Air-pollutant-mediated disruption of the sinonasal epithelial cell barrier function was reversed by activation of the Nrf2 pathway.[33] Mice with Nrf2 deficiency were more sensitive and more likely to develop an asthmatic-type response after chlorine exposure.[34] Also, in another mouse study, Nrf2 activation reduced allergic asthma in mice through an enhanced airway epithelial cytoprotective function.[35]

More important and relevant, though, are the human studies. Sulforaphane improved the bronchoprotective response in asthmatic patients.[36] This was shown to be acting via Nrf2 activation: targets of Nrf2 were upregulated proportionally to the observed bronchoprotective response. A sulforaphane-rich broccoli sprout extract also reduced the nasal allergic response to diesel exhaust particles in humans.[37] We can argue reasonably strongly that the Nrf2 herbs – but especially broccoli sprouts – improve barrier function in general.

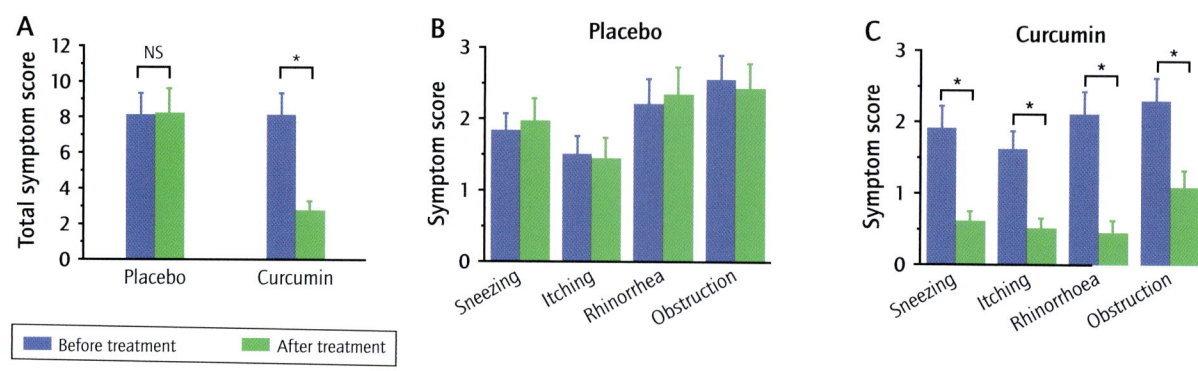

Figure 12.5 Curcumin as an antiallergic phytochemical.[38] RCT ($n = 241$): patients with AR received either placebo or oral curcumin (500 mg/day) for 2 months. Curcumin alleviated nasal symptoms and congestion.

Curcumin is another Nrf2-priming phytochemical that shows antiallergic and anti-inflammatory activity. Results from a recent RCT in AR are provided in **Figure 12.5**.

As can be seen from the figure, overall, symptoms dropped from baseline for treatment with curcumin only, with no change shown by the placebo. This included all the different types of symptoms in AR, such as sneezing, itching, rhinorrhoea, and blockage or obstruction. Curcumin also exerted diverse immunomodulatory effects, including suppression of IL-4, IL-8, and tumour necrosis factor α, and increased production of IL-10.

12.1.7 FHT for atopy

12.1.7.1 FHT for enhancing barriers

Given that the body's barriers each have physical, immune, and ecological components, all three aspects need to be considered as part of any strategy for barrier enhancement.

Relevant herbs are as follows:

- Innate immunity is the key immunological component of body barriers and must be boosted with Echinacea root, Astragalus, and medicinal mushrooms
- Physical barrier integrity can be enhanced in the following ways:
  - for skin, using herbs like gotu kola (topical and internal) and Calendula (topical) and avoiding harsh detergents

- for mucous membranes, anticatarrhal herbs (eyebright, ribwort for upper respiratory, mullein for lower) will improve integrity but, above all, golden seal, the mucous membrane trophorestorative
- cytoprotective herbs: the Nrf2 pathway improves barrier integrity, as detailed above

12.1.7.2 FHT treatment modules for atopy

In terms of FHT for atopy, in addition to the specific herbs indicated for each individual condition, the concept of treatment modules is highly relevant. We know that innate immunity is important, as are healthy barriers. Gut dysbiosis is another important consideration, and we might wish to lower the impact of toxin exposure. How can all this be properly managed, without compromising efficacy? The answer to this conundrum is the FHT concept of treatment modules. A selected module can be applied for a given time period to address a chosen objective and then, depending on the patient response, either continued or changed to a different one.

For example, the bowel flora/barrier protocol (see Chapter 8) can be combined with a high-fibre diet and avoidance of gluten (because of the negative effects of gluten on the barrier). Phellodendron and/or golden seal can be used for weeding in children. This can be applied for 6–10 weeks and then either continued, if progress is still ongoing, or switched to a different treatment module.

Relevant treatment modules for atopy are summarised as follows:

- Bowel flora/barrier protocol ⇒ for 6–10 weeks with a high-fibre diet and no gluten. Continue with just a barrier probiotic and/or slippery elm. Children's variant with Phellodendron and/or golden seal for weeding.
- Lower immune danger with willow bark, bioavailable curcumin, other Nrf2 herbs, and medicinal mushrooms ⇒ for 8 weeks.
- Detoxify with Nrf2 herbs, especially broccoli sprouts, bioavailable curcumin, rosemary, and garlic ⇒ for 8–12 weeks.
- Boost innate immunity with Echinacea root, Astragalus, and medicinal mushrooms ⇒ 8 weeks, or ongoing.

These are the four key treatment modules for atopy. A fifth module, recommended only for asthma, is a barrier protocol that is specific for the lungs (see Section 12.2.4, but also touched on in Section 12.1.7.1).

12.2 FHT and asthma

12.2.1 The asthma mosaic

While it is true to say that asthma in children has peaked in countries like Australia, the worldwide prevalence of asthma is still increasing.[39] By 2025, there will be 100 million people with asthma. Asthma is a mosaic disease that is well suited to the framework of FHT (see **Figure 12.6**).[40]

Since asthma is a mosaic disease, the protective and risk factors at play listed in the figure will vary according to the individual patient. Interestingly,

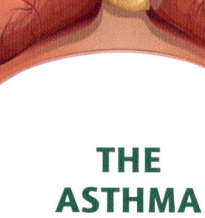

Protective factors

Household:
- Being the younger sibling

Birth and nursing:
- Natural birth
- Breast feeding

Farm living:
- Agriculture
- Pig/cattle farming
- Unpasteurised milk consumption
- Constant stay in animal sheds
- Silage

Microbiological exposures:
- Diverse and healthy microbiota (including members of the FLVR groups)
- Foodborne pathogens (e.g.: HAV, *H. pylori*)
- High burden helminth infections (e.g.: *A. lumbricoides*, *T. trichiura*)

Higher socioeconomic status:
- Better access to doctors/treatments
- Increased education level
- Lower stress

Other environmental factors:
- Healthy diet
- Low pollution rates
- Exercise

THE ASTHMA MOSAIC

Risk factors

Household:
- Asthma history in the family

Birth and nursing:
- Caesarean section
- Formula feeding

Farm living:
- Sheep farming
- Pressed or loose hay

Urban living:
- Altered dietary practices
- Community associated infections

Microbiological exposures:
- Dysbiotic microbiota
- Respiratory viral infections (e.g.: RV, RSV)
- Bacterial pathogens (e.g.: *M. catarrhalis*, *S. pneumoniae*)
- Lower burden helminth infections (e.g.: *T. canis*)

Lower socioeconomic status:
- Increased smoking rates
- Higher stress

Other environmental factors:
- Smoking
- Obesity
- Use of antibiotics

Figure 12.6 The asthma mosaic: protective and risk factors.[41] [HAV = hepatitis A virus; FLVR = four bacterial genera, *Faecalibacterium*, *Lachnospira*, *Rothia*, and *Veillonella*; RV = rhinovirus; RSV = respiratory syncytial virus.]

mainstream research is now recognising that individuals can have different pictures of asthma. The terms *endotype* and *phenotype* have been adopted to describe, respectively, the classes of this individual causation and expression (see Section 12.2.2).

Asthma has been defined as a chronic inflammatory disorder of the airways characterised by:[42]

- variable and recurring respiratory symptoms
- airflow limitation or obstruction
- bronchial hyper-responsiveness

In other words, the key issues are acute inflammation, which causes the acute attacks, and chronic inflammation – with nonspecific airway hyper-reactivity – that drives the underlying disease. Eventually, especially in certain phenotypes, airway remodelling leads to a persistent airflow obstruction and subsequent reinforcement of the chronicity of the disease.

If we look at histological samples from asthmatic lungs, we find that there is a host of indicators of chronic inflammation involving a range of inflammatory cells releasing a plethora of inflammatory mediators,[43] all leading to the classic histological findings of microvascular leakage, mucus hypersecretion, bronchoconstriction, and airway hyper-reactivity that you see in asthma. Hence, asthma is clearly a multifactorial mosaic disease, in terms of both the factors that drive its development and the many cells and inflammatory mediators that are involved its pathology and perpetuate its chronicity.

It should come as no surprise, then, that a group of authors recently asserted that targeting a single molecule or pathway in asthma benefits very few patients.[44] Unfortunately, that is still the trend in modern drug research for asthma. Pharmaceutical research is constantly looking for smart drugs for asthma that will target this or that pathway, typically using antibodies or receptor blockers. But what the above authors are suggesting is that this is a costly and, ultimately, a futile endeavour. They posit that the findings from multiple lines of research confirm not only that the pathogenesis of severe asthma is variable between patients (so if you have a smart drug that just targets one pathway, it will be ineffective for those people for whom that pathway is not relevant), but, even more importantly, that each molecular defect or imbalance on its own is likely to contribute little in each patient. This paper tends to validate the FHT approach to asthma, and we can even boldly assert that such a multifactorial approach is more evidence-based in this context than is current mainstream medicine.

12.2.2 Endotype and phenotype in the asthma mosaic

As alluded to above, there is a recognition now that there are two types of asthma patients in terms of the main inflammatory cell involved (the endotype):[45] either the classical Th2-driven asthma, involving eosinophils as the main inflammatory cell, or the more newly recognised Th17-driven asthma, involving neutrophils.

Specifically, for Th2-driven eosinophilic asthma, the airway space becomes dominated by eosinophils and Th2 cells, with more of these cells also found within the lung tissue. Plasma cells are also present and are responsible for the production of allergen-specific IgE. For Th17-driven neutrophilic asthma, the dominant cell types are the Th17 cells and the neutrophils they recruit. Eosinophils, Th2 cells, and IgE are absent. Other cell types, including B cells, mast cells, and basophils, may also be present, depending on the endotype.

In other words, the Th2 endotype is more allergic, while the Th17 endotype is more inflammatory. They do both have aspects of inflammation, but the Th17 endotype is primarily inflammatory. You may have come across this distinction in the past, labelled with terms "extrinsic" and "intrinsic" asthma, respectively. In order to achieve the optimal benefit from herbal treatments, it is important that herbal clinicians identify these endotypes in patients.

Endotype describes what is happening at the cellular level. The phenotype is how this is expressed in a person in terms of symptoms and clinical characteristics.[46] Various ways of phenotyping asthma have been proposed. For example, one approach is in terms of the airway response: either a remodelling phenotype or an inflammatory phenotype. Even better is the classification table from the advanceweb website (see **Table 12.2**).[47]

In terms of phenotypes, as can be seen in the table, each endotype is assigned three phenotypes, making six phenotypes in all. Some of these can obviously be diagnosed by the patient's history, but the neutrophilic type is best confirmed by a sputum analysis. Does phenotyping for asthma inform FHT choices? Yes, it definitely does (see later in this chapter).

Table 12.2 Endotype versus phenotype in asthma[48]

Endotype	Phenotype	Clinical features	Pathobiology and biomarkers
Th2 asthma	early onset allergic	allergic symptoms and comorbidities	specific ; Th2 cytokines, thick subbasement membrane
	late onset eosinophilic	sinusitis, less allergic	corticosteroid-refractory eosinophilia; IL-5
	exercise-induced	mild, intermittent with exercise	mast-cell activation; Th2 cytokines
Non-Th2 asthma	obesity-related (late-onset)	primarily women, very symptomatic	oxidative stress
	neutrophilic	low FEV1	sputum neutrophilia, Th17 pathway, IL-8
	smoking-related	passive or active smoking, deteriorating FEV1	decreased FeNO

Note. FeNO = fractional exhaled nitric oxide; FEV1 = forced expiratory volume in 1 second.

12.2.3 Herbs and asthma

Moving on to an examination of herbal treatments for asthma, we should begin with the *British Herbal Pharmacopeia* (1983), which shows the Western herbs traditionally indicated for asthma (see **Table 12.3**).[49] The first observation we can make is that several of these herbs are difficult to access now, either because of regulatory restriction or because they have gone out of favour. But two key herbs still widely used today – Euphorbia and Grindelia – are described as spasmolytic and expectorant. While these are very important actions in asthma, the suggested approach is incomplete. As highlighted in the introduction to this chapter, we are now much better informed about what we can use, so while this information is still important, it misses the mosaic of all those complex factors.

From both traditional and biomedical sources, the key pieces in the asthma mosaic can be listed as follows:[50]

- gut, oral, sinus, and lung microbiome
- gut and respiratory barrier
- internal and external toxins, and immune danger
- chronic, unresolving inflammation and oxidative damage
- imbalanced immune responses
- overactive allergic responses
- poor digestive function
- gastro-oesophageal reflux
- chronic rhinosinusitis (mostly nonallergic and/or aspirin-sensitive asthma)
- mucus-forming diet and salt intake (barrier)
- exacerbating infections, especially viral infections in children
- stress and hormonal issues

A mucus-forming diet does play a role (although this is controversial in mainstream thinking). Such a diet includes mainly dairy intake (from any animal), but gluten and other factors such as dietary salt intake may also play a part. Dietary salt impairs the respiratory barrier. I can still remember the naturopathy classes I attended in the 1970s, when I was studying in Melbourne at the Southern School. Lecturer Alf Jacka highlighted the importance of reducing salt in a person's diet if they were asthmatic or suffered from hay fever. We now understand that as a barrier issue.

What is the role of gastro-oesophageal reflux in asthma? It has been suggested that acid causes irritation in the lower oesophagus, which promotes

Table 12.3   Major herbs for asthma according to the BHP 1983

Herb	Action
Datura	spasmolytic
Drosera	bronchodilator, expectorant
Ephedra	bronchodilator (antiallergic)
Euphorbia	spasmolytic, expectorant
Grindelia	antispasmodic, expectorant
Lobelia	spasmolytic, expectorant
Polygala	expectorant, diaphoretic
Urginea	expectorant

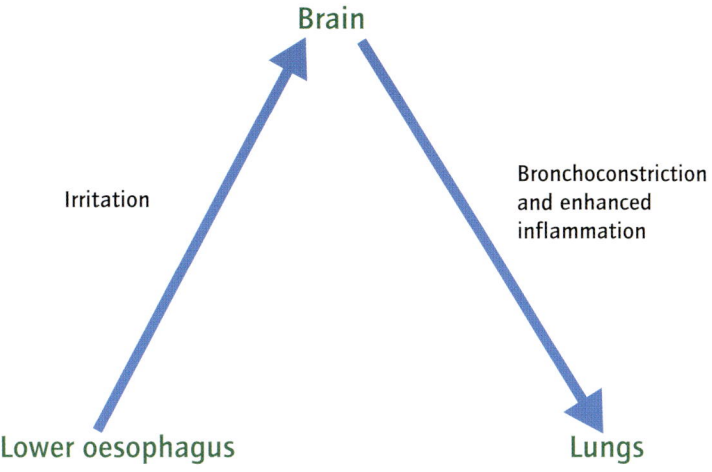

Figure 12.7 A vagal reflex.

a reflex carried by the vagus nerve to the brain and back to the lungs (see **Figure 12.7**).

This results in a reflex bronchoconstriction and enhanced inflammation. Herbal clinicians have understood this reflex for a long time, because they have employed it in the reverse aspect over the centuries: by soothing the stomach and lower oesophagus with demulcent herbs that, then, by reflex, initiate a soothing and anti-inflammatory effect in the lungs (see **Figure 12.8**). This phenomenon is known as reflex demulcency.

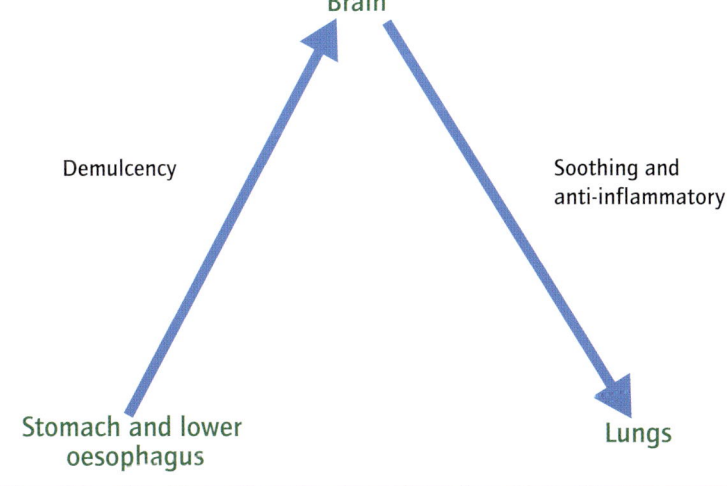

Figure 12.8 Reflex demulcency

Hence, any chronic asthmatic patient, especially one with a persistent cough, should be assessed for reflux (and it might be silent reflux). The key treatment should, then, contain demulcent herbs.

12.2.3.1 Clinical aside

A patient has suffered an acute respiratory viral infection and is coughing repeatedly, even after having largely recovered. The infection is gone, but the cough persists for weeks afterwards. One reason behind this is that the coughing has weakened the lower oesophageal sphincter, and the person is experiencing silent reflux. Every time they lie down, the reflux stimulates those pathways described above. A good way to stop this is a herbal demulcent mix. One example is meadowsweet, licorice (high in glycyrrhizin), and marshmallow root glycetract in a ratio 15:15:70. The dose is 4 mL, taken undiluted as often as is required.

A longstanding patient developed a viral infection and had a very bad persistent cough for weeks afterwards, to the point where she could not sleep. In a consultation focused on other issues, this was mentioned only because I inquired about her sleep. I proposed a trial of the above formula. Her response was:

"Oh, Kerry, I've been going to you for ages and I really trust you as a therapist, but you're wasting my time because I've tried everything. I've been to my doctor, I've asked the pharmacist, I've literally tried everything, and nothing has worked."

My response was to offer it at no charge, and when she returned a month later, her opening words were:

"Oh, by the way, I have to apologise to you. It worked from the first dose and I slept very well."

12.2.3.2 Herbal clinical trials in asthma

There have been relatively few clinical trials of herbs for asthma. Earlier trials on Ginkgo show its value due to inhibition of platelet activating factor (PAF), one of the inflammatory factors implicated in asthma.[51] In one early clinical trial using Boswellia for asthma, it is shown to be particularly useful for exercise-induced asthma.[52] More recently, a trial using *Pelargonium sidoides* root extract for 5 days prevented asthma attacks during upper respiratory viral infections in children.[53]

12.2.4 Developing FHT protocols for asthma

When treating an asthma patient using FHT guidelines, we first need to look at environment and lifestyle, and that begins with diet.[54] The diet should be low in inflammatory impact – hence for example, fried food should be avoided. Also, the diet should be lower in omega-6 fatty acids, high in fibre, and, obviously, should avoid key allergens (gluten, dairy). Breathing techniques are important – such as, for example, the Buteyko method. Yoga also has valuable breathing techniques. Air quality improvement is vital, and this can be achieved with the use of high-quality air filters that remove allergens and fine particulate matter. Home allergen elimination should be addressed: this includes dust mite, mould, cockroaches, and certain pets.

Moving on to herbal strategies, **Table 12.4** lists the FHT goals, actions, and key herbs for asthma. The key herbs for asthma and reasons for their use are outlined in **Table 12.5**.

The key treatment modules in asthma are as follows:

1. bowel flora/barrier protocol with a high-fibre diet and no gluten ⇒ for 6–8 weeks
2. immune danger ↓ with willow bark, bioavailable curcumin, Nrf2 herbs, and medicinal mushrooms ⇒ for 8 weeks
3. detoxify with Nrf2 herbs, especially broccoli sprouts, bioavailable curcumin, rosemary, and garlic ⇒ for 8–12 weeks
4. innate immunity ↑ with Echinacea root, Astragalus, and medicinal mushrooms ⇒ 8 weeks or ongoing
5. lung barrier ↑ with golden seal, mullein, and expectorant herbs ⇒ 8 weeks or ongoing

Table 12.6 illustrates how phenotyping can inform FHT asthma strategies. Together, Tables 12.4, 12.5, and 12.6 can be used to translate the required herbal actions into the most effective herb selections. The above treatment modules can also be selected, as dictated by the case.

Table 12.4 FHT goals, actions, and key herbs for asthma

Goal	Required actions	Herbs
Control the allergic response	antiallergic	▹ Baical skullcap, Albizia, Nigella
Control acute respiratory infection	diaphoretic, immune enhancing, etc.	▹ Echinacea, Andrographis, ginger, yarrow, etc.
Reduce inflammation	anti-inflammatory, reflex demulcent	▹ Ginkgo, Bupleurum, turmeric, marshmallow root, Boswellia
Clear the airways	expectorant	▹ Elecampane, fennel, Adhatoda
Relax bronchial smooth muscle	bronchospasmolytic	▹ Elecampane, Grindelia, Coleus
Allay debilitating cough	expectorant, demulcent, antitussive	▹ Elecampane, marshmallow root, Bupleurum, licorice
Treat sinusitis	anticatarrhal, antiallergic, immune enhancing, etc.	▹ eyebright, Andrographis, golden seal, golden rod
Increase gastric acid	bitter tonic, digestive	▹ gentian, Andrographis
Control reflux	antispasmodic, demulcent, antacid, mucoprotective	▹ meadowsweet, marshmallow root, licorice
Eliminate infection	immune enhancing, antiviral, antibacterial	▹ Echinacea root, Andrographis
Reduce the physical effects of stress	adaptogen	▹ Astragalus, Siberian ginseng
Reduce anxiety and tension	sedative and nervine tonic	▹ valerian, St John's wort, kava
Boost the hypothalamic-pituitary-adrenal axis	tonic, adrenal tonic	▹ Withania, Rehmannia, licorice
Balance immunity	immune modifying, immune depressant	▹ Echinacea root, Hemidesmus,
Improve cytoprotection and barrier	Nrf2 priming healing	▹ Ginkgo, rosemary, turmeric, grape seed, gotu kola
Improve the health of mucous membranes	anticatarrhal, mucous membrane trophorestorative, lymphatic, depurative	▹ eyebright, golden seal, mullein

Table 12.5 Key herbs and their beneficial qualities for asthma

Herb	Action
▹ Nigella ▹ Baical skullcap ▹ Albizia	antiallergic; anti-inflammatory
▹ bioavailable curcumin	anti-inflammatory; detox; Nrf2
▹ Ginkgo ▹ Boswellia	anti-inflammatory
▹ Echinacea root ▹ Pelargonium	balance immunity
▹ willow bark	anti-inflammatory; lower immune danger
▹ medicinal mushrooms	boost innate immunity, dectin-1 effects
▹ Adhatoda ▹ Elecampane	dilate airways; clear lungs
▹ broccoli sprouts	Nrf2 effects; boost barrier; detox

Table 12.6 Targeting phenotype in asthma

Phenotype	Action
Early onset/allergic	antiallergic, anti-inflammatory, immunity
Late onset/eosinophilic	antiallergic, anti-inflammatory, sinus, ↑ barrier, stealth pathogens?
Exercise-induced	antiallergic, anti-inflammatory, ↑ barrier
Obesity/late onset	weight loss, ↑ Nrf2, anti-inflammatory
Neutrophilic	↑ air quality, ↑ barrier, immunity, anti-inflammatory, stealth pathogens?
Smoking-related, air pollution	↓ exposure, ↑ barrier, detox, ↑ Nrf2

12.3 Allergic rhinitis

Allergic rhinitis (AR), or hay fever, is characterised by sneezing, nasal pruritus, airflow obstruction, and a mostly clear nasal discharge.[55] It is caused by IgE-mediated reactions against inhaled allergens and involves mucosal inflammation driven by Th2 cells. Key allergens include seasonal pollens and perennial indoor allergens: dust mites, pets, pests, and some moulds.

Sensitisation to indoor allergens usually precedes sensitisation to pollens. Viral respiratory infections occur frequently in young children, so it can be difficult to diagnose AR in the first 2 or 3 years of life. The prevalence of AR peaks at 20–50 years then gradually diminishes.

AR is a systemic allergic disease associated with numerous multi-morbid disorders. The co-morbidities of AR overlap substantially with asthma (the unified airway concept).[56] Hence, in the case of patients with AR and asthma, we must treat both, not just the one or the other, because asthma feeds the AR, and, more particularly, the AR feeds the asthma. The association between asthma and rhinitis has been recognised since the pioneering study by Brydon, which showed that the majority of 1,000 asthmatics also had rhinitis, which preceded the asthma in 45% of cases. Other comorbidities of AR include eczema, food allergies, eosinophilic oesophagitis, conjunctivitis, chronic middle ear effusions, rhinosinusitis, adenoid hypertrophy, olfaction disorders, obstructive sleep apnoea, and disordered sleep.[57]

12.3.1 Barrier and other causative factors in AR

The skin barrier hypothesis (atopic march), immune system issues, barrier issues with the nasal mucosa, and a host of environmental factors, including exposure to allergens and noxious inhalants, are all relevant in the cause and progression of AR. In terms of genetic factors, the filaggrin gene is one of the risk factors that has been highlighted (in connection with the atopic march theory). **Figure 12.9** outlines key factors behind the development and chronicity of AR.[58]

As mentioned above, barrier integrity has been proposed as an important factor in protecting against AR. Barrier-enforcing measures, as achieved by nasal administrations of cellulose powder and microemulsions, have been shown to have symptom-reducing effects in AR.[59] One of the key issues thought to damage the respiratory barrier in AR is air pollution. Again, the value of having a home air filter – for example, for clearing diesel exhaust particles that are damaging to the mucosa – should be emphasised. Mast cells are deep in the upper respiratory mucosa and hence will not react to inhaled allergens unless the barrier is damaged.

Figure 12.10 provides a schematic diagram of diesel exhaust particle (DEP)-induced tight junction (TJ) disruption and resultant exacerbation

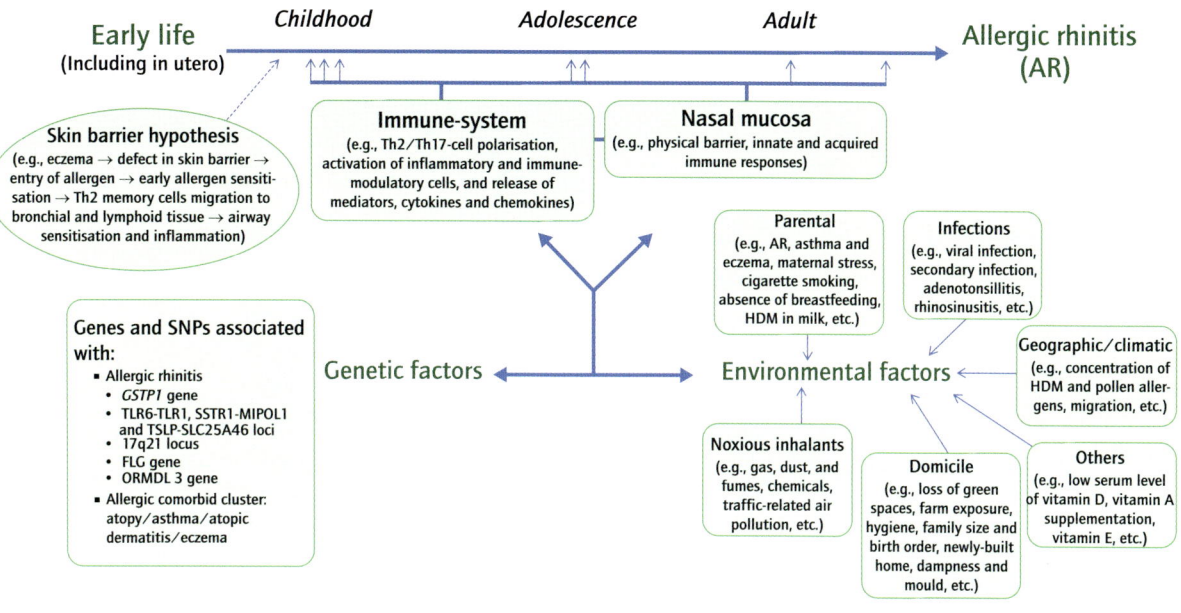

Figure 12.9 Recent developments in the AR mosaic. [HDM = house dust mite; FLG = filaggrin; SNPs = single nucleotide polymorphisms.]

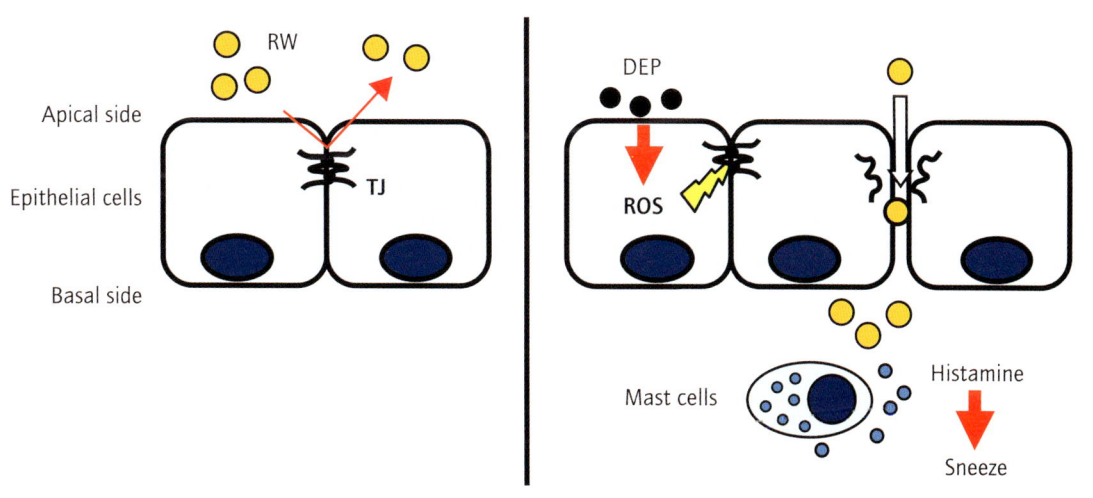

Figure 12.10 Barrier disruption in AR.[60] [DEP = diesel exhaust particle; ROS = reactive oxygen species; RW = ragweed pollen; TJ = tight junction.]

of AR. Without DEP exposure, the penetration of allergens is prevented by the TJ barrier. Nasal TJ are disrupted by reactive oxygen species production when nasal mucosa are exposed to DEP. This disruption allows allergens to penetrate into the subepithelial tissue, resulting in increased inflammation and sneezing.

12.3.2 Developing FHT protocols for AR

For AR management, in terms of environment and lifestyle, the diet should be low in inflammatory activity (as outlined for asthma above). Ensure adequate exercise, saline nasal irrigation, air quality improvement with potential use of air filters, and home allergen elimination: dust mite, mould, cockroaches, cats.

Key herbs and reasons for using for AR are outlined in **Table 12.7**. The treatment modules provided for atopy are also relevant to any FHT strategy for this disorder.

Table 12.7 Key herbs and corresponding actions for allergic rhinitis

Herb	Action
▹ Nigella ▹ Baical skullcap ▹ Albizia ▹ nettle leaf	anti-allergic, anti-inflammatory
▹ bioavailable curcumin	anti-inflammatory, Nrf2, detox
▹ Echinacea root ▹ Astragalus	balance immunity
▹ willow bark	anti-inflammatory, ↓ immune danger
▹ medicinal mushrooms	↑ innate immunity, dectin-1 effects
▹ golden seal ▹ eyebright ▹ ribwort	↑ upper respiratory barrier
▹ broccoli sprouts	Nrf2, ↑ barrier, detox

References

1. Burbank AJ, Sood AK, et al. Environmental determinants of allergy and asthma in early life. *J Allergy Clin Immunol*. 2017 Jul; **140**(1): 1–12. doi:10.1016/j.jaci.2017.05.010. PMID: 28673399.
2. Platts-Mills TA. The allergy epidemics: 1870–2010. *J Allergy Clin Immunol*. 2015 Jul; **136**(1): 3–13. doi:10.1016/j.jaci.2015.03.048. PMID: 26145982.
3. Cabezas-Cruz A, Hodžić A, Román-Carrasco P, et al. Environmental and molecular drivers of the α-gal syndrome. *Front Immunol*. 2019 May 31; **10**: 1210. doi:10.3389/fimmu.2019.01210.
4. Platts-Mills TA. The allergy epidemics: 1870–2010. *J Allergy Clin Immunol*. 2015 Jul; **136**(1): 3–13. doi:10.1016/j.jaci.2015.03.048. PMID: 26145982.
5. Brandt EB, Myers JM, Ryan PH, et al. Air pollution and allergic diseases. *Curr Opin Pediatr*. 2015 Dec; **27**(6): 724–735. doi:10.1097/MOP.0000000000000286. PMID: 26474340.
6. Mostafalou S, Abdollahi M. Pesticides: an update of human exposure and toxicity. *Arch Toxicol*. 2017 Feb; **91**(2): 549–599. doi:10.1007/s00204-016-1849-x. PMID: 27722929.
7. Strassle PD, Smit LAM, Hoppin JA. Endotoxin enhances respiratory effects of phthalates in adults: results from NHANES 2005–6. Environ Res. 2018 Apr; **162**: 280–286. doi:10.1016/j.envres.2018.01.017. PMID: 29407759.
8. Brown SW, Liu B, Taioli E. The relationship between tobacco smoke exposure and airflow obstruction in US children: analysis of the National Health and Nutrition Examination Survey (2007–2012). *Chest*. 2018 Mar; **153**(3): 630–637. doi:10.1016/j.chest.2017. PMID: 29037529.
9. Kubo A, Nagao K, Amagai M. Epidermal barrier dysfunction and cutaneous sensitization in atopic diseases. *J Clin Invest*. 2012 Feb; **122**(2): 440–447. doi:10.1172/JCI57416. PMID: 22293182. [p 440]
10. Tsang M, Guy RH. Effect of aqueous cream BP on human stratum corneum in vivo. *Br J Dermatol*. 2010; **163**(5): 954–958. doi:10.1111/j.1365-2133.2010.09954.x.
11. Czarnowicki T, Krueger JG, Guttman-Yassky E. Novel concepts of prevention and treatment of atopic dermatitis through barrier and immune manipulations with implications for the atopic march. *J Allergy Clin Immunol*. 2017 Jun; **139**(6): 1723–1734. doi:10.1016/j.jaci.2017.04.004. PMID: 28583445.
12. Shaker M, Murray RGP, Mann JA. The ins and outs of an "outside-in' view of allergies: atopic dermatitis and allergy prevention. *Curr Opin Pediatr*. 2018; **30**(4): 576–581. doi:10.1097/MOP.0000000000000646.
13. Czarnowicki T, Krueger JG, Guttman-Yassky E. Novel concepts of prevention and treatment of atopic dermatitis through barrier and immune manipulations with implications for the atopic march. *J Allergy Clin Immunol*. 2017 Jun; **139**(6): 1723–1734. doi:10.1016/j.jaci.2017.04.004. PMID: 28583445.
14. *Ibid*.
15. Lowe AJ, Leung DYM, et al. The skin as a target for prevention of the atopic march. *Ann Allergy Asthma Immunol*. 2018 Feb; **120**(2): 145–151. doi:10.1016/j.anai.2017.11.023. PMID: 29413338.
16. Stoelzel K, Bothe G, Chong PW, Lenarz M. Safety and efficacy of Nasya/Prevalin in reducing symptoms of allergic rhinitis. *Clin Respir J*. 2014; **8**(4): 382–390. doi:10.1111/crj.12080.
17. Matzinger P. The evolution of the danger theory. Interview by Lauren Constable, Commissioning Editor. *Expert Rev Clin Immunol*. 2012 May; **8**(4): 311–317. doi:10.1586/eci.12.21. PMID: 22607177. [p 315]

18. Gon Y, Hashimoto S. Role of airway epithelial barrier dysfunction in pathogenesis of asthma. *Allergol Int.* 2018 Jan; **67**(1): 12–17. doi:10.1016/j.alit.2017.08.011. PMID: 28941636.
19. Dzidic M, Abrahamsson TR, Artacho A, et al. Aberrant IgA responses to the gut microbiota during infancy precede asthma and allergy development. *J Allergy Clin Immunol.* 2017 Mar; **139**(3): 1017–1025. doi:10.1016/j.jaci.2016.06.047. PMID: 27531072.
20. Stiemsma LT, Reynolds LA, et al. The hygiene hypothesis: current perspectives and future therapies. *Immunotargets Ther.* 2015 Jul 27; **4**: 143–157. doi:10.2147/ITT.S61528. PMID: 27471720.
21. Rook GA. The hygiene hypothesis and the increasing prevalence of chronic inflammatory disorders. *Trans R Soc Trop Med Hyg.* 2007 Nov; **101**(11): 1072–1074. doi.10.1016/j.trstmh.2007.05.014. PMID: 17619029.
22. Rook GA, Lowry CA, Raison CL. Hygiene and other early childhood influences on the subsequent function of the immune system. *Brain Res.* 2015 Aug 18; 1617: 47–62. doi:10.1016/j.brainres.2014.04.004. PMID: 24732404.
23. Platts-Mills TA. The allergy epidemics: 1870–2010. *J Allergy Clin Immunol.* 2015 Jul; **136**(1): 3–13. doi:10.1016/j.jaci.2015.03.048. PMID: 26145982.
24. *Ibid.*
25. *Ibid.*
26. Lambrecht BN, Hammad H. The immunology of the allergy epidemic and the hygiene hypothesis. *Nat Immunol.* 2017 Sep 19; **18**(10): 1076–1083. doi:10.1038/ni.3829. PMID: 28926539.
27. Adami AJ, Bracken SJ. Breathing better through bugs: asthma and the microbiome. *Yale J Biol Med.* 2016 Sep 30; **89**(3): 309–324. PMID: 27698615.
28. Mitre E, Susi A, Kropp LE, Schwartz DJ, Gorman GH, Nylund CM. Association between use of acid-suppressive medications and antibiotics during infancy and allergic diseases in early childhood. *JAMA Pediatr.* 2018 Jun 4; **172**(6): e180315. doi:10.1001/jamapediatrics.2018.0315. PMID: 29610864.
29. Morgan M. Major therapeutic activity of Nigella seed. *A Phytotherapist's Perspective.* 2012; **153**: 1–3. Available from: https://mediherb.com.au
30. Ansari MA, Ansari NA, Junejo SA. Montelukast versus *Nigella sativa* for management of seasonal allergic rhinitis: a single blind comparative clinical trial. *Pak J Med Sci.* 2010; **26**(2): 249–254. Available from: http://www.pjms.com.pk/issues/aprjun2010/pdf/article01.pdf
31. *Ibid.*
32. Salem AM, Bamosa AO, Qutub HO, et al. Effect of *Nigella sativa* supplementation on lung function and inflammatory mediators in partly controlled asthma: a randomized controlled trial. *Ann Saudi Med.* 2017 Jan–Feb; **37**(1): 64–71. doi:10.5144/0256-4947.2017.64. PMID: 28151459.
33. London NR Jr, Tharakan A, Rule AM, et al. Air pollutant-mediated disruption of sinonasal epithelial cell barrier function is reversed by activation of the Nrf2 pathway. *J Allergy Clin Immunol.* 2016 Dec; **138**(6): 1736–1738. doi:10.1016/j.jaci.2016.06.027. PMID: 27576127.
34. Ano S, Panariti A, Allard B, et al. Inflammation and airway hyperresponsiveness after chlorine exposure are prolonged by Nrf2 deficiency in mice. *Free Radic Biol Med.* 2017 Jan; 102: 1–15. doi:10.1016/j.freeradbiomed.2016.11.017. PMID: 27847240.
35. Sussan TE, Gajghate S, Chatterjee S, et al. Nrf2 reduces allergic asthma in mice through enhanced airway epithelial cytoprotective function. *Am J Physiol Lung Cell Mol Physiol.* 2015 Jul 1; **309**(1): L27–36. doi:10.1152/ajplung.00398.2014. PMID: 25957295.
36. Brown RH, Reynolds C, Brooker A, et al. Sulforaphane improves the bronchoprotective

response in asthmatics through Nrf2-mediated gene pathways. *Respir Res.* 2015 Sep 15; **16**: 106. doi:10.1186/s12931-015-0253-z. PMID: 26369337.
37. Heber D, Li Z, Garcia-Lloret M, et al. Sulforaphane-rich broccoli sprout extract attenuates nasal allergic response to diesel exhaust particles. *Food Funct.* 2014 Jan; **5**(1): 35–41. doi:10.1039/c3fo60277. PMID: 24287881.
38. Wu S, Xiao D. Effect of curcumin on nasal symptoms and airflow in patients with perennial allergic rhinitis. *Ann Allergy Asthma Immunol.* 2016 Dec; **117**(6): 697–702. doi:10.1016/j.anai.2016.09.427. PMID: 27789120.
39. Loftus PA, Wise SK. Epidemiology of asthma. *Curr Opin Otolaryngol Head Neck Surg.* 2016 Jun; **24**(3): 245–249. PMID: 26977741.
40. van Tilburg BE, Arrieta MC. Hygiene hypothesis in asthma development: is hygiene to blame? *Arch Med Res.* 2017 Dec 7; **48**(8): 717–726. doi:10.1016/j.arcmed.2017.11.009. PMID: 29224909.
41. Ibid.
42. Bousquet J, Jeffery PK, et al. Asthma. From bronchoconstriction to airways inflammation and remodeling. *Am J Respir Crit Care Med.* 2000 May; **161**(5): 1720–1745. doi.10.1164/ajrccm.161.5.9903102. PMID: 10806180.
43. Bone KM, Mills SY. *Principles and Practice of Phytotherapy: Modern Herbal Medicine*, 2nd ed. Elsevier, UK, 2013, pp 250–260.
44. Chang A, Bossé Y. Targeting single molecules in asthma benefits few. *Trends Mol Med.* 2016 Nov; **22**(11): 935–945. PMID: 27692867.
45. Adami AJ, Bracken SJ. Breathing better through bugs: asthma and the microbiome. *Yale J Biol Med.* 2016 Sep 30; **89**(3): 309–324. PMID: 27698615.
46. Saglani S, Lloyd CM. Novel concepts in airway inflammation and remodelling in asthma. *Eur Respir J.* 2015 Dec; **46**(6): 1796–804. doi:10.1183/13993003.01196-2014. PMID: 26541520.
47. http://advanceweb.com/web/AstraZeneca/focus_on_copd_issue12/focus_on_copd_issue12_overview_of_asthma_phenotypes.html; Holgate ST, Wenzel S, Postma DS, Weiss ST, Renz H, Sly PD. Asthma. *Nat Rev Dis Primers.* 2015 Sep 10; **1** (1): 15025. doi: 10.1038/nrdp.2015.25. PMID: 27189668.
48. Ibid.
49. British Herbal Medicine Association's Scientific Committee. *British Herbal Pharmacopoeia.* BHMA, Cowling, 1983.
50. Bone KM, Mills SY. *Principles and Practice of Phytotherapy: Modern Herbal Medicine*, 2nd ed. Elsevier, UK, 2013, pp 250–260.
51. Ibid., pp 613–614.
52. Ibid., p 446.
53. Tahan F, Yaman M. Can the Pelargonium sidoides root extract EPS® 7630 prevent asthma attacks during viral infections of the upper respiratory tract in children?. *Phytomedicine.* 2013; **20**(2): 148–150. doi:10.1016/j.phymed.2012.09.022.
54. Garcia-Larsen V, Del Giacco SR, Moreira A, et al. Asthma and dietary intake: an overview of systematic reviews. *Allergy.* 2016; **71**(4): 433–442. doi:10.1111/all.12800. PMID: 26505989.
55. Wheatley LM, Togias A. Clinical practice. Allergic rhinitis. *N Engl J Med.* 2015 Jan 29; **372**(5): 456–463. doi:10.1056/NEJMcp1412282. PMID: 25629743.
56. Cingi C, Gevaert P, Mosges, et al. Multi-morbidities of allergic rhinitis in adults: European Academy of Allergy and Clinical Immunology Task Force Report. *Clin Transl Allergy.* 2017 Jun 1; **7**: 17. doi:10.1186/s13601-017-0153-z. PMID: 28572918.
57. Ibid.
58. Ng CL, Wang DY. Latest developments in allergic rhinitis in Allergy for clinicians

and researchers. *Allergy.* 2015 Dec; **70**(12): 1521–1530. doi:10.1111/all.12782. PMID: 26443244.
59. Andersson M, Greiff L, Ojeda P, Wollmer P. Barrier-enforcing measures as treatment principle in allergic rhinitis: a systematic review. *Curr Med Res Opin.* 2014; **30**(6): 1131–1137. doi:10.1185/03007995.2014.882299.
60. Fukuoka A, Yoshimoto T. Barrier dysfunction in the nasal allergy. *Allergol Int.* 2018; **67**(1): 18–23. doi:10.1016/j.alit.2017.10.006 PMID: 29150353.

13

FHT for immune and respiratory health: viral infections

We are hearing the word resilience often these days. Building resilience, which is the ability to adapt well to adversity, trauma, tragedy, threats, noxious agents, virulent pathogens, and other significant sources of stress is now of paramount importance. Today it can no longer be just a case of papering over our health weaknesses, because, as we are seeing every day now, they leave us vulnerable. The take home lesson of the COVID-19 pandemic and its sequelae is that true resilience is fundamentally underpinned by robust health. There is no better place to start building resilience in this context than with our immune system. Do herbs have a significant role to play here? You might agree they can – but which herbs and how do we best use them? Can we credibly extend this role of herbs to helping with the fight against the many challenges to our respiratory health, including SARS-CoV-2?

Grasping relevant, traditional, and evidence-based insights into building immune health and resisting respiratory infections is vital for patients' health and wellbeing and will also indeed, in uncertain times, grow the success of adept clinicians. But we need to apply good science and be able to make judicious recommendations, confident that we are doing no harm. A key aspect is to adopt the stepwise structured approach of FHT for our protocols. This is a powerful therapeutic approach that will optimise the use of the information in this chapter. In fact, knowing the best herb choices to deliver a range of identified FHT outcomes will enhance the three clinical **R**s: therapeutic **R**each, **R**eputation, and, above all, **R**esults.

13.1 Key immune herbs for respiratory infections

It is now clear that we are approaching a crisis point with infection control. So, what can we offer? What is the **key** herbal action when treating or preventing any type of infection? The answer, **immune enhancement**, is playing precisely to the strengths of FHT. Immune enhancement with herbs is **the** frontline therapy: it is fundamental to herbal infection control and treatment. Any treatment that relies only on herbs that might be thought to attack viruses, without at the same time providing immune support, will be relatively useless. (For more on this topic, see Chapter 9.)

The important immune herbs for infections are as follows:

Major immune herbs

- Echinacea root
- Andrographis
- medicinal mushrooms (including reishi, shiitake, and maitake)

Other immune herbs

- holy basil
- Pelargonium
- myrrh
- elderberry
- adaptogenic/tonic herbs, but especially Astragalus, Eleutherococcus, and Tinospora

(Also see Chapter 9.)

13.1.1 Echinacea root

Echinacea root, if of high quality, has much to often offer the modern herbal clinician, but it is a herb that is misunderstood and largely underestimated. One common misunderstanding is that the plant possesses clinically relevant antiviral and antibacterial activities. The probable reality is that Echinacea root is only indirectly active against pathogens via the facilitation of the host's immune response. Direct antimicrobial activity is, most probably, a trivial experimental finding of little clinical relevance (see Section 9.5.3).

Adding to the confusion over Echinacea, there are multiple commercial products using different species, plant parts, and manufacturing methods. This reflects on the debate over which phytochemicals in Echinacea are responsible for its immune activity. Some think it is all due to the polysaccharides, and therefore that water-based (aqueous) extracts that do not contain any alkylamides are preferable. We only have a basic understanding of Echinacea's precise effects on the immune response, and this drives the polarity over what Echinacea products should contain to make them work. But there have been number of intriguing recent developments.

If that is not enough, there are many myths about how Echinacea should and should not be used: the Echinacea rules and regulations. Now there is another one coming through: an increased risk of cytokine storm (see Section 13.2).

We first learnt about Echinacea from native American tribes; their use of this herb was then adopted by the Eclectic physicians (see Chapter 4). The Eclectics, like the native Americans, preferred the root of Echinacea, especially as an ethanolic extract rich in alkylamides. By 1921, Echinacea (specifically the root of *E. angustifolia*) was by far the most popular treatment prescribed by Eclectic physicians. In fact, its sales completely dwarfed the next-best-selling herb, which, interestingly, was fringe tree.[1] Echinacea had achieved this status in just 36 years, no doubt partly fuelled by the Spanish flu pandemic.

An important piece of research that I was involved in was a human pharmacokinetic study on Echinacea root in an effort to understand what was absorbed after oral doses. It is these absorbed phytochemicals that will probably be responsible for its activity. This was a study in 11 healthy individuals: blood samples were taken over 12 hours after a single dose of Echinacea root extract.[2] The only Echinacea-related compounds that could be identified in the human plasma after oral doses were the alkylamides, and they were there in approximately the same ratio as that in the initial product. So, if we want a relevant model for test-tube research on how Echinacea acts on immune cells, then we should obviously be testing the alkylamides.

What do the alkylamides do in such experiments? One fascinating finding is that they strongly bind to a key cannabinoid receptor: CB2. They are, in fact, phytocannabinoids inducing subtle and complex modulation of immune function. Interestingly, they do not exert pro-inflammatory effects by driving pro-inflammatory cytokines: rather, they display anti-inflammatory activity. There is other research that shows that the alkylamides probably enhance the preparedness of immune cells for cytokine signalling (see Section 13.2). They also inhibit the breakdown of endocannabinoids, extending their effects in the body and possibly up-regulating dendritic cell maturation.

All this speaks to the innate side of immune function: the alkylamides potentially prime innate immune responses. As part of this, they support natural killer (NK) cell numbers and their activity and viability. There is also a suggestion that they can help to counter immunosenescence, which impacts innate immunity in particular.

What about the clinical evidence for Echinacea? In a Cochrane review published in 2014, the authors noted the conundrum we have already flagged, that most consumers, and even clinicians, are unaware that the products available under the "Echinacea" banner differ appreciably in their composition. This variability in products used in clinical trials was said to confound any systematic review and meta-analysis (although this has been done by others). The Cochrane review still went ahead and assessed the evidence that Echinacea preparations are effective and safe compared to placebo in the prevention and treatment of the common cold. Of 7 treatment trials on cold duration, only one showed a significant effect for Echinacea versus placebo. In contrast, while most prevention trials were inconclusive, a post-hoc pooling of their results suggested a relative risk reduction of 10–20%.[3] Here, for the first time, we see a shift in the evidence, supporting the contention that Echinacea is more effective as a preventative.

Supporting this finding, a meta-analysis published one year later concluded that the use of Echinacea extracts was associated with reduced risk – prevention – of recurrent respiratory infections (relative risk, RR 0.649; $p \leq 0.0001$). **Ethanolic extracts** (likely to be higher in alkylamides) from Echinacea appeared to provide superior effects to those of pressed juices, and **increased dosing** during acute episodes further enhanced these effects.[4]

One of the key myths about Echinacea that has worked against its adoption as a preventative treatment for infections is that it can only be consumed for short periods of time – a matter of days – before it "wears out" the immune response. After some forensic investigation, it appears that this myth had arisen from an early German clinical study on *E. purpurea* root – a study that has been widely misinterpreted as demonstrating that Echinacea causes immune system tachyphylaxis if taken for more than a few days. A cursory examination of the figures published in this paper might lead to the conclusion that the use of Echinacea for more than a few days depletes the phagocytic response. This would, however, be a misinterpretation of the results. The arrows at the bottom of those figures indicate the application of the test dose, which was administered for only the first 5 days. While the Echinacea was given, phagocytic activity remained high. Only when the Echinacea was stopped did the phagocytic activity decline to normal levels – a typical washout effect.[5]

In fact, the study demonstrated the following:

- Phagocytic activity remained higher than normal while Echinacea was given.
- Oral doses of Echinacea stimulated phagocytic activity more than did injected doses.
- When Echinacea was stopped, phagocytic activity remained well above normal for a few days, indicating that far from causing depletion, there was a residual stimulating effect when Echinacea was stopped.
- Phagocytic activity returned to normal only after the Echinacea had been stopped – that is, there was no depleting effect where the activity dropped to less than normal (as might be expected if continuous use of Echinacea **depletes** immune function, as some claim).

It was previously thought that, because our innate immune responses are just receptor-based, with the pattern recognition receptors, innate immunity could not be conditioned to respond more efficiently. But now we are realising that, via epigenetic mechanisms, it can be. Many immune herbs, including Echinacea root, might actually train the innate immune system with repeated dosing to make it more responsive. Scientists are investigating certain vaccines, like BCG (Bacillus Calmette–Guérin vaccine) for tuberculosis, in exactly this regard, but the effect does wear off, as the BCG is given just the one time. We can take Echinacea root daily and perhaps train our innate immunity to give a heightened response every day.

There is further discussion on the mode of action and clinical use of Echinacea root in relation to the misguided concerns over its potential to trigger cytokine storm in Section 13.2.3.1.

13.1.2 Other immune herbs

Other immune herbs worthy of further study include holy basil, Pelargonium, and Tinospora. (For more details on myrrh, see Section 9.5.2, and the corresponding monograph in *Principles and Practice of Phytotherapy*.)

Holy basil is widely used in India for the prevention and treatment of respiratory viral infections. In a small proof-of-principle clinical trial, only 1 of 7 children receiving holy basil had a recurrence of infection over a 6-month period, compared to 10 of 11 children in the placebo group.[6] Results for a cross-over RCT ($n = 22$) demonstrated that holy basil significantly increased the immune response of healthy volunteers as compared to placebo (increase in T-helper cells, NK cells, and interferon gamma). The daily dose was 2 g dried leaf for 4 weeks.[7]

Pelargonium sidoides root originally came from South Africa, but it has become very popular in Europe for the treatment of acute respiratory infections, especially in children. Despite good clinical evidence, its mode of action is not fully understood, although it probably works in part by favourably influencing the immune response. Meta-analysis of four placebo-controlled trials involving adults found that a liquid preparation of *Pelargonium sidoides* root significantly reduced bronchitis symptom scores by Day 7.[8] Positive clinical trial outcomes are also seen for the common cold, acute bacterial maxillary sinusitis, acute sinusitis and acute exacerbation of chronic recurrent sinusitis, and acute tonsillopharyngitis.[9] Higher doses gave better results in a common cold trial.[10] In athletes submitted to intense running, secretory immunoglobulin A levels in saliva were increased, while IL-15 and IL-6 in serum were decreased.[11]

Tinospora cordifolia (guduci) is a succulent, climbing shrub that sends out long thread-like aerial roots. Almost all parts of the plant are used traditionally in Ayurveda, with the stem having the most applications. In patients with obstructive jaundice undergoing surgery, Tinospora stem improved the survival rate and increased polymorphonuclear leukocyte functioning. The stem improved recovery in patients with tuberculosis and had a greater effect on viral elimination in asymptomatic carriers of hepatitis B surface antigen than did placebo. Modest effects for preventing chemotherapy-induced leukopenia in breast cancer patients were achieved by taking Tinospora stem extract. In children experiencing frequent infections, Tinospora stem significantly reduced symptoms and increased IgG levels compared to baseline values.[12]

This research suggests that a key role for Tinospora is for infection prevention and the early stages of infection. This preventative role also applies to the other tonic/adaptogenic herbs, such as Astragalus, Eleutherococcus, Withania, and Korean ginseng. For example, regular intake of KRG (Korean red ginseng) for 12 weeks was investigated in a double blind RCT in 100 healthy volunteers to assess its impact on acute respiratory illness (ARI). The primary efficacy end-point was the number of ARIs reported. Fewer people in the KRG group reported contracting at least one ARI than did those in the placebo group (12 [24.5%] vs 22 [44.9%], $p = 0.034$).[13]

13.2 Herbs and cytokine storm risk

During the height of the COVID-19 pandemic, there was an urgent and concerted search for repurposed drugs that might improve the chances of survival. Doctors in acute care were observing a particular pathophysiology or clinical manifestation and responding as best they could in the evidence vacuum, using the drugs and equipment they had at their disposal. This was certainly medicine by the seat of one's pants.

In contrast, in those torrid times, all we seemed to be hearing about herbs was negative. You can't give this, you can't give that, and don't you dare claim they will help, because there is no evidence!

The fundamental, often ignored point was that while there was – and still is – little direct evidence for or against herb use in the fight against SARS-CoV-2, the FHT system allows us to draw on past experiences with other infections, viruses, pandemics, and known risk factors. This is neither misinformed nor unethical: it is, in fact, identical to what the frontline doctors were doing with their drugs and procedures. The key word here is functional, because understanding a health problem in terms of function, with all its ramifications, will always map out a credible and robust approach to treatment. Undue speculation, on the other hand, especially about obscure herbs, should be avoided at all costs.

Specifically, in the debate over the role of herbs in acute respiratory infections, concerns have been raised that certain herbs acting on the immune system might deleteriously enhance the cytokine response, leading to cytokine storm. These concerns are **not supported** by a detailed analysis of the published scientific and traditional literature (see Section 13.2.2).

In the following exploration of this issue, a few pivotal insights into best practice FHT for acute respiratory infections are additionally outlined.

13.2.1 What are cytokines?

Cytokines are a large group of molecules comprising proteins, peptides, and glycoproteins that are secreted by specific cells of the immune system. They are signalling molecules that mediate and regulate both immunity and inflammation. Cytokine is a general term: other group names, based on function, cell of secretion, or target of action, are used. For example, cytokines made by lymphocytes can also be referred to as lymphokines, and interleukins are made by one leukocyte and act on other leukocytes. Chemokines are cytokines with chemotactic activities. Interferons are named for their ability to indirectly interfere with viral infection.[14]

In essence, cytokines and chemokines are soluble proteins secreted by immune cells that enable the passage of information between immune cells and participate in cell activation, cell growth, migration, and differentiation. They are a large part of the grammar of the immune system – that is, the way it talks to itself and orchestrates an immune response or the resolution of a response. Cell–cell interaction is also important, but here, as well, **the message is often conveyed by particular cytokines**.[15]

Recent advances in the understanding of innate immunity show that the activation of the innate immune system is essential for subsequent adaptive immune responses, including specific antibody production and cytotoxic T lymphocyte activation, which play a key role in fighting viral infection.[16] Cytokines are key for facilitating the initiation of the adaptive immune response.

Put another way, cytokines are, in effect, the language of the immune system, and they play a critical communicative role in initiating and sustaining both the innate and the adaptive immune responses to an invading pathogen. Just because an agent – such as a medicinal plant – facilitates cytokine signalling release in the early stages of an immune response, this does not necessarily mean that it will drive that cytokine response to an excessive level in the later rampant stage of the infection. In other words, improving efficiency does not imply subsequent overproduction. The opposite is more likely to be true (see Section 13.2.2).

13.2.2 Defining cytokine storm

Exuberant immune responses induced by the later stages of an infection have been described as a "cytokine storm" and are associated with excessive levels of proinflammatory cytokines and widespread tissue damage.[17] A range of pathogens have been observed to cause this response, but the reasons why the cytokine storm affects only certain individuals during an infection and not others are not fully understood. The term "cytokine storm" was first used in 1993 to describe the effects of graft-versus-host disease. In 2003, cytokine storm was shown to be associated with severe reactions to influenza viruses and, subsequently, to various viral, bacterial, or fungal infections. While there is no agreed definition of what a cytokine storm is exactly, it is characterised by a marked severity of infection due to an activation cascade that leads to an auto-amplification of cytokine production.[18] It is in fact an **autotoxicity** induced by the pathogen.

It is worthwhile to explore how a cytokine storm develops during a viral infection. It has been proposed that our response to a respiratory virus occurs in three stages:

1. Stage I, an asymptomatic incubation period with or without detectable virus
2. Stage II, a non-severe symptomatic period with the presence of virus
3. Stage III, a severe respiratory symptomatic stage with a high viral load [19]

During the incubation and non-severe stages, a specific adaptive immune response is required to eliminate the virus and to prevent disease progression to the severe stage. This, in turn, requires a dynamic innate immune response, which will, of course, involve the efficient local release of cytokines as signalling agents. Therefore, any strategies that boost immune responses at the early stages are regarded as important.[20] If they are efficient, then Stage III will not occur.

When a protective immune response is impaired, the virus will propagate, and massive destruction of affected tissues may occur. In this event, damaged host cells induce chaotic innate inflammatory responses in the lungs that are largely mediated by proinflammatory macrophages and granulocytes, and a cytokine storm results.[21] In other words, a cytokine storm is a late-stage manifestation of the viral disease that occurs only when the immune system fails to contain the virus. It is not the manifestation of an overactive immune response directly targeted at the infection – in fact, it is quite the opposite. Surely this argues for the intensive use of immune support during Stages I (late stage prevention) and II (early acute management) to avoid its occurrence?

13.2.3 Concerns over cytokine storm risk for specific herbs

While cytokine storm was first linked to a viral infection in only 2003, it has clearly been a feature of such infections since time immemorial. Hence, we are not dealing with a new phenomenon when it comes to observations about herbs and their role to prevent and reduce infection. There is no suggestion from traditional Western herbal writings – including those of well-documented groups such as the Eclectics (who accumulated considerable experience during the Spanish flu pandemic[22]) – that the use of immune herbs aggravated viral infections. Also, a range of traditional Chinese formulations (several containing the immune herb Astragalus) have been used extensively in China during various recent viral epidemics, including COVID-19, with no suggestion that they exacerbated cytokine storm.

13.2.3.1 Echinacea

First it should be pointed out that, as noted above, the key role of Echinacea root is for infection prevention. In the modern prescribing context, it plays a secondary role during the actual viral infection. Antiviral herbs such as licorice and sweet wormwood (the latter in pulsed doses) and, more importantly, other immune herbs such as Andrographis and holy basil, become more relevant in acute phase management – although Ellingwood very much regarded Echinacea as a frontline remedy during all acute infections (see below). Hence, concerns about cytokine storm and Echinacea are not really that relevant to its current best clinical use.

But even given this, there is no evidence that Echinacea root will inappropriately stimulate the cytokine response during an acute viral infection and cause harm.

From the Echinacea root monograph in *Principles and Practice of Phytotherapy* (2nd edition):[23]

> Cytokine antibody arrays were used to investigate changes in pro-inflammatory cytokines released from human bronchial epithelial cells exposed to a rhinovirus.[24] Virus infection stimulated the release of at least 31 cytokine-related molecules and most of these were **reversed** by simultaneous exposure to the Echinacea extracts. The lipophilic extract of *E. purpurea* root was less active than the expressed juice of the aerial parts in this regard. However, in uninfected cells these cytokines were stimulated by Echinacea, with the lipophilic extract being more active.
>
> There is still much to understand about the way Echinacea root impacts the human immune system. Each *in vitro* study by its nature can provide just a narrow insight into a few specific aspects of immune function, with any clinical relevance potentially confounded by bioavailability, dosage issues, and local tissue factors. The *in vitro* studies probably of most relevance are the ones investigating alkylamides, since these compounds have proven bioavailability.
>
> Research has been particularly insightful into one aspect of the mode of action of Echinacea alkylamides.[25] A lipophilic extract of *E. purpurea* strongly stimulated TNF-alpha mRNA synthesis in peripheral monocytes, but not TNF-alpha protein production. In other words, the Echinacea-induced new TNF-alpha transcripts (mRNA) were not translated into TNF-alpha itself. When monocytes were treated with LPS (lipopolysaccharide or endotoxin, a powerful stimulator of the immune system) TNF-alpha protein production was substantially increased. However, co-incubation of monocytes with LPS and Echinacea extract resulted in a strong **inhibition** of this effect of LPS. Investigation over a longer time-span revealed that the lipophilic

Echinacea extract, via interaction with CB2 receptors, modulated and prolonged TNF-alpha production following immune stimulation. The results of this study suggest that Echinacea acted more as a modulator or facilitator of the immune response, rather than as an immune stimulant. In resting monocytes it prepared them for a quicker immune response by inducing TNF-alpha mRNA. However, in overstimulated monocytes (as in the case of LPS [or viral damage that induces cytokine storm]) it first reduced, and then extended their response in terms of TNF-alpha production. In particular, these key findings challenge the concept that traditional Echinacea extracts will "overstimulate and wear out" the immune system if taken continuously. [bold added for emphasis]

So, on the evidence we have to date, a lipophilic extract of Echinacea root rich in alkylamides will prime the immune response before virus exposure but will then tone it down and sustain it once the virus takes hold: this is the exact opposite of the misinformed concerns based on a superficial and one-dimensional analysis of the published literature.

Interestingly, the Eclectic physician Ellingwood actually noted the value of a lipophilic extract of Echinacea root for conditions that seem quite akin to cytokine storm (we now know that **sepsis** is typically characterised by an initial intense inflammatory response or cytokine storm) when he wrote, in in 1919:[26]

> It is the remedy for blood poisoning, if there is one in the *Materia Medica*. Its field covers acute auto-infection, slow progressive blood taint, faults of the blood from imperfect elimination of all possible character, and from the development of disease germs within the blood. It acts equally well, whether the profound influence be exerted upon the nervous system, as in puerperal **sepsis** and uremia . . .
>
> In **pleuritis**, in **bronchitis**, in peritonitis, especially pelvic peritonitis from **sepsis**; in hepatitis and nephritis and cystitis **always at the beginning of the acute stage** before much structural change has occurred, it may be given, and will retard and often throw off the attack. [bold added for emphasis]

and again:

> I am convinced that success in certain cases depends upon the fact that the patient must have at times, a sufficiently large quantity of this remedy in order to produce full antitoxic effects on the virulent infections. I would therefore emphasize the statement which I have previously made that it is

perfectly safe to give *echinacea* in massive doses – from two drams to half an ounce every two or three hours – for a time at least, when the system is overwhelmed with these toxins.

and:

In septic peritonitis it (Bryonia) may be given alternately with *aconite*, or *aconite* and *echinacea*, **the latter remedy directly controlling the sepsis**. [bold added for emphasis]

13.2.3.2 Astragalus

In traditional Chinese medicine (TCM), Astragalus is generally contraindicated in acute infections, except where there is chi deficiency. However, as mentioned above, it has been used in TCM formulations to treat recent viral epidemics but is more often included in preventative formulations.[27] As per the TCM guidelines, Astragalus is particularly indicated for prevention when a person has compromised immunity and/or resilience.

Hence, Astragalus can be safely taken for prevention but is best stopped once acute symptoms develop (unless there is advice to the contrary from a skilled TCM practitioner). There is no suggestion from any research that its use only prior to an infection will increase the risk of cytokine storm once an infection takes hold (and the Astragalus has been subsequently stopped). In fact, this is extremely unlikely.

In one clinical trial, Astragalus (by injection) **reduced** inflammatory cytokines.[28] This was in patients undergoing heart valve replacement (HVR). Astragalus was found to decrease the inflammatory cytokines TNF-α and IL-8 and increase the level of the anti-inflammatory cytokine (IL-10), thereby exerting an anti-inflammatory activity in patients after HVR.

13.2.3.3 Elderberry

The use of the black elderberry (*Sambucus nigra*) during acute respiratory viral infections is relatively new, arising from research conducted in the 1970s. Initial investigations revealed antiviral activity, and this remains a research focus.[29] However, later research has indicated a potential role for the herb in enhancing immune responses, especially cytokine production.[30]

Meta-analysis certainly supports its benefit when administered during acute viral infections.[31]

The exact mode of action of elderberry is not fully understood, and since its bioavailable components have not been determined (other than the polyphenolics, which have relatively low bioavailability), *in vitro* studies need to be interpreted with great caution. As noted above (and in Chapter 9), by their nature *in vitro* studies on a herb can provide just a narrow insight into a few specific aspects of immune function, with any clinical relevance potentially confounded by bioavailability, dosage issues, and local tissue factors.

Hence, what we can glean from clinical studies is bound to be more reliable. One such trial in 473 patients (including many with confirmed influenza A and/or B) found that a combination of elderberry and Echinacea given for 10 days as soon as possible after symptoms developed was as effective as the antiviral drug oseltamivir.[32] There was no suggestion of harmful effects or induction of cytokine storm (the authors used the term "septic shock" to flag this possibility). In fact, adverse events were higher in the antiviral drug group. No hospitalisations were reported during the investigational period in either treatment group.

In another large trial involving 312 economy-class passengers travelling from Australia to an overseas destination, participants took elderberry continuously from 10 days before flying overseas until 5 days after arriving at the travel destination.[33] Most cold episodes occurred in the placebo group (17 vs 12); however, the difference was not significant ($p = 0.4$). Placebo group participants did have a significantly longer duration of cold-episode days (117 vs. 57, $p = 0.02$), and the average symptom score over these days was also significantly higher (583 vs. 247, $p = 0.05$). These data suggest a significant reduction of cold duration and severity in air travellers, but not of incidence. The herbal treatment was well tolerated, with no serious adverse events.

These and other human trial results strongly imply that concerns over what is essentially a food precipitating a life-threatening adverse event during an infection (cytokine storm) are merely theoretical.

13.2.3.4 Medicinal mushrooms

As is the case with Astragalus, the main role of medicinal mushrooms, such as reishi, maitake, and shiitake, is for infection prevention and they can be discontinued during acute infection onset to make way for other higher-priority treatments. Research suggests that the branched chain beta-glucan polymers found in the fruiting bodies of various mushroom species seem particularly adapted to heightening immune vigilance against potential pathogens.

The interaction of mushroom beta-glucans with immune cells involves distinct pathways, especially as revealed by the recent discovery of the dectin-1 receptor. Innate immune cells express pattern recognition receptors (PRRs) such as dectin-1, Toll-like receptors, and mannose receptors on their cell surfaces. These PRRs recognise pathogens by binding to highly conserved pathogen-associated molecular patterns such as beta-glucan (from fungi), mannan, and lipopolysaccharide (LPS). The immunomodulating activities of innate immune cells are augmented by the binding of beta-glucans to dectin-1 expressed by macrophages or dendritic cells. Upon binding beta-glucan, innate immune cells then activate adaptive immune cells such as B and T lymphocytes or NK cells by secreting various cytokines.[34] But as before, these cytokines are acting as signalling agents and are released only in low and localised amounts.

Interaction of mushroom beta-glucans with the dectin-1 receptor may even be able to "train" the innate immune response, as mentioned above for Echinacea.[35] Trained (innate) immunity (TI) can be induced by a variety of stimuli, of which BCG and beta-glucan have been particularly studied. Both BCG (via NOD2 signalling) and beta-glucan (via dectin-1) can induce epigenetic changes that lead to TI. Interestingly, because of the discovery of TI, BCG is currently being investigated as a prevention for an acute respiratory viral infection (COVID-19) among 4,000 healthcare workers.[36] There is clearly no concern about triggering a cytokine storm with this powerful agent, presumably because its role, like that of the medicinal mushrooms, is preventative.

13.2.4 Herbs and fever management

One aspect that seems to have been largely overlooked when discussing herbs for managing viral infections is the important role of diaphoretic herbs in Stage II. Their appropriate use could prove to be critical in preventing the development of cytokine storm. (See a more complete discussion of diaphoretics in Chapter 1 and in *Principles and Practice of Phytotherapy*.)

A diaphoretic is an agent that literally is used to promote sweating, and in the context of a fever, diaphoretic herbs were used to manage the febrile phase of an infection. In modern herbal practice, diaphoretic herbs are still considered appropriate in fever management, including remedies such as *Mentha × piperita* (peppermint), Achillea (yarrow), Sambucus (elder flowers), Matricaria (chamomile), Tilia (lime flowers), and *Asclepias tuberosa* (pleurisy root). Their objective is to help to facilitate the fever as a "slow burn" (usually in the range of 100–102°F or 37.8–38.9°C), ensuring that this important physiological response is supported but kept at a level that is comfortable, restorative, and not harmful to the person. They work best when taken hot, as in an infusion or decoction.

In the classical model of pathogenesis, induction of fever is mediated by the release of pyrogenic cytokines such as tumour necrosis factor (TNF), IL-1, IL-6, and interferons into the bloodstream in response to exogenous pyrogens from infecting agents.[37] These are the same cytokines that are largely responsible for cytokine storm. Hence, diaphoretic herbs might well reduce the risk of developing cytokine storm during an infection.

This might be disregarded as idle speculation, except for the Eclectic experience with diaphoretic herbs during the Spanish flu pandemic, where they were regarded as key remedies. Drawing from just one of the many testaments to the value of diaphoretic herbs from that time, as reviewed by Abascal and Yarnell:[38]

> One physician, who saw 10–35 patients with influenza per day during the epidemic began treatment by mixing 2 teaspoons of boneset and 1 teaspoon of pleurisy root tinctures in a cup of hot water. This was given immediately with a second dose 15 minutes later, a third dose half an hour later, and a fourth dose an hour after the first dose. He reported that this treatment typically reduced a fever of 103–104°F by 3–4° in a few hours. Yet another physician reported that boneset was always a significant remedy in influenza.

We now know that boneset contains low levels of toxic pyrrolizidine alkaloids, so other diaphoretic herbs (see the above list and in Chapter 1) should be used instead.

13.2.5 Herbs and cytokine storm risk: summary

Concerns over herbs and cytokine storm risk do not differentiate between the initial role of cytokines during an infection as immune signalling agents and their later role in promoting an inflammatory response. Cytokine storm in particular is a chaotic, intense, unregulated response to massive necrotic tissue destruction that is unlikely to be capable of further augmentation by any agent, much less a relatively benign medicinal plant.

Neither traditional use, nor clinical trials, nor modern pharmacology (when interpreted in the appropriate context) support any concerns about common immune herbs increasing the risk of cytokine storm during an infection. In fact, the opposite is more likely to be the case, since these herbs will support a focused initial immune response, including enhanced cytokine signalling, and thereby reduce the risk of any infection progressing to the Stage-III development of cytokine storm.

Herbs are best given in combination, and such informed use of herbal prescribing can lower the risk of any side effects and improve clinical outcomes. In the context of reducing the risk of cytokine storm once an infection has taken hold, the potentially valuable role for the inclusion of diaphoretic herbs in the treatment protocol needs to be given due attention.

13.3 Clinically relevant antiviral herbs

The clinically relevant antiviral herbs are St John's wort, licorice, *Artemisia annua*, and turmeric as bioavailable curcumin (see Chapter 9). Given their broad activity, they are likely to be active against many respiratory viruses (and in several instances such activity has been demonstrated *in vitro* and *in vivo*). It should be kept in mind that St John's wort and licorice are active only against viruses that have a lipid envelope, such as herpesviruses and coronaviruses.

Generally, there is only a call to use antiviral herbs in respiratory infections when the virus is highly contagious or might potentially cause severe infection (due to the vulnerability of the patient and/or the virulence of the virus). Influenza and coronaviruses are two examples where this would be relevant.

13.4 FHT immune protocols for infection prevention

- Echinacea root is the principal herb for prevention, with a focus on products/preparations that contain adequate levels of alkylamides.
- Andrographis can play a role here, but in rare cases long-term use can cause loss of taste and allergic reactions, so its use is best reserved for the management of acute episodes.
- Respiratory viruses often gain entry via the mouth or throat, so a liquid herbal throat spray or gargle twice a day will assist with prevention. Herbs of value here include myrrh, Echinacea root, Calendula, sage, and green tea.
- If the virus is highly contagious or might potentially cause severe infection (due to the vulnerability of the patient and/or the virulence of the virus), then several of the clinically relevant antiviral herbs listed above should be taken for prevention. The best ones are St John's wort, licorice and bioavailable curcumin. *Artemisia annua* is not suitable for prevention, as it should only be taken for up to 7 days at a time (see Chapter 9). Other traditional antiviral herbs such as Thuja can also be considered.
- Medicinal and dietary mushrooms can be used, especially for people with weaker immunity, or the vulnerable
- Adaptogenic/tonic herbs including Astragalus, Eleutherococcus, Withania, Tinospora, and Korean ginseng can be given in addition to all the above if a person is immune-depleted or compromised, has a low white cell count, or experiences frequent recurrent respiratory infections. Adrenal support with licorice and Rehmannia can be a valuable support for these herbs, especially if the person is anxious and/or stressed.
- Other herbs that can be considered for prevention include elderberry, Pelargonium, holy basil, golden seal, and garlic. They are probably most useful, however, when taken in the early stages of the infection. But, most importantly of all:
- At the first sign of an infection threatening, or if the patient has encountered an infected person, temporarily double or triple the dose of Echinacea root until the threat subsides, perhaps with increased doses of the other herbal strategies above.

(See the appropriate monographs in *Principles and Practice of Phytotherapy* for more information about adequate dosing for the above.)

13.5 FHT protocols for respiratory infections

At the initial development of symptoms, select from the following until the condition resolves and for a further 24–48 hours:

- Provide acute immune support with appropriate higher doses of Andrographis, Echinacea root, and holy basil, supported by Pelargonium and elderberry.
- For fever management, use hot diaphoretic herbal teas (peppermint, elder flowers, chamomile, or yarrow) and formulations with pleurisy root. These can be combined with warming herbs such as ginger and cayenne to enhance their effectiveness. Other diaphoretics, such as lime flowers, can be considered.

Further support to be considered:

- If the virus is highly contagious or might potentially cause severe infection (due to the vulnerability of the patient and/or the virulence of the virus), then a selection of clinically relevant antiviral herbs is indicated, as follows: *Artemisia annua* (for up to 7 days, then take 7 days off; repeat if necessary), St John's wort, licorice, and bioavailable curcumin.
- Garlic, golden seal, and/or medicinal mushrooms are further options, especially for mucous membrane protection and resistance.
- To soothe the throat, a liquid herbal throat spray or gargle can be given, as needed. Herbs of value here include myrrh, Echinacea root, Calendula, sage, marshmallow root, and green tea.
- If the immune response is overactive, consider bioavailable curcumin to modulate the inflammatory response (which has the additional advantage that it is antiviral).

For supporting the lungs (if the virus takes hold there):

- During any dry, unproductive cough phase, respiratory demulcents such as marshmallow root glycetract should be considered. This combines well with a small quantity of licorice (see Chapter 12).

- Expectorant herbs, which include Elecampane (*Inula helenium*), thyme (*Thymus vulgaris*), licorice and other saponin-containing herbs, Adhatoda, Foeniculum (fennel), Pimpinella (aniseed), and Marrubium (white horehound) can be prescribed throughout the course of the infection to allay cough, loosen tenacious sputum, clear the lungs, and provide a more soothing mucus flow.
- Anticatarrhal herbs, especially mullein (Verbascum), ribwort (*Plantago lanceolata*), and golden seal, may be indicated when the sputum is particularly copious or if a productive cough lingers. These will be needed most when a secondary bacterial infection takes hold.
- Antibacterial herbs, such as Elecampane, thyme, and garlic, should be considered if a secondary bacterial infection takes hold.
- Respiratory spasmolytics with expectorant activity, such as Adhatoda, Grindelia, and Elecampane, should also be prescribed if there is a debilitating cough.
- Mucolytic herbs, such as garlic and horseradish, may also be required to help loosen tenacious sputum. These will be needed most if a secondary bacterial infection takes hold.

13.6 Special considerations for respiratory viral epidemics/pandemics

Over the past 100 years or so, humanity has been afflicted by several epidemics and potential or actual pandemics involving respiratory viral infections. The viruses involved have all been strains of influenza A or coronaviruses. They include H1N1 (Spanish influenza), H1N1v (swine flu), H3N2 (Hong Kong flu), H5N1 (bird flu), SARS-CoV (SARS), MERS CoV (Middle East respiratory syndrome, MERS), and SARS-CoV-2 (COVID-19). These viruses have the potential to cause considerable morbidity and mortality, and hence require additional considerations in terms of FHT.

The following exploration focuses on COVID-19, as it is the most recent challenge, but many of the issues examined apply to the diseases caused by other dangerous and contagious respiratory viruses in these families.

What is a fundamental lesson from the COVID-19 pandemic, one that few in our health care systems seem to be talking about? It demonstrates that we have a piecemeal system of "disease care" that leaves us exposed and vulnerable to a novel infectious threat and then struggles to find ways out of the conundrum, still clinging to the "pill (or jab) for every ill" paradigm.

COVID-19 forces us to confront the most brutally honest and vitally important question: that we are, on the whole, a sick species, with overall resilience- and immune systems that are badly compromised by our modern way of life. It reveals that governments are prepared to spend trillions of dollars on social, economic, and medical remediation of the impact of a virus, but **all** after the fact. It demonstrates the inherent complacency and shortsightedness of a system of health care that pays only token attention to – and expenditure on – disease prevention and improving community health, and will no doubt continue to do so, despite the now glaring, and ultimately costly, deficiencies in this approach.

13.6.1 COVID-19 vulnerabilities

Studies from several countries indicate that age is a significant risk factor for hospitalisation and death from COVID-19 infection. For example, New York City (NYC) data showed that 70% of all deaths were in people aged 65 years or above.[39] Also from NYC data, the hospitalisation rate per 100,000 population for those 75-year-olds and older was around 3 times that for the 45–64 age bracket, and the corresponding death rate was more than 8 times that of the younger cohort.

A number of comorbidities also appear to increase the risk of hospitalisation and death. A study from California of hospitalised patients (median age 61 years) observed the following incidences of comorbidities: hypertension, 43.5%, diabetes, 31.3%, chronic kidney disease, 12.7%, chronic obstructive pulmonary disease or asthma, 7.4%, congestive heart failure, 5.8%, liver cirrhosis, 5.6%, and cancer, 4.8%.[40] This was supported by a study from NYC, that found, additionally, that 41.7% of hospitalised patients were obese.[41] **Figure 13.1** shows death rates of COVID-19 patients with pre-existing conditions supplied by the Chinese Centre for Disease Control and Prevention.[42] The same comorbidities have been linked to increased risk of death from COVID-19 in several other studies.

In the United Kingdom, age, sex (male), obesity, and underlying illness emerged as risk factors for severe COVID-19 or death, according to a

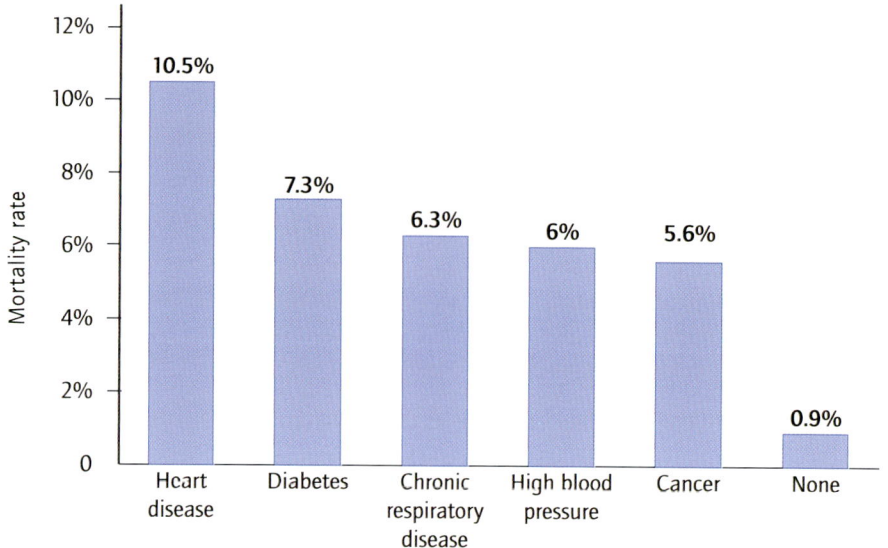

Figure 13.1 Death rates in China of COVID-19 patients with pre-existing conditions. [Source: Chinese Center for Disease Control and Prevention.]

large cohort study published by *The BMJ* (22 May 2020).[43] The risk of death increased in the over 50s, especially those who were male, obese, and/or those with underlying heart, lung, liver, and kidney disease. As the largest prospective observational study reported worldwide at the time of publication, the article provided a comprehensive picture of the characteristics of patients hospitalised in the UK with COVID-19 and their outcomes.[44]

A retrospective study of 1,591 patients with COVID-19 (median age 63 years) requiring treatment in an intensive care unit (ICU) in the Lombardy region of Italy revealed that 68% had at least one comorbidity and 49% had prior hypertension.[45]

Comorbidities probably play a causal role in increasing the risk of more severe COVID-19 disease. In support of this, a Chinese study found that people with type 2 diabetes whose blood sugar was well controlled fared much better than did those with more poorly controlled blood sugar.[46] The senior author, Hongliang Li of Renmin Hospital of Wuhan University, said:

> We were surprised to see such favourable outcomes in [the] well-controlled blood glucose group among patients with COVID-19 and pre-existing type 2 diabetes.

Considering that people with diabetes had much higher risk for death and various complications, and there are no specific drugs for COVID-19, our findings indicate that controlling blood glucose well may act as an effective auxiliary approach to improve the prognosis of patients with COVID-19 and pre-existing diabetes.[47]

13.6.2 COVID-19 late-stage pathological features

It is not the intention in this section to imply that FHT will be appropriate for the late-stage, life-threatening scenarios that can ensue from COVID-19 infection, including cytokine storm. Rather, this exploration aims to understand these clinical phenomena with a view to providing appropriate support in the early stages of infection, to avoid them happening in the first place.

Figure 13.2 provides a basic timeline for severe COVID-19 infection.[48] As can be seen from the figure, severe disease requiring hospitalisation typically does not begin until around 6 to 7 days after the first onset of symptoms. Cytokine storm, as indicated by ARDS (acute respiratory disease syndrome) and intensive care admission typically occurs at 9–11 days.

As already discussed in Section 13.2, what is abundantly clear from this timeline is that the dangerous complications, including cytokine storm, are late-stage manifestations of the infection. If the immune system can largely resolve the infection in the first 5 or 6 days, then severe disease will not follow. This is the strongest argument for supporting immune responses, both prior to and in the early stages of infection.

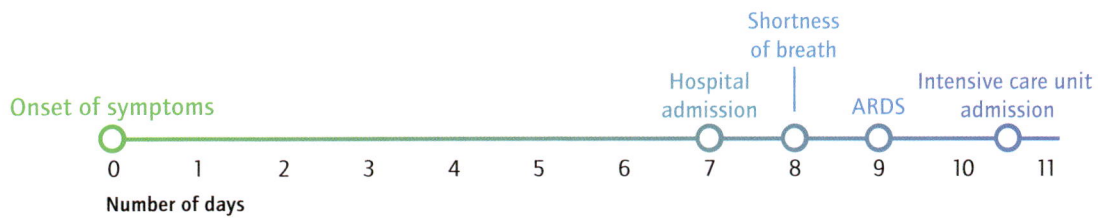

Figure 13.2 A basic timeline for severe COVID-19 infection. Number of days is the median time from onset of symptoms, including fever (in 98% of patients), cough (75%), myalgia or fatigue (44%), and others. [ARDS = acute respiratory disease syndrome.]

In fact, sophisticated computer modelling of the disease course suggests that problems may arise when the adaptive immune response kicks in too soon.[49] Using the "target cell-limited model", a common mathematical model developed to understand the dynamics of viral infections, researchers examined how immune responses work in COVID-19 patients, compared to patients who have influenza. The influenza virus is typically a fast-moving infection that attacks target cells on the surface of the upper respiratory system and kills almost all the target cells within 2–3 days. The death of these cells deprives the virus of more targets to infect and allows the innate immune response time to clear the body of almost all the virus before the adaptive system comes into play. But COVID-19, which targets surface cells throughout the respiratory system including in the lungs, has an average incubation of about 6 days and a much slower disease progression. Mathematical modelling suggests that the adaptive immune response may kick in before the target cells are depleted, slowing down the infection and interfering with the innate immune response's ability to kill off most of the virus quickly.[50] "The danger is, as the infection keeps going on, it will mobilise the whole of the adaptive immune response with its multiple layers", said Weiming Yuan, associate professor in the Department of Molecular Microbiology and Immunology at the Keck School of Medicine of USC, and co-corresponding author of the study. "This longer duration of viral activity may lead to an overreaction of the immune system, called a cytokine storm, which kills healthy cells, causing tissue damage."[51]

The interaction of the innate and the adaptive immune responses might also explain why some COVID-19 patients experience two waves of the disease, first seeming to get better before eventually getting much worse. While the authors advocated the counterintuitive idea of a short regimen of an immunosuppressant drug applied early in the disease process to improve outcomes, another safer strategy might be to ensure that an adequate innate immune response is present when the virus first takes hold.

Another key feature of advanced COVID-19 infection is a state of increased reactivity of the patient's blood. This has been termed COVID-19-associated haemostasis abnormality (CAHA).[52] Of note are the occurrence of microthrombi, large blood clots, and increased blood viscosity. These serve to amplify tissue damage and thereby fuel the counterproductive immune response to such damage (cytokine storm).

The growing evidence strongly suggests that some of the clinical features of COVID-19 infection (like hypoxemia) are driven by a localized thrombotic phenomenon where both platelets and endothelium come together to initiate thrombosis. Endothelial cells constitute almost a third of the cells in the alveolar component of the lungs and have the key receptors for the SARS-CoV-2 including the angiotensin-converting enzyme-2 receptors.[53]

Enhanced platelet inhibition has been shown to improve hypoxaemia in patients with severe COVID-19 and hypercoagulability.[54] High fibrinogen levels associated with increased blood viscosity have also been implicated.[55]

13.6.3 COVID-19: how do the vulnerabilities and pathological features inform treatment?

The above discussion suggests several additional strategies that might help the vulnerable patient avoid serious complications from COVID-19 infection. The rationalisations behind these are as follows:

1. The slow disease progression and critical role of the innate immune response suggests supporting barrier defences (gut and respiratory), including innate immunity itself.
2. The link to hypertension, T2D, and kidney disease, together with the occurrence of microthrombi, suggests enhancing endothelial and microcirculatory function and improving blood quality.
3. The link to obesity and T2D suggests addressing non-resolving inflammation and up-regulating Nrf2.
4. The link to advanced age suggests addressing immunosenescence and boosting the HPA axis response to enhance resilience with ageing.
5. The link to heart and kidney disease, as well as the need to boost innate immune function, suggests boosting mitochondrial function and dynamics.
6. The demonstration that better glycaemic control in T2D reduces the risk of severe infection suggests addressing metabolic imbalances and lowering insulin resistance.

13.6.4 Additional FHT interventions for the vulnerable COVID-19 patient

Based on all the above, the suggested strategies/goals for the vulnerable patient are **additional to** the FHT protocols for respiratory infections provided in Section 13.5. They will also be largely relevant for patients who are vulnerable to other potentially severe respiratory viral infections, such as influenza A (which is known to trigger heart attacks, by way of example).

These additional FHT interventions for the vulnerable COVID-19 patient are:

- Support the HPA axis to counter the deleterious effects of the biological stress caused by the infection; especially consider adaptogenic herbs that have an immune provenance, such as Astragalus, Tinospora, and Eleutherococcus (see Chapter 2).
- Compensate for the effects of ageing on the immune system (see Section 13.4).
- Enhance mitochondrial function and biogenesis (see Chapters 2, 6, and 11).
- Boost macrocirculatory, microcirculatory, and endothelial health; improve blood quality (see Chapters 2 and 5).
- Resolve deleterious non-resolving inflammation and support Nrf2 (see Chapters 2 and 6).
- Enhance natural defensive barriers (see Chapters 2 and 12).
- Address metabolic imbalances, especially targeting blood sugar and blood pressure (see Chapter 11).
- Support the affected tissues (for lungs, see this chapter and Chapter 12; for heart and kidneys, see Chapter 2).

Further reading

For more details on the research on Andrographis as an immune herb during respiratory viral infections, and on research on the mode of action of Echinacea root, see the corresponding monographs in the following:

Bone KM, Mills SY. *Principles and Practice of Phytotherapy: Modern Herbal Medicine*, 2nd edition. UK: Elsevier, 2013.

References

1. Lloyd JU. *Echinacea Angustifolia*. Lloyd Brothers, Cincinnati, 1923. In: Bauer R, Wagner H. *Echinacea: Handbuch für Ärzte, Apotheker und andere Naturwissenschaftler*. WVG, Stuttgart, 1990, p 16.
2. Matthias A, Addison RS, Penman KG, Dickinson RG, Bone KM, Lehmann RP. Echinacea alkamide disposition and pharmacokinetics in humans after tablet ingestion. *Life Sci*. 2005 Sep 2; **77**(16): 2018–2029. PMID: 15919096.
3. Karsch-Völk M, Barrett B, Kiefer D, et al. Echinacea for preventing and treating the common cold. *Cochrane Database Syst Rev*. 2014 Feb 20; **2**(2): CD000530. doi:10.1002/14651858.CD000530.pub3. PMID: 24554461.
4. Schapowal A, Klein P, Johnston SL. Echinacea reduces the risk of recurrent respiratory tract infections and complications: a meta-analysis of randomized controlled trials. *Adv Ther*. 2015; **32**(3): 187–200. doi:10.1007/s12325-015-0194-4.
5. Jurcic K, Melchart D, Holzmann M, et al. Zwei Probandenstudien zur Stimulierung der Granulozytenphagozytose durch Echinacea-Extrakt-haltige Präparate. *Zeitschrift für Phytotherapie*. 1989; **10**: 67–70.
6. Wagner H (Ed). *Immunomodulatory Agents from Plants*. Birkauser Verlag, Basel, 1999.
7. Mondal S, Varma S, Bamola VD, et al. Double-blinded randomized controlled trial for immunomodulatory effects of Tulsi (*Ocimum sanctum* Linn.) leaf extract on healthy volunteers. *J Ethnopharmacol*. 2011; **136**(3): 452–456. doi:10.1016/j.jep.2011.05.012.
8. Agbabiaka TB, Guo R, Ernst E. Pelargonium sidoides for acute bronchitis: a systematic review and meta-analysis [published correction appears in *Phytomedicine*. 2009 Aug; **16**(8):798–799]. *Phytomedicine*. 2008; **15**(5): 378–385. doi:10.1016/j.phymed.2007.11.023.
9. Morgan M. Pelargonium: medicinal root from South Africa. *A Phytotherapist's Perspective*. 2009 April; **122**: 1–2. Available from: https://mediherb.com.au
10. Riley DS, Lizogub VG, Zimmermann A, et al. Efficacy and tolerability of high-dose pelargonium extract in patients with the common cold. *Altern Ther Health Med*. 2018 Mar; **24**(2): 16–26. PMID: 29055287.
11. Luna LA Jr, Bachi AL, Novaes e Brito RR, et al. Immune responses induced by Pelargonium sidoides extract in serum and nasal mucosa of athletes after exhaustive exercise: modulation of secretory IgA, IL–6 and IL–15. *Phytomedicine*. 2011 Feb 15; **18**(4): 303–308. doi:10.1016/j.phymed.2010.08.003. PMID: 20850953.
12. Morgan M. Major therapeutic activity of Tinospora. *A Phytotherapist's Perspective*. November 2018; **242**. Available from: https://mediherb.com.au
13. Lee CS, Lee JH, Oh M, et al. Preventive effect of Korean red ginseng for acute respiratory illness: a randomized and double-blind clinical trial. *J Korean Med Sci*. 2012; **27**(12): 1472–1478. doi:10.3346/jkms.2012.27.12.1472.
14. https://www.sinobiological.com/resource/cytokines/cytokine-function
15. Furman D, Davis MM. New approaches to understanding the immune response to vaccination and infection. *Vaccine*. 2015; **33**(40): 5271–5281. doi:10.1016/j.vaccine.2015.06.117.
16. Koyama S, Ishii KJ, Coban C, Akira S. Innate immune response to viral infection. *Cytokine*. 2008; **43**(3): 336–341. doi:10.1016/j.cyto.2008.07.009.
17. Guo XJ, Thomas PG. New fronts emerge in the influenza cytokine storm. *Semin Immunopathol*. 2017 Jul; **39**(5): 541–550. doi:10.1007/s00281-017-0636-y. PMID: 28555383.
18. Chousterman BG, Swirski FK, Weber GF. Cytokine storm and sepsis disease pathogenesis. *Semin Immunopathol*. 2017 Jul; **39**(5): 517–528. doi:10.1007/s00281-017-0639-8. PMID: 28555385.

19. Shi Y, Wang Y, Shao C, Huang J, Gan J, Huang X, et al. COVID-19 infection: the perspectives on immune responses. *Cell Death Differ.* 2020 Mar 23 [Epub ahead of print]. doi:10.1038/s41418-020-0530-3. PMID: 32205856.
20. Guo XJ, Thomas PG. New fronts emerge in the influenza cytokine storm. *Semin Immunopathol.* 2017 Jul; **39**(5): 541–550. doi:10.1007/s00281-017-0636-y. PMID: 28555383.
21. Ibid.
22. Abascal K, Yarnell E. Herbal treatments for pandemic influenza: learning from the eclectics' experience. *Alternative and Complementary Therapies* 2006 Oct; **12**(5): 214–221 doi:10.1089/act.2006.12.214.
23. Bone KM, Mills SY. *Principles and Practice of Phytotherapy: Modern Herbal Medicine*, 2nd edition. UK, Elsevier, 2013. [p 530]
24. Sharma M, Arnason JT, Burt A, Hudson JB. Echinacea extracts modulate the pattern of chemokine and cytokine secretion in rhinovirus-infected and uninfected epithelial cells. *Phytother Res.* 2006 Feb; **20**(2): 147–152. PMID: 16444669.
25. Gertsch J, Schoop R, Kuenzle U, Suter A. Echinacea alkylamides modulate TNF-alpha gene expression via cannabinoid receptor CB2 and multiple signal transduction pathways. *FEBS Lett.* 2004 Nov 19; **577**(3): 563–569. PMID: 15556647.
26. Ellingwood F. *American Materia Medica: Therapeutics and Pharmacognosy.* 1919. [pp 183, 183, 87]
27. Luo H, Tang QL, Shang YX, Liang SB, Yang M, Robinson N, Liu JP. Can Chinese medicine be used for prevention of corona virus disease 2019 (COVID-19)? A review of historical classics, research evidence and current prevention programs. *Chin J Integr Med.* 2020 Feb 17. doi:10.1007/s11655 020-3192-6. PMID: 32065348.
28. Wang F, Xiao MD, Liao B. [Effect of Astragalus on cytokines in patients undergoing heart valve replacement]. *Zhongguo Zhong Xi Yi Jie He Za Zhi.* 2008 Jun; **28**(6): 495–498. [Chinese.] PMID: 18655554.
29. Vlachojannis JE, Cameron M, Chrubasik S. A systematic review on the sambuci fructus effect and efficacy profiles. *Phytother Res.* 2010 Jan; **24**(1): 1–8. [Review.] doi:10.1002/ptr.2729. PMID:19548290.
30. Torabian G, Valtchev P, Adil Q, Dehghani F. Anti-influenza activity of elderberry (*Sambucus nigra*). *Journal of Functional Foods* 2019; **54**: 353–360. doi.org/10.1016/j.jff.2019.01.031.
31. Hawkins J, Baker C, Cherry L, Dunne E. Black elderberry (*Sambucus nigra*) supplementation effectively treats upper respiratory symptoms: a meta-analysis of randomized, controlled clinical trials. *Complement Ther Med.* 2019 Feb; **42**: 361–365. doi:10.1016/j.ctim.2018.12.004. PMID: 30670267.
32. Rauš K, Pleschka S, Klein P, Schoop R, Fisher P. Effect of an echinacea-based hot drink versus oseltamivir in influenza treatment: a randomized, double-blind, double-dummy, multicenter, noninferiority clinical trial. *Curr Ther Res Clin Exp.* 2015 Apr 20; **77**: 66–72. doi:10.1016/j.curtheres.2015.04.001. PMID: 26265958.
33. Tiralongo E, Wee SS, Lea RA. Elderberry supplementation reduces cold duration and symptoms in air-travellers: a randomized, double-blind placebo-controlled clinical trial. *Nutrients.* 2016 Mar 24; **8**(4): 182. doi:10.3390/nu8040182. PMID: 27023596.
34. Lee DH, Kim HW. Innate immunity induced by fungal β-glucans via dectin–1 signaling pathway. *Int J Med Mushrooms.* 2014; **16**(1): 1–16. PMID: 24940900.
35. van der Meer JW, Joosten LA, Riksen N, Netea MG. Trained immunity: a smart way to enhance innate immune defence. *Mol Immunol.* 2015 Nov; **68**(1): 40–44. doi:10.1016/j.molimm.2015.06.019. PMID: 26597205.
36. https://www.ausdoc.com.au/news/aussie-team-trial-tb-vaccine-against-covid19
37. Netea MG, Kullberg BJ, Van der Meer JW. Circulating cytokines as mediators of fever. *Clin Infect Dis.* 2000 Oct; **31**(Suppl 5): S178–184. PMID: 11113021.

38. Abascal K, Yarnell E. Herbal treatments for pandemic influenza: learning from the eclectics' experience. *Alternative and Complementary Therapies* 2006 Oct; **12**(5): 214–221 doi:10.1089/act.2006.12.214. [p 217]
39. https://www1.nyc.gov/site/doh/covid/covid-19-data.page
40. Myers LC, Parodi SM, Escobar GJ, Liu VX. Characteristics of hospitalized adults with COVID-19 in an integrated health care system in California. *JAMA*. 2020 [published online ahead of print, 2020 Apr 24]; **323**(21): 2195–2198. doi:10.1001/jama.2020.7202.
41. Richardson S, Hirsch JS, Narasimhan M, et al. Presenting characteristics, comorbidities, and outcomes among 5700 patients hospitalized with COVID-19 in the New York City area. [published correction appears in doi:10.1001/jama.2020.7681]. *JAMA*. 2020 [published online ahead of print, 2020 Apr 22]; **323**(20): 2052–2059. doi:10.1001/jama.2020.6775.
42. https://www.businessinsider.com.au/coronavirus-death-rates-preexisting-conditions-heart-disease-cancer-2020-2?r=US&IR=T
43. https://www.sciencedaily.com/releases/2020/06/200601101308.htm
44. Docherty AB, Harrison EM, Green CA, et al. Features of 20 133 UK patients in hospital with covid-19 using the ISARIC WHO Clinical Characterisation Protocol: prospective observational cohort study. *BMJ*. 2020 May 22; **369**: m1985. doi:10.1136/bmj.m1985.
45. Grasselli G, Zangrillo A, Zanella A, et al. Baseline characteristics and outcomes of 1591 patients infected with SARS-CoV–2 admitted to ICUs of the Lombardy region, Italy. *JAMA*. 2020 [published online ahead of print, 2020 Apr 6]; **323**(16): 1574–1581. doi:10.1001/jama.2020.5394.
46. Zhu L, She ZG, Cheng X, et al. Association of blood glucose control and outcomes in patients with COVID-19 and pre-existing type 2 diabetes. *Cell Metab*. 2020; **31**(6): 1068–1077.e3. doi:10.1016/j.cmet.2020.04.021.
47. https://www.sciencedaily.com/releases/2020/05/200501120102.htm
48. https://www.thelancet.com/infographics/coronavirus
49. Du SQ, Yuan W. Mathematical modeling of interaction between innate and adaptive immune responses in COVID-19 and implications for viral pathogenesis. *J Med Virol*. 2020 [published online ahead of print, 2020 May 1]. doi:10.1002/jmv.25866.
50. https://www.technologynetworks.com/tn/news/covid-19-progression-may-be-impacted-by-immune-response-timing-334276?utm_campaign=NEW%E2%80%A6
51. *Ibid.*
52. Thachil J, Srivastava A. SARS-2 coronavirus-associated hemostatic lung abnormality in COVID-19: is it pulmonary thrombosis or pulmonary embolism? *Semin Thromb Hemost*. 2020 [published online ahead of print, 2020 May 12]. doi:10.1055/s-0040-1712155.
53. *Ibid.*
54. Viecca M, Radovanovic D, Forleo GB, Santus P. Enhanced platelet inhibition treatment improves hypoxemia in patients with severe COVID-19 and hypercoagulability. A case control, proof of concept study. *Pharmacol Res*. 2020 [published online ahead of print, 2020 May 23]; **158**: 104950. doi:10.1016/j.phrs.2020.104950.
55. Maier CL, Truong AD, Auld SC, Polly DM, Tanksley CL, Duncan A. COVID-19-associated hyperviscosity: a link between inflammation and thrombophilia?. *Lancet*. 2020; **395**(10239): 1758–1759. doi:10.1016/S0140-6736(20)31209-5.

14

FHT strategies for IBS and SIBO

It seems that everyone you talk to has a problem with their digestion these days. Poor diet, stress, entrenched dysbiosis, drug side effects, and a compromised intestinal wall barrier are all contributing to this growing and undeclared contagion. Two of the most common digestive problems are irritable bowel syndrome (IBS) and small intestinal bacterial overgrowth (SIBO). Research is now suggesting that they are linked to each other and even to other gastrointestinal conditions, such as functional dyspepsia and gastro-oesophageal reflux disease. Given the number and complexity of the underlying factors behind these disorders, how do we get the best outcomes from herbal prescribing for our patients?

Keeping up with relevant new evidence-based insights into these gut maladies is essential for patients' health and wellbeing and helps to underpin our success as clinicians. Adopting a mosaic disease FHT model that embraces, rather than fears, the complexity becomes a powerful therapeutic tool in this quest. A key part of this is knowing the best herbs to use to deliver the range of desired actions.

Perhaps you are somewhat confused by all the new information, the different theories and perspectives and, indeed, treatments, for these conditions. You might even be reflecting that there may not be any good, effective herbal approaches for treating such challenging disorders, and the only answer appears to be highly restrictive diets.

Information on SIBO and IBS is growing rapidly. In 2019, 987 papers were published on PubMed about IBS. This is equivalent roughly to the combined number from 1990 to 2000 inclusive. For SIBO there are now around 100 papers a year.

In this chapter, the following are reviewed:

- IBS and SIBO: what they are, and what main factors are at play
- the relationship between SIBO and IBS, and with other gut disorders and beyond
- corrective FHT strategies for both SIBO and IBS
- revisiting the bowel flora protocol (BFP) in the context of SIBO and IBS.

14.1 Irritable bowel syndrome (IBS)

14.1.1 IBS diagnosis and definition

Gastroenterologists appear to like travelling to pleasant places for working holidays. And Rome seems to be a city they prefer. They periodically visit Rome, meeting to set the different criteria for IBS. The most recent consensus resulted in the Rome IV Diagnostic Criteria published in 2016 (see **Table 14.1**). According to these criteria, IBS can be diagnosed when a patient complains of **recurrent abdominal pain** associated with two or more of the following:

1. defecation
2. a change in the frequency of defecation
3. a change of stool appearance

There are some differences in diagnostic criteria of IBS in adults, children, and adolescents, which are not shown in the table.

The main differences between the Rome Criteria III from 2006 and Rome Criteria IV from 2016 can be readily seen in Table 14.1.[1] First, the term "discomfort" was removed, because it is not easy to distinguish pain from discomfort. Also, this term has been differently understood across several languages. Symptoms should appear at least four days per month, not one day per week, as it was before. Changes in stool consistency no longer need to be linked to pain onset, but only associated with pain presence.

In addition, pain relief after defecation has been replaced by pain related to defecation. Patients with constipation and abdominal pain should be first

Table 14.1 IBS diagnosis according to the Rome criteria

Rome III Criteria (2006) [Adults]	Rome IV Criteria (2016) [Adults]
Recurrent abdominal pain or discomfort with onset at least 6 months prior to diagnosis, associated with 2 or more of the following, at least 3 days per month in the last 3 months	Recurrent abdominal pain with onset at least 6 months prior to diagnosis, associated with 2 or more of the following, at least 1 day per week in the last 3 months
▹ improvement with defaecation ▹ onset associated with a change in frequency of stool ▹ onset associated with a change in form (appearance) of stool	▹ related to defaecation ▹ associated with a change in frequency of stool ▹ associated with a change in form (appearance) of stool

treated for the constipation only. If constipation treatment reduces the severity of symptoms, then functional constipation should be diagnosed, rather than IBS.

Also (not shown in the table), the current criteria allow the clinician to limit the number of diagnostic tests and replace the previously used term "no evidence for organic disease" with "after appropriate medical evaluation the symptoms cannot be attributed to another medical condition".

The important aspect to emphasise with both Rome criteria is that pain – specifically, abdominal pain – must be present. Pain is the defining symptom. A person who has diarrhoea with no pain does not meet the diagnosis of IBS.

Intrinsic in the Rome criteria are different patterns in stool frequency. This is reflected in the three IBS subtypes:[2]

1. IBS-C: predominantly constipation
2. IBS-D: predominantly diarrhoea
3. IBS-M: a mixed pattern of the above

One study examined the role of symptoms, psychological criteria, and biomarkers in the diagnosis of IBS. This was a meta-analysis of 22 studies in 7,106 people.[3] It was observed that, in general, biomarkers (they considered 11 of them) performed no better than symptom-based criteria. However, faecal calprotectin at <10 mg/L was deemed useful for diagnosis. Faecal calprotectin indicates the migration of neutrophils into the intestinal mucosa and hence is a marker of immune-based inflammation (as in inflammatory bowel disease,

IBD). So, if this level is high, then this helps to differentiate between IBS and IBD. The review concluded that combining symptoms with biomarkers (especially faecal calprotectin) appears more effective and may represent a way forward in IBS diagnosis.

14.1.2 IBS incidence and aetiological factors

A recent high-level review concluded that IBS is one of the most common disorders of gut–brain interaction, estimated to affect around 1 in 10 people globally. Although the prevalence rates seem to differ between countries, the magnitude of the effect of IBS – in terms of cost and quality of life – seems comparable around the world.[4] The authors suggested that the pathophysiology of IBS is complex and the role of risk factors, such as genetics, diet, and the microbiome, might vary depending on the geographical location. They also suggested that, as developing countries increasingly adopt a Western diet and lifestyle, we might see a corresponding increase in IBS prevalence rates – a trend that might also reflect an increasing awareness of the condition.

In terms of an overview of IBS and the aetiological factors involved, one review classified identified factors as host factors, luminal factors (occurring actually inside the gastrointestinal lumen, including the microbiome), and factors external to the person, which the authors called environmental factors. Specifically, these were as follows:[5]

1. **Host factors:**
   - altered gastrointestinal motility
   - visceral hypersensitivity
   - altered gut–brain interactions
   - increased intestinal permeability
   - gut mucosal immune activation

2. **Luminal factors:**
   - dysbiosis
   - neuroendocrine mediators
   - bile acids

3. **Environmental factors:**
   - psychosocial distress

- food
- medications
- supplements
- antibiotics
- enteric infection

Psychosocial distress could possibly have been better defined a host factor.

Some of these issues are explored in more detail in further sections. While the authors were comprehensive with their review, we can identify a few additional factors from the published literature. These include female hormonal fluctuations: often IBS is worse premenstrually.[6] The potential role of proton pump inhibitor drugs as an environmental factor should also be specifically flagged.[7] And finally, of course, is the contribution of SIBO to IBS (discussed later in this chapter).

14.1.3 Central sensitivity syndrome and IBS

IBS is considered to be part of a class of disorders that can be grouped under the heading of central sensitivity syndrome (CSS). These are functional somatic-type disorders and syndromes. A marked overlap of many functional disorders and syndromes in patients had been noted in the 1980s and 1990s. These were originally grouped and described as functional somatic syndrome,[8] but it was Yunus who later proposed that CSS was a better description.[9] According to Yunus, conditions that were covered by this term included chronic fatigue syndrome, fibromyalgia, primary dysmenorrhea, IBS, tension-type headache, migraine, interstitial cystitis, temporomandibular joint dysfunction, multiple chemical sensitivity, and restless legs syndrome.[10]

CSS ties in with the observed phenomenon of visceral hyperalgesia in IBS. In other words, the gut wall of a person with IBS appears to be more sensitive to pain than that of someone who does not have IBS. This is possibly due to this central sensitisation phenomenon, where a top-down response from the brain in response to a bottom-up signal from gut nervous tissue amplifies the pain signal to one that is disproportionate to the degree of original gut wall stretching.

What is behind this CSS phenomenon? The answer is thought to be neuroinflammation or, more specifically, "neuroendocrine immune dysfunction".

What causes CSS? Many of the same factors that have been implicated in IBS are thought to lead to CSS,[11] as can be seen in **Figure 14.1**. There are also a few additional considerations, with poor sleep being a factor that we need to especially consider in IBS.

Treating for CSS does not necessarily need to be given great emphasis in the initial stages of any therapeutic strategy for IBS. But if there is a difficult or non-responsive case, and especially if the IBS is comorbid with fibromyalgia or chronic fatigue or other CSS conditions, then it is probably worthwhile to consider an FHT strategy to reduce neuroinflammation and thereby central

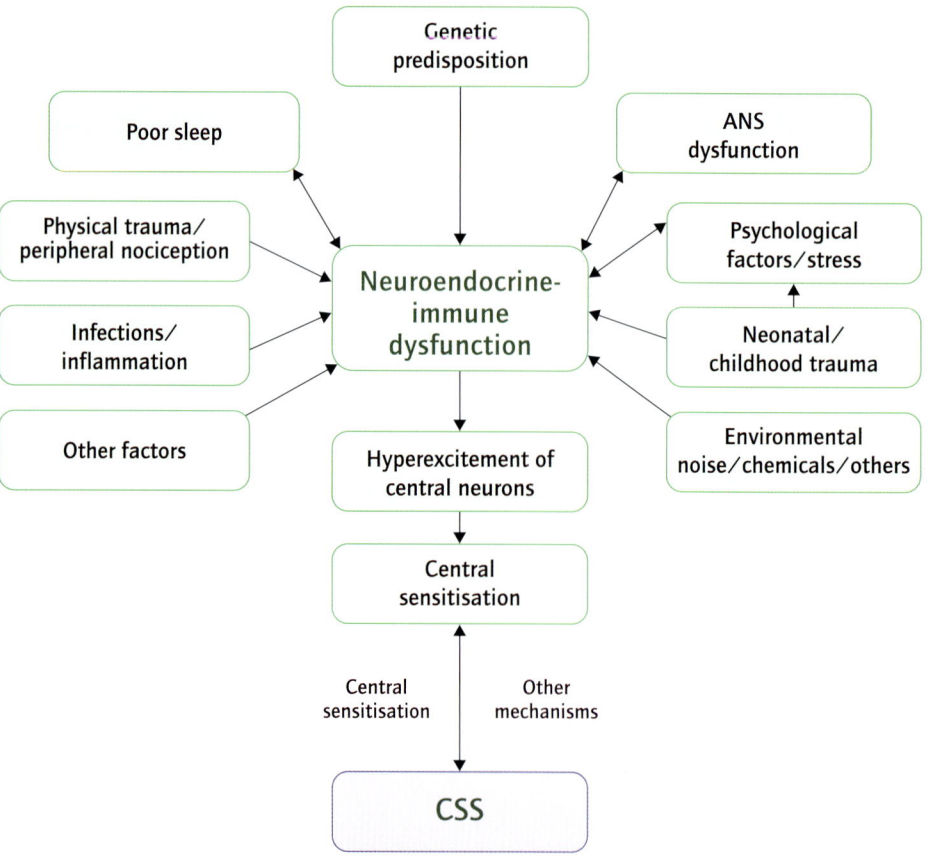

Figure 14.1 Factors and events leading to CSS. [ANS = autonomic nervous system; CSS = central sensitivity syndrome]

sensitisation. The likelihood from ample lines of evidence is that the more severe the IBS symptoms, the more likely is it that CSS is a dominant factor.

14.1.4 A deeper exploration of selected factors behind IBS

14.1.4.1 Gut microbiome

Although several studies comparing the gut microbiota composition in patients with IBS with that of healthy people have failed to provide consistent results, some key findings have emerged. These include:

- an increase in the *Firmicutes:Bacteroidetes* ratio
- decreases in *Lactobacilli* and *Bifidobacteria* populations
- increases in *Streptococci* and *Ruminococcus* species.[12]

Gut microbiota modulate key pathophysiological mechanisms underlying IBS, such as gastrointestinal motility and sensation, disrupted gut–brain axis, immune activation (with low-grade non-resolving inflammation), and compromised intestinal barrier function. Composition of gut microbiota is also affected by known IBS risk factors, such as host genetics, stress, diet, antibiotic usage, and early childhood experience.

A systematic review and meta-analysis of 13 articles assessed the molecular signature of the intestinal microbiota of 360 IBS patients and 268 healthy controls.[13] Down-regulation of bacterial colonisation, including *Lactobacilli*, *Bifidobacteria* and *F. prausnitzii*, was observed in IBS patients, particularly in diarrhoea-predominant IBS (IBS-D). The authors of this study suggested microbiota changes participate in the pathogenesis of IBS and may underlie the efficacy of probiotic supplements. Methanogenic microbiota were associated with IBS with constipation (IBS-C).

In addition, the dysbiosis might also be a presence or excess of the wrong bacteria. One review concluded that the incidence and prevalence of post-infection (PI) IBS varies between 9 and 10%.[14] A bacterial aetiology was most frequent, but post-viral and parasitic cases have also been reported.

A systematic review and meta-analysis of 45 studies, comprising 21,421 individuals with enteritis followed for 3 months to 10 years, found that more than 10% of patients with infectious enteritis develop IBS later.[15] The risk of IBS was 4-fold higher than in individuals who did not have infectious enteritis, although there was heterogeneity among the studies analysed. Women, particularly those with severe enteritis, are at increased risk for developing IBS, as are individuals with psychological distress and users of antibiotics during the enteritis. Of patients with enteritis caused by protozoa or parasites, 41.9% developed IBS. This compares strikingly with patients with enteritis caused by bacterial infection, of whom only 13.8% developed IBS.

14.1.4.2 Bile acid

Bile acid diarrhoea (BAD) is usually seen in patients with ileal Crohn's disease or ileal resection. However, 25–50% of patients with functional diarrhoea or IBS-D also show evidence of BAD.[16] It is further estimated that 1% of the population may suffer from BAD. Causes of BAD include a deficiency in fibroblast growth factor 19 (FGF-19), a hormone produced in enterocytes that regulates hepatic bile acid (BA) synthesis. Other potential causes include genetic variations that affect proteins involved in the enterohepatic circulation of bile acids and their synthesis, and variations in the TGR5 receptor that mediates the actions of bile acid on colonic secretion and motility. BAs enhance mucosal permeability, induce water and electrolyte secretion, and accelerate colonic transit partly by stimulating propulsive high-amplitude colonic contractions. Supporting evidence for the role of BAD in IBS-D is the finding that there is an increased proportion of primary BAs in the stool of patients.

14.1.4.3 Enteroendocrine dysfunction

Several types of endocrine cells are abnormal in all segments of the gastrointestinal tract of IBS patients. These enteroendocrine cells interact and integrate with each other, with the enteric nervous system, and with the afferent and efferent nerve fibres of the central nervous system – in particular the autonomic nervous system. They regulate several functions of the gastrointestinal tract, including sensation, motility, secretion, absorption, local immune defence, and food intake (by affecting appetite).[17]

Abnormalities in enteroendocrine cells are considered to play a major role in the development of symptoms in IBS and therefore represent potential targets for treatment. In particular, several of these cells express receptors for bitter phytochemicals, and their function can be favourably influenced by the intake of bitter herbs (see the incretin effect in Chapter 11).

14.1.4.4 Unresolving inflammation

Studies demonstrate a chronic, low-grade inflammation in patients with IBS. In one study, a total of 242 IBS patients and 244 healthy controls (HC) were compared for serum levels of the inflammatory marker high-sensitivity C-reactive protein (hs-CRP).[18] Median hs-CRP levels in the IBS group were significantly higher than in HC (1.80 vs. 1.20, $p < 0.006$). Levels were highest in IBS-D patients with greater disease severity. Hs-CRP levels mildly correlated with symptom severity ($p = 0.009$); this correlation was stronger for the IBS-D patients. IBS was a significant independent predictor for higher hs-CRP levels, whereas other pain and psychological comorbidities were not.

14.1.4.5 Barrier issues

Many patients with inflammatory bowel disease experience IBS symptoms. It has been suggested that a common linking factor could be damage to the intestinal barrier.[19] One study found that oral 5-hydroxytryptophan induced alterations in mucosal serotonin metabolism.[20] In healthy controls, a reinforcement of the intestinal barrier was seen, whereas such a reaction was absent in IBS patients. This could indicate the presence of a serotonin-mediated mechanism aimed to reinforce intestinal barrier function, which seems to be dysfunctional in IBS patients.

Exposure to non-steroidal anti-inflammatory drugs (NSAIDs) – which damage the intestinal barrier – has been linked to IBS.[21]

14.1.4.6 Functional dyspepsia

Functional dyspepsia (FD) and IBS exhibit a substantial overlap, and often one condition cannot be addressed without treating the other. The essential difference between the two is anatomic: IBS relates to the colon, and the pain is perceived largely in that part of the body; in the case of functional dyspepsia, it is the upper gastrointestinal tract that is affected, and, typically, symptoms occur with food intake.

Two subtypes of FD are recognised:[22]

1. postprandial distress syndrome (PDS): indigestion after meals and early satiety
2. epigastric pain syndrome (EPS): epigastric pain and epigastric burning, which can be confused with a peptic ulcer or gastro-oesophageal reflux

The overlap of IBS with FD has been examined in several studies, and there are examples of the evidence supporting this. In a Swedish study of people with IBS, 87% also fulfilled the dyspepsia criteria.[23] A Chinese study found that some half of patients with IBS had FD,[24] and in a Korean study patients with an IBS–FD overlap had more severe symptoms and higher depression scores.[25]

It is important to note this differentiation between IBS and FD, because several herbal trials have been conducted in people with FD, or in cohorts with FD and IBS not differentiated. But because of the considerable overlap between these two key conditions, this does not invalidate the relevance of these trial results to the treatment of IBS.

14.1.5 IBS treatments

14.1.5.1 Drug treatments for IBS

The main drugs used in the treatment of IBS are listed in **Table 14.2**.[26] When there is a medical condition that is treated by about 20 different drugs addressing a dozen or so different targets, what does that tell us? It suggests that the treatment is piecemeal, symptomatic, and probably not very effective in many cases. It further suggests that the "magic bullet" approach struggles with such an incompletely understood mosaic disease with many potential targets for treatment. It is interesting to note that enteric-coated peppermint oil makes the list in the table, because there is high-level evidence that it reduces abdominal pain in IBS due to its well-documented spasmolytic activity.[27]

Table 14.2 Drugs used to treat IBS

Condition	Drug	Mechanism of action
Constipation	Tegaserod	$5\text{-}HT_4$-receptor agonist
	Prucalopride	$5\text{-}HT_4$-receptor agonist
	Lubiprostone	luminally acting prostanoid
	Linaclotide	luminally acting guanylate cyclase-c agonist
	Elobixibat	highly selective inhibitor of the ileal bile acid transporter
	PEG (polyethylene glycol)	osmotic laxative
Diarrhoea	Loperamide	synthetic peripheral μ-opioid agonist
	Eluxadoline	mixed μ-opioid agonist and δ-opioid receptors antagonist
	Ondansetron	$5\text{-}HT_3$ antagonist
	Alosetron	$5\text{-}HT_3$ antagonist
	Asimadoline	κ-opioid receptor agonist
	Rifaximin	broad-spectrum, poorly absorbed antibiotic
	Mesalazine	intestinal anti-inflammatory
Abdominal pain	Trimebutine	antispasmodic agents
	Mebeverine	
	Amitriptyline	tricyclic antidepressant
	Citalopram	SSRI (serotonin reuptake inhibitor)
	peppermint oil	
	probiotics, prebiotics, synbiotics	

14.1.5.2 Diet treatments for IBS

The low FODMAPs diet was developed in Australia at Monash University, and it has swept the world. It has certainly been very successful for the management of IBS, but it does have its limitations. And, interestingly, those limitations have been highlighted by the FODMAPs pioneers themselves in order to clarify its value and purpose.

FODMAP is an acronym for "Fermentable Oligo-, Di-, Mono-saccharides and Polyols". The key principle of the diet is avoiding foods high in specific short-chain carbohydrates (FODMAPs) that tend to be malabsorbed because they are either:

- indigestible (fructo- and galacto-oligosaccharides, that are then fermented by gut flora; and lactose in those with hypolactasia) *or*
- slowly absorbed from the small intestine (fructose in excess of glucose, and polyols like sorbitol and mannitol)

The diet is practised in three steps:

1. **Exclusion phase**, during which strict adherence to the diet is important to determine response (expectation is 70%)
2. **Reintroduction phase:** foods are re-introduced to determine the degree of restriction needed to maintain a satisfactory symptom level (75% of responders can reduce restrictions considerably)
3. **Ongoing personalised diet**, where well-tolerated FODMAPS are included, while still restricting the ones that are poorly tolerated

The high FODMAP foods to be avoided are outlined in **Table 14.3**.[28]

The FODMAPS pioneers emphasise that the diet is not:[29]

- good for health (some FODMAPs are prebiotics)
- meant for the long term
- a "cure" for the underlying pathophysiology of IBS
- a diagnostic tool

For those for whom the FODMAPs diet is too difficult, a reduced fructose diet can be implemented, as per **Table 14.4**.[30] This diet improved symptoms in around half of tested patients with IBS.

Avoiding gluten may also be a useful strategy, especially in IBS-D. A dietitian-led gluten-free diet (GFD) provided sustained benefit in one RCT involving 45 patients with IBS-D.[31] Furthermore, gluten intake was shown to alter gut barrier function in these patients with IBS-D, particularly in those who were HLA-DQ2/8-positive. (HLA-DQ2 is the most common of the two main coeliac disease susceptibility genes; HLA-DQ8 is the other.)

Table 14.3 High FODMAP foods and low FODMAP alternatives

Food category	High FODMAP foods	Low FODMAP food alternatives
Vegetables	▷ artichoke, asparagus, cauliflower, garlic, green peas, leeks, mushrooms, onions, sugar snap peas	▷ aubergine/eggplant, beans (green), bok choy, capsicum (bell pepper), carrot, cucumber, lettuce, potato, tomato, zucchini
Fruits	▷ apples, apple juice, cherries, dried fruit, mango, nectarines, peaches, pears, plums, watermelon	▷ cantaloupe, grapes, kiwi fruit (green), mandarin, orange, pineapple, strawberries
Dairy and alternatives	▷ cow's milk, custard, evaporated milk, ice cream, soy milk (made from whole soybeans), sweetened condensed milk, yoghurt	▷ almond milk, brie/camembert cheese, feta cheese, hard cheeses, lactose-free milk, soy milk (made from soy protein)
Protein sources	▷ most legumes/pulses, some marinated meats/poultry/seafood, some processed meats	▷ eggs, firm tofu, plain cooked meats/poultry/seafood, tempeh
Breads and cereal products	▷ wheat/rye/barley-based breads, breakfast cereals, biscuits and snack products	▷ corn flakes, oats, quinoa flakes, quinoa/rice/corn pasta, rice cakes (plain), sourdough spelt bread, wheat/rye/barley-free breads
Sugars/sweeteners and confectionery	▷ high-fructose corn syrup, honey, sugar-free confectionery	▷ dark chocolate, maple syrup, rice malt syrup, table sugar
Nuts and seeds	▷ cashews, pistachios	▷ macadamias, peanuts, pumpkin seeds, walnuts

Another RCT in 72 IBS patients found a large number to be sensitive to gluten.[32] Overall, the symptomatic improvement was statistically different in the gluten group compared with the placebo (gluten-free) group, with improvement in 25.7% (9 patients) and 83.8% (31 patients), respectively ($p < 0.001$).

A 6-week GFD in 41 patients with IBS-D reduced the IBS Symptom Severity Score (IBSSSS) by ≥ 50 points in 71% (29 patients) overall.[33] The mean total IBSSSS decreased from 286 before the diet to 131 points after 6 weeks on the diet ($p < 0.001$); the reduction was similar in each HLA-DQ group. However, HLA-DQ2/8-negative participants had a greater reduction in abdominal distention ($p = 0.04$). Both HLA-DQ2/8-negative and -positive

Table 14.4 Elements of a reduced fructose diet

Food item	In moderation	Use sparingly	Avoid
Fruit/berries	▷ lemons, raspberries, blueberries		▷ all other types of fruit and berries
Vegetables	▷ most vegetables, avocado	▷ tomato purée	▷ carrots, legumes, boiled potatoes
Meat/fish/eggs	▷ 100% ground beef ▷ fish with no additives	▷ caviar, mackerel in tomato sauce ▷ anchovies, herring	
Milk products	▷ white/brown cheeses, cream, sour cream	▷ cheeses with fruit added	▷ fruit yoghurt, ice cream, puddings
Grain products	▷ bread, pasta, rice, white flour		▷ sweet bakery, cereals
Miscellaneous	▷ margarine, oils, mayonnaise, nuts	▷ dressings, ketchup	▷ sweets, chocolates
Drinks	▷ water, milk, tea, coffee, light soda, light fructose drinks	▷ light orange juice	▷ juice, nectar, sodas, fructose drinks, milk with sugar or fructose added

patients had marked mean improvements in hospital anxiety and depression scores, fatigue impact score, and Short Form-36 results (a measure of quality of life), although HLA-DQ2/8-positive participants had a greater reduction in depression.

From meta-analysis, soluble (but not insoluble) fibre, such as psyllium, has been shown to benefit IBS in general and will have particular benefit for IBS-C.[34]

14.1.5.3 Herbal treatments for IBS

An open study on 553 dyspeptic patients found that after 6 weeks of treatment with an average dose of about 7 g/day of globe artichoke (*Cynara cardunculus* var *scolymus*) leaves, symptoms improved in a clinically relevant and statistically significant ($p < 0.001$) manner. The therapeutic efficacy of the standardised extract was rated by physicians as excellent or good in 87% of patients. Substantial improvement was recorded for the following symptoms:

vomiting, nausea, abdominal pain, constipation, flatulence, belching, and fat intolerance.[35]

Healthy patients with self-reported functional dyspepsia ($n = 516$), as assessed via the Nepean Dyspepsia Index and the State-Trait Anxiety Inventory, were randomly allocated 320 or 640 mg/day of globe artichoke extract for 2 months in an open study.[36] In both dosage groups there was a significant reduction of all dyspeptic symptoms, with an average reduction of 40% in the Global Dyspepsia Score compared with baseline values. A follow-up *post hoc* analysis of the data was later conducted to assess the subset of patients with IBS symptoms ($n = 208$).[37] Analysis revealed that there was a significant fall in IBS incidence of 26.4% ($p < 0.001$) after the herbal treatment, with a significant shift away from alternating constipation and diarrhoea ($p < 0.001$).

In a 28-day RCT of a globe artichoke/ginger combination in 126 patients with FD, there was a significant reduction in symptoms versus placebo, including bloating, epigastric pain, and nausea.[38] Doses used were equivalent to about 2 and 1 g/day, respectively.

A 30-day RCT of deglycyrrhizinised licorice (4.1 g/day root equivalent) in 50 patients with FD observed significant reductions in FD symptoms versus placebo.[39]

The traditional Chinese formula known as Si-Ni-San (SNS) containing Zhi Shi (immature bitter orange), Bupleurum, paeony, and licorice was more effective in IBS patients when compared to conventional therapy (meta-analysis of 16 trials).[40]

Treatment with a standardised globe artichoke extract (equivalent to 8.6 g/day dried leaf) reduced the severity of symptoms of patients with IBS in a post-marketing surveillance study. The overall effectiveness of the herb was rated favourably by both physicians and patients. In fact, 96% of patients rated the herb as better than or at least equal to previous therapies.[41]

An 8-week RCT of 800 mg/day berberine in 192 IBS-D sufferers found typical symptoms such as diarrhoea, pain, and defecation frequency to be significantly reduced.[42]

Boswellia in a lecithin-based delivery form improved IBS, particularly when compared to symptomatic drug treatments.[43] The study included 69 otherwise healthy participants with a mild level of IBS who completed a 6-month follow-up period. In total, 34 were assigned to the standard management group: diet and, if needed, spasmolytic drugs; 35 were assigned to supplementation with Boswellia and the drugs as needed.

The high-level evidence supporting enteric-coated peppermint oil for pain and spasm in IBS has been noted above, with positive assessment from several meta-analyses.[44]

14.1.6 FHT strategies for IBS

The FHT goals, actions, and key herbs for IBS are as follows:

- improve gastrointestinal motor function: spasmolytic herbs, especially chamomile, ginger, Corydalis, peppermint, fennel, and cramp bark.
- balance nervous system function: anxiolytic and nervine tonic herbs for reducing stress and improving sleep, particularly valerian, kava, passionflower, and skullcap.
- manage barrier and inflammation issues: anti-inflammatory, antiallergic, and gut-barrier-promoting herbs, especially turmeric and/or curcumin, chamomile, Baical skullcap, golden seal, meadowsweet, and licorice.
- improve the gastric acid barrier, enteroendocrine dysfunction, and overall digestion with bitter herbs – gentian, wormwood and feverfew – and ginger and chen pi.
- balance any symptoms association with the menstrual cycle with chaste tree.
- regulate bowel function with mild laxative herbs for IBS-C, such as Rehmannia and licorice.
- in extreme cases with strong psychological symptoms and marked visceral hyperalgesia: focus more centrally and treat for neuroinflammation with anti-inflammatory herbs such as Boswellia and bioavailable curcumin (see also Chapter 2).
- enhance bile release and flow with choleretic and cholagogue herbs – globe artichoke, milk thistle, dandelion root – with ginger for IBS-C; but avoid in IBS-D.
- gentle fibre for IBS-C, using demulcent herbs such as slippery elm and marshmallow root.
- address SIBO, if present (see Section 14.2).
- work on improving dysbiosis and gut wall integrity as per the following information.

Since both dysbiosis and a dysfunctional gut barrier have been implicated in IBS, the best strategy to engage is the modified version of the BFP with the focus on gut wall healing. This is fully described in Chapter 8, but some additional comments are worth noting here.

Since high-dose berberine has been shown to be of value in IBS-D, it might represent the best option for weeding in that subset of IBS (as, say, Phellodendron). This BFP bowel/barrier protocol is best combined with a gluten-free diet in IBS (given the diet trials above and because of the negative effects of gluten on the barrier). The herbs recommended for gut wall healing – namely licorice (can be deglycyrrhizinised), chamomile, and meadowsweet – will be very useful for other reasons in IBS, as outlined in the FHT strategies above.

14.2 Small intestinal bacterial overgrowth

14.2.1 Definition, assessment, and symptoms

SIBO is a heterogeneous syndrome, defined as the presence of an increased number and/or abnormal type of bacteria in the distal small intestine. The classic presentation has been steatorrhea, malabsorption, abdominal bloating, and weight loss, but this is actually infrequent. More commonly, now, patients with a diagnosis of SIBO report bloating, flatulence, abdominal pain, and diarrhoea (just as for IBS).[45]

The human gastrointestinal microflora is a complex ecosystem of approximately 400 bacterial species. Because the small intestine is the site of digestion and the absorption of food, bacterial flora are largely excluded. This has the consequence of preventing unwanted nutrient competition with the host and abnormal entry of bacteria across the more permeable epithelium of the small intestine. In addition, gas production from bacterial fermentation of food is thereby minimised.[46]

There are several endogenous defence mechanisms for preventing bacterial overgrowth in the small intestine: gastric acid secretion, good intestinal motility, intact ileo-caecal valve function, immunoglobulins, and the bacteriostatic properties of pancreatic and biliary secretion. In keeping with this understanding, the complex aetiology of SIBO is usually associated with disorders of protective antibacterial mechanisms (such as achlorhydria, pancreatic exocrine insufficiency, immunodeficiency syndromes), anatomical abnormalities (such as small intestinal obstruction, diverticula, fistulae, surgical blind loop, previous ileo-caecal resections), and/or motility disorders (e.g., scleroderma, autonomic neuropathy in diabetes mellitus, post-radiation enteropathy, small intestinal pseudo-obstruction). In some patients more than one factor may be involved. The gold standard for diagnosing SIBO is still microbial investigation of jejunal aspirates; however, non-invasive hydrogen and methane breath tests using glucose or lactulose as the test probe are more commonly used.[47]

Complicating the picture further is the finding that small intestinal fungal overgrowth (SIFO), which would probably test negative on a breath test, has also been described recently. A study was performed on 150 patients with persistent gastrointestinal complaints and negative endoscopy/radiology tests.[48] They completed a validated symptom questionnaire and underwent 24-hour ambulatory antro-duodeno-jejunal manometry (ADJM). Simultaneously, a duodenal aspirate was obtained for aerobic, anaerobic, and fungal culture. Bacterial growth $\geq 10^3$ cfu (colony-forming units)/mL, or similar fungal growth, was considered evidence for SIBO/SIFO. It was found that 63% of patients had overgrowth. Of these, 40% had SIBO, 26% had SIFO, and the remaining 34% had mixed SIBO/SIFO. SIBO was predominately due to *Streptococcus, Enterococcus, Klebsiella,* and *E. coli*. SIFO was due to *Candida spp.* (*albicans or torulopsis*). Of the 150 patients, 53% (80 patients) had dysmotility issues, and 43% (65 patients) had used proton pump inhibitor drugs (PPIs). PPI use ($p = 0.0063$) and dysmotility ($p = 0.0003$) were independent significant risk factors ($p < 0.05$) for overgrowth. Symptom profiles were similar for those with or without SIBO/SIFO.

14.2.1.1 Testing for SIBO

The use of tests to diagnose SIBO is the subject of considerable debate and controversy.

The 2017 Hydrogen and Methane-Based Breath Testing in Gastrointestinal Disorders: The North American Consensus (a panel of 17 experts) proposed the following:[49]

- SIBO diagnosis is *suggested* when there is an increase in H_2 (hydrogen) of ≥20 ppm over baseline within the first 90 minutes of the test, with either lactulose or glucose as the test probe
  OR
- when there is an increase in CH_4 (methane) of ≥10 ppm at any time point of the test following lactulose or glucose

One review highlighted the many issues that can confound the current tests for SIBO. These are summarised in **Table 14.5**. Based on their review, the authors concluded that[50]

> There are significant limitations in the tests clinically available to diagnose SIBO, small bowel aspirates, and breath tests. . . . As a result, there is currently no true gold standard for its diagnosis.

14.2.2 SIBO: does it really exist, or is it overdiagnosed?

Despite the increase in interest in the role of the gut microbiome in health and disease and the recognition for over 50 years that an excess of colonic-type flora in the small intestine can lead to a malabsorption syndrome, small intestinal overgrowth remains poorly defined. This lack of clarity owes much to the difficulties that arise in attempting to arrive at consensus regarding its

Table 14.5 Potential limitations of diagnostic testing for small intestinal bacterial overgrowth

Small bowel aspirates or culture	Breath testing
invasive and costly	requires proper preparation
bacterial colonisation may be patchy or located in more distal aspects of the small bowel	false positive tests may be seen with chronic lung disease and in smokers
improper handling of samples	glucose may not detect bacterial overgrowth in the more distal portions of the small bowel
contamination may occur from oropharyngeal flora	lactulose shortens orocecal transit time
controversy regarding diagnostic cut-off	wide variation in interpretation and diagnostic criteria

diagnosis. As noted above, there is currently no gold standard, and the commonly available methodologies (the culture of jejunal aspirates and a variety of breath tests) suffer from considerable variations in their performance and interpretation, leading to variations in the prevalence of overgrowth in a variety of clinical contexts.[51]

Debate is also fuelled by the fact that this is a heterogenous condition. At one extreme there is no doubt that SIBO can be a serious medical condition, associated with several comorbidities as well as genuine malabsorption with weight loss. But in many cases the label SIBO is applied to people with mild functional symptoms, who could perhaps just as validly be diagnosed as having IBS.

This debate has been fuelled – and perhaps settled, according to some workers in the field – by recent key publications that have received widespread attention. In particular, there was the 2018 study by Sundin and colleagues:[52] Eighteen patients reporting symptoms consistent with SIBO underwent a glucose breath test. On a later day, the jejunal lumen of each person was sampled via aspiration during enteroscopy. Jejunal aspirates were cultured on aerobic and anaerobic media. DNA was extracted from the same samples and analysed by quantitative pan-bacterial PCR amplification of 16S ribosomal rRNA genes, which provides a culture-independent bacterial cell count. Combined bacterial colony counts ranged from 5.7×10^3 to 7.9×10^6 cfu/mL. DNA-based yields ranged from 1.5×10^5 to 3.1×10^7 bacterial genomes per mL. Microbial viability ranged from 0.3% to near 100%. There was no significant correlation of the glucose breath test results with either the number of bacterial colonies (cfu counts) or with the DNA-based bacterial cell counts. Instead, higher readings in the hydrogen-methane breath test were actually significantly correlated with a **lower** viability of jejunal bacteria. The authors concluded that the glucose-based hydrogen and methane breath test is not sensitive to the overgrowth of jejunal bacteria. However, a positive breath test may indicate altered jejunal function and microbial dysbiosis.

In the editorial commentary on this work, it was proposed that the sole function of breath tests is to detect carbohydrate malabsorption, and that they are incapable of defining SIBO.[53]

An even more convincing re-examination of the SIBO conundrum was published in 2019. In this study, 126 symptomatic patients (21% male) underwent oesophago-gastro-duodenoscopy (EGD) with duodenal aspirate collection. The major symptoms that led to this investigation of small bowel bacterial counts included diarrhoea (45%), abdominal pain (28%), and bloating (13%).[54] Of the 126 patients, 66 (52%) tested positive for SIBO. Interestingly, there was a positive correlation between a positive SIBO diagnosis (by aspirate and culture) and recent antibiotic exposure (odds ratio of 4.2).

But the fascinating finding from this study was that a SIBO diagnosis based on duodenal aspirate culture reflected an overgrowth of anaerobic bacteria that did not correspond with patient symptoms and might even be the result of dietary preferences. On the other hand, qualitative changes in small intestinal microbial composition (as determined by bacterial DNA analysis) were significantly correlated with symptomatic patients. Specifically, small intestinal microbial communities from symptomatic patients were characterised by significantly lower phylogenetic alpha diversity (localised species diversity), richness (the number of species), and evenness (the similarity of the population size of each of the species present).

Additional work in the study found that asymptomatic healthy people consuming a high-fibre diet commonly met the diagnostic criteria (aspirate and culture) for SIBO. When these people were switched to a high-sugar, low-fibre diet, IBS-like symptoms were induced, together with decreased small intestinal microbial diversity and increased small intestinal permeability.

In the title of their sentinel paper, the authors suggested a new term to describe this phenomenon: small intestinal microbial dysbiosis (SIMD).

For the sake of simplicity, and mindful that most of the cited research has used breath testing for diagnosis, the term SIBO is used in this chapter, but bearing in mind that many cases labelled as SIBO – probably the majority – are, in fact, either SIMD or a variant of IBS. Despite the complexity and debate, the key message here is in fact very simple: for patients with a SIBO diagnosis, the main focus of treatment should be on correcting dysbiosis.

14.2.3 SIBO protective and risk factors

It is important to identify and treat the underlying issues causing a diagnosis of SIBO.[55] The natural protective factors and the circumstances that undermine these were mentioned above. The following discussion goes into more detail, being mindful of the limitations of the SIBO diagnosis explored above.

Table 14.6 SIBO risk factors

Category	Risk factor
Anatomical	▹ small-bowel obstruction ▹ adhesions ▹ small-bowel diverticula ▹ fistula ▹ postsurgical anatomical alteration
Dysmotility	▹ primary dysmotility (i.e., gastroparesis) ▹ Parkinson's disease ▹ scleroderma ▹ hypothyroidism ▹ diabetes mellitus ▹ gastroparesis ▹ narcotic medications
Alteration in pH	▹ achlorhydria ▹ proton pump inhibitors ▹ advanced age
Immune system	▹ immunoglobulin A deficiency ▹ combined variable immunodeficiency ▹ human immunodeficiency virus

The key risk factors for SIBO – grouped into four key categories: anatomical, dysmobility, alteration in pH, and immune system – are listed in **Table 14.6**.[56] Protective factors are listed in **Table 14.7**.[57] The most important physiological mechanisms protecting against SIBO are considered to be small bowel motility and gastric acid. This strongly correlates with the study of SIBO/SIFO cited above.

Table 14.7 SIBO protective factors

Protective factor
▹ gastric acid ▹ pancreatic enzymes ▹ bile acids ▹ cholecystectomy ▹ motility ▹ migrating motor complex ▹ biofilm ▹ secretory immunoglobulin A

Regarding impaired motility, 39% of gastroparesis patients tested positive for SIBO using the breath test.[58] SIBO is frequently found in patients with progressive familial intrahepatic cholestasis.[59] It has also been strongly linked to hypothyroidism, which slows intestinal transit.[60]

Prolonged transit enhances serum bile acid levels via bacterial overgrowth and increased ileal reabsorption, contributing to gallstone disease.[61] If fat is not being fully absorbed in the small intestine, it reaches the ileum. The normal physiological response is then to apply the ileal brake to slow transit and facilitate the absorption of this fat. But this application of the ileal brake to slow transit increases the risk for SIBO and enhances bile acid reabsorption, thereby creating a vicious cycle, with the slowing of small intestinal motility leading to further small intestinal bacterial colonisation and increased fat malabsorption.[62]

The contribution of ileocaecal valve dysfunction to digestive disorders has long been recognised by natural therapists. Ileocaecal valve dysfunction was significantly associated with SIBO in two small studies and linked to higher symptom scores.[63,64] In a 2017 study of 30 symptomatic patients, those with SIBO were found to have significantly lower ileocaecal junction pressure, prolonged small bowel transit time, and a higher gastrointestinal pH when compared to those without the disorder.[65]

14.2.4 SIBO comorbidities

As might be expected from the above, there is a considerable overlap between the diagnoses of IBS and SIBO. A meta-analysis found that patients with IBS were more likely to have SIBO than healthy subjects, as determined using the glucose hydrogen breath test (HBT) or jejunal aspirate culture, but not using the lactulose HBT.[66] Patients with IBS-D had SIBO more often. Some 4–78% of patients with IBS and 1–40% of controls have SIBO. Such wide variations might result from population differences, IBS diagnostic criteria, and, most importantly, methods to diagnose SIBO.[67] SIBO was again associated with IBS-D in a recent study and linked to higher *Prevotella* abundance.[68]

There are several significant comorbidities linked to SIBO, but whether they are cause or effect remains unclear in many instances:

- chronic pancreatitis[69]
- restless legs syndrome[70]
- deep vein thrombosis[71]
- kidney stones[72]
- Crohn's disease[73]
- functional dyspepsia[74]
- gall stones[75]
- fatty liver[76]
- osteoporosis[77]
- erosive oesophagitis[78]
- visceral fat[79]
- rosacea[80]

However, a causal role is probably quite likely for gall stones, chronic liver disease, and rosacea.[81]

14.2.5 Diet and SIBO

One review concluded:[82]

- The role of dietary changes in the management of SIBO is poorly understood. Carbohydrate intolerance is common in SIBO, and carbohydrate may act as a primary substrate for bacteria and provide a rich environment for bacterial growth.
- Thus, carbohydrate restriction (such as lactose restriction) may theoretically be of benefit in SIBO in some individuals; this has, however, not been subjected to rigorous study.
- Similarly, the much more involved low FODMAP diet may have merit in the treatment of SIBO, particularly for patients with irritable bowel symptoms.
- The role of a low FODMAP diet in SIBO deserves further study. It is generally agreed that the clinical symptoms of SIBO, which are not specific to SIBO, may improve with avoidance of fermentable foods.

At the time of writing there has been only one clinical trial of a diet therapy for SIBO, published in 2004.[83] This was an open label trial in 93 people with "IBS" and a positive lactulose breath test (LBT). They were placed on a

14-day elemental diet, and 80% (74/93) returned a normal LBT by Day 15. Those who had successfully normalised their breath test experienced a 66% improvement in bowel symptoms, compared to just 12% of those who did not normalise ($p < 0.001$).

Some therapists have proposed diets for SIBO based on their clinical observations. Here are two popular examples:

> - the SIBO Specific Diet, designed by Dr Allison Siebecker, which combines the low FODMAP diet and a specific carbohydrate diet (SCD)[84]
> - the SIBO Bi-Phasic Diet, designed by Dr Nirala Jacobi, which has a reduce-and-repair phase (4–6 weeks) followed by a remove-and-restore phase (4–6 weeks)[85]

Neither dietary approach has been assessed in a clinical trial.

14.2.6 Evidence for herbal treatments for SIBO

In contrast to IBS, there is only one clinical trial of a Western herbal formulation for the treatment of SIBO, published in 2014.[86] Patients positive for newly diagnosed SIBO by LBT ($n = 104$) were offered either rifaximin (1,200 mg daily) or herbal therapy for 4 weeks, with a repeat LBT post-treatment. Of the 37 patients who received herbal therapy, 46% (17) had a negative follow-up LBT, compared to 34% (23/67) of rifaximin users; of the rifaximin non-responders, 57.1% (8/14) had a negative LBT after completing rescue herbal therapy. The herbal protocol was quite complex but did contain substantial doses of berberine and essential oils of thyme and oregano.

14.2.7 FHT strategies for SIBO

FHT for SIBO has as its main focus:

1. reducing microbial burden/dysbiosis in the small intestine via oral herbal preparations;

    AND

2. addressing any underlying risk factors that might cause or exacerbate the disorder, or lead to a relapse;

AND

3   correcting general gastrointestinal dysbiosis;

AND

4   supporting all the above with appropriate dietary changes (low refined carbohydrates; possibly low FODMAPs)

Or another way to put this:[87]

1   elimination/modification of the underlying causes
2   induction of remission (antimicrobials and diet)
3   maintenance of remission (promotility treatments, dietary modifications, repeat or cyclical antimicrobials)

Given the uncertainty over the diagnostic tests for SIBO, a "test-by-treating" approach is a useful strategy. This entails the initial emphasis on broad-spectrum (active against bacteria AND fungi) antimicrobial herbs.

As a consequence, the FHT goals, **actions,** and key herbs for SIBO are the following:

- **immune support:** especially Echinacea root and Andrographis
- **antibacterial and antifungal herbs:** berberine herbs, oregano oil, garlic (allicin-releasing), myrrh, sage, and tannin herbs such as pomegranate hulls (ingested away from alkaloids such as berberine): *all these are the pivotal herbal treatments*
- gentle biofilm strategies (see Chapter 9)
- **choleretic and cholagogue herbs** to increase bile flow and reduce transit time: globe artichoke, dandelion root, milk thistle
- **anti-inflammatory herbs** to reduce the impact of inflammation: chamomile, licorice, turmeric (curcumin)
- mucoprotection and healing with **demulcent** and **barrier-supporting herbs**: licorice, meadowsweet, chamomile, golden seal
- improving gastric acid with **bitter herbs**
- increasing transit and improving gastric acid with ginger (especially), Coleus, chen pi
- **spasmolytic herbs** for pain and dysmotility: chamomile, chen pi, fennel, cramp bark, ginger, Corydalis
- correct dysbiosis: the BFP, but with a twist! (see **Box 14.1**)
- probiotics and gentle prebiotics (cautiously).

> **Box 14.1 BFP example for SIBO: 10–20-day cycle**
>
> | Weed | Feed |
> |---|---|
> | **5–10 days** | **5–10 days** |
> | ▸ Andrographis: 3 g twice a day
▸ Phellodendron: 4.8 g twice a day
▸ anise oil: 375 mg twice a day
▸ oregano oil: 225 mg twice a day | ▸ probiotic: once or twice a day
▸ a gentle prebiotic fibre like slippery elm: 1.5 g twice a day |
> | **only first 5 days:** | **at least 2 hours away from probiotic:** |
> | ▸ myrrh: 1 g twice a day | ▸ rosemary: 1 g twice a day
▸ green tea: 4 g twice a day
▸ grape seed: 6 g twice a day
▸ turmeric: 2 g twice a day |
>
> For best results, about 3–4 cycles are recommended.
>
> Base protocol can be adapted to the needs of each patient. More antimicrobial activity can be added with extra berberine (Phellodendron), plus synergists, garlic, biofilm strategy, tannins.

Further reading

Bone KM, Mills SY. *Principles and Practice of Phytotherapy: Modern Herbal Medicine*, 2nd edition. UK: Elsevier, 2013.

References

1. Oświęcimska J, Szymlak A, Roczniak W, Girczys-Połedniok K, Kwiecień J. New insights into the pathogenesis and treatment of irritable bowel syndrome. *Adv Med Sci.* 2017; **62**(1): 17–30. doi:10.1016/j.advms.2016.11.001.
2. Schoenfeld PS. Advances in IBS 2016: a review of current and emerging data. *Gastroenterol Hepatol (NY).* 2016; **12**(8, Suppl 3): 1–11.
3. Sood R, Gracie DJ, Law GR, Ford AC. Systematic review with meta-analysis: the accuracy of diagnosing irritable bowel syndrome with symptoms, biomarkers and/or psychological markers. *Aliment Pharmacol Ther.* 2015; **42**(5): 491–503. doi:10.1111/apt.13283.
4. Black CJ, Ford AC. Global burden of irritable bowel syndrome: trends, predictions and risk factors. *Nat Rev Gastroenterol Hepatol.* 2020 [published online ahead of print, 2020 Apr 15]. doi:10.1038/s41575-020-0286-8.

5. Chey WD, Kurlander J, Eswaran S. Irritable bowel syndrome: a clinical review. *JAMA.* 2015; **313**(9): 949–958. doi:10.1001/jama.2015.0954.
6. Jane ZY, Chang CC, Lin HK, Liu YC, Chen WL. The association between the exacerbation of irritable bowel syndrome and menstrual symptoms in young Taiwanese women. *Gastroenterol Nurs.* 2011; **34**(4): 277–286. doi:10.1097/SGA.0b013e3182248708.
7. Schmulson MJ, Frati-Munari AC. Bowel symptoms in patients that receive proton pump inhibitors. Results of a multicenter survey in Mexico. [Síntomas intestinales en pacientes que reciben inhibidores de bomba de protones (IBP). Resultados de una encuesta multicéntrica en México.] *Rev Gastroenterol Mex.* 2019; **84**(1): 44–51. doi:10.1016/j.rgmx.2018.02.008.
8. Wessely S, Nimnuan C, Sharpe M. Functional somatic syndromes: one or many? *Lancet* 1999; **354**(9182): 936–939. PMID: 10489969.
9. Yunus MB. Central sensitivity syndromes: a unified concept for fibromyalgia and other similar maladies. *J Ind Rheum Dis.* 2000; **8**: 27–33.
10. Yunus MB. Fibromyalgia and overlapping disorders: the unifying concept of central sensitivity syndromes. *Semin Arthritis Rheum.* 2007 Jun; **36**(6): 339–356. PMID: 17350675.
11. *Ibid.*
12. Bhattarai Y, Muniz Pedrogo DA, Kashyap PC. Irritable bowel syndrome: a gut microbiota-related disorder?. *Am J Physiol Gastrointest Liver Physiol.* 2017; **312**(1): G52–G62. doi:10.1152/ajpgi.00338.2016.
13. Liu HN, Wu H, Chen YZ, Chen YJ, Shen XZ, Liu TT. Altered molecular signature of intestinal microbiota in irritable bowel syndrome patients compared with healthy controls: a systematic review and meta-analysis. *Dig Liver Dis.* 2017; **49**(4): 331–337. doi:10.1016/j.dld.2017.01.142.
14. Schmulson M, Bielsa MV, Carmona-Sánchez R, et al. Microbiota, gastrointestinal infections, low-grade inflammation, and antibiotic therapy in irritable bowel syndrome: an evidence-based review. *Rev Gastroenterol Mex.* 2014; **79**(2): 96–134. doi:10.1016/j.rgmx.2014.01.004.
15. Klem F, Wadhwa A, Prokop LJ, et al. Prevalence, risk factors, and outcomes of irritable bowel syndrome after infectious enteritis: a systematic review and meta-analysis. *Gastroenterology.* 2017; **152**(5): 1042–1054.e1. doi:10.1053/j.gastro.2016.12.039.
16. Camilleri M. Bile Acid diarrhea: prevalence, pathogenesis, and therapy. *Gut Liver.* 2015; **9**(3): 332–339. doi:10.5009/gnl14397.
17. El-Salhy M, Gundersen D. Diet in irritable bowel syndrome. *Nutr J.* 2015 Apr 14; **14**: 36. doi:10.1186/s12937-015-0022-3.
18. Hod K, Ringel-Kulka T, Martin CF, Maharshak N, Ringel Y. High-sensitive C-reactive protein as a marker for inflammation in irritable bowel syndrome. *J Clin Gastroenterol.* 2016; **50**(3): 227–232. doi:10.1097/MCG.0000000000000327.
19. Qin X. Damage of the mucus layer: the possible shared critical common cause for both inflammatory bowel disease (IBD) and irritable bowel syndrome (IBS). *Inflamm Bowel Dis.* 2017; **23**(2): E11–E12. doi:10.1097/MIB.0000000000001010.
20. Keszthelyi D, Troost FJ, Jonkers DM, et al. Serotonergic reinforcement of intestinal barrier function is impaired in irritable bowel syndrome. *Aliment Pharmacol Ther.* 2014; **40**(4): 392–402. doi:10.1111/apt.12842.
21. Keszthelyi D, Dackus GH, Masclee GM, Kruimel JW, Masclee AA. Increased proton pump inhibitor and NSAID exposure in irritable bowel syndrome: results from a case-control study. *BMC Gastroenterol.* 2012 Sep 5; **12**: 121. doi:10.1186/1471-230X-12-121.
22. Asano H, Tomita T, Nakamura K, et al. Prevalence of gastric motility disorders in patients with functional dyspepsia. *J Neurogastroenterol Motil.* 2017; **23**(3): 392–399. doi:10.5056/jnm16173.

23. Agréus L, Svärdsudd K, Nyrén O, Tibblin G. Irritable bowel syndrome and dyspepsia in the general population: overlap and lack of stability over time. *Gastroenterology.* 1995; **109**(3): 671–680. doi:10.1016/0016-5085(95)90373-9.
24. Wang A, Liao X, Xiong L, et al. The clinical overlap between functional dyspepsia and irritable bowel syndrome based on Rome III criteria. *BMC Gastroenterol.* 2008 Sep 23; **8**: 43. doi:10.1186/1471-230X-8-43.
25. Choi YJ, Kim N, Yoon H, et al. Overlap between irritable bowel syndrome and functional dyspepsia including subtype analyses. *J Gastroenterol Hepatol.* 2017; **32**(9): 1553–1561. doi:10.1111/jgh.13756.
26. Oświęcimska J, Szymlak A, Roczniak W, Girczys-Połedniok K, Kwiecień J. New insights into the pathogenesis and treatment of irritable bowel syndrome. *Adv Med Sci.* 2017; **62**(1): 17–30. doi:10.1016/j.advms.2016.11.001.
27. Alammar N, Wang L, Saberi B, et al. The impact of peppermint oil on the irritable bowel syndrome: a meta-analysis of the pooled clinical data. *BMC Complement Altern Med.* 2019 Jan 17; **19**(1): 21. doi:10.1186/s12906-018-2409-0.
28. https://www.monashfodmap.com/3_step_fodmap_diet
29. https://www.ausdoc.com.au/author/professor-peter-gibson
30. Berg LK, Fagerli E, Myhre AO, Florholmen J, Goll R. Self-reported dietary fructose intolerance in irritable bowel syndrome: proposed diagnostic criteria. *World J Gastroenterol.* 2015; **21**(18): 5677–5684. doi:10.3748/wjg.v21.i18.5677.
31. Vazquez-Roque MI, Camilleri M, Smyrk T, et al. A controlled trial of gluten-free diet in patients with irritable bowel syndrome-diarrhea: effects on bowel frequency and intestinal function. *Gastroenterology.* 2013; **144**(5): 903–911.e3. doi:10.1053/j.gastro.2013.01.049.
32. Shahbazkhani B, Sadeghi A, Malekzadeh R, et al. Non-celiac gluten sensitivity has narrowed the spectrum of irritable bowel syndrome: a double-blind randomized placebo-controlled trial. *Nutrients.* 2015 Jun 5; **7**(6): 4542–4554. doi:10.3390/nu7064542.
33. Aziz I, Trott N, Briggs R, North JR, Hadjivassiliou M, Sanders DS. Efficacy of a gluten-free diet in subjects with irritable bowel syndrome-diarrhea unaware of their HLA-DQ2/8 genotype. *Clin Gastroenterol Hepatol.* 2016; **14**(5): 696–703.e1. doi:10.1016/j.cgh.2015.12.031.
34. Nagarajan N, Morden A, Bischof D, et al. The role of fiber supplementation in the treatment of irritable bowel syndrome: a systematic review and meta-analysis. *Eur J Gastroenterol Hepatol.* 2015; **27**(9): 1002–1010. doi:10.1097/MEG.0000000000000425.
35. V. Fintelmann. Antidyspeptische und lipidsenkende Eigenschaften von Artischockenblätterextrakt. Ergebnisse klinischer Untersuchungen zur Wirksamkeit und Verträglichkeit von Hepar-SL forte an 553 Patienten *Z. Allg. Med.* 1996; **72**(Suppl. 2): 3–19.
36. Marakis G, Walker AF, Middleton RW, Booth JC, Wright J, Pike DJ. Artichoke leaf extract reduces mild dyspepsia in an open study. *Phytomedicine.* 2002; **9**(8): 694–699. doi:10.1078/094471102321621287.
37. Bundy R, Walker AF, Middleton RW, Marakis G, Booth JC. Artichoke leaf extract reduces symptoms of irritable bowel syndrome and improves quality of life in otherwise healthy volunteers suffering from concomitant dyspepsia: a subset analysis. *J Altern Complement Med.* 2004; **10**(4): 667–669. doi:10.1089/acm.2004.10.667.
38. Giacosa A, Guido D, Grassi M, et al. The effect of ginger (*Zingiber officinalis*) and artichoke (*Cynara cardunculus*) extract supplementation on functional dyspepsia: a randomised, double-blind, and placebo-controlled clinical trial. *Evid Based Complement Alternat Med.* 2015; **2015**: 915087. doi:10.1155/2015/915087.
39. Raveendra KR, Jayachandra, Srinivasa V, et al. An extract of *Glycyrrhiza glabra* (GutGard) alleviates symptoms of functional dyspepsia: a randomized, double-blind, placebo-controlled study. *Evid Based Complement Alternat Med.* 2012; **2012**: 216970. doi:10.1155/2012/216970.
40. Ling W, Li Y, Jiang W, Sui Y, Zhao HL. Common mechanism of pathogenesis in gastro-

intestinal diseases implied by consistent efficacy of single Chinese medicine formula: a PRISMA-compliant systematic review and meta-analysis. *Medicine (Baltimore)*. 2015; **94**(27): e1111. doi:10.1097/MD.0000000000001111.

41. Walker AF, Middleton RW, Petrowicz O. Artichoke leaf extract reduces symptoms of irritable bowel syndrome in a post-marketing surveillance study. *Phytother Res*. 2001; **15**(1): 58–61. doi:10.1002/1099-1573(200102)15:1<58::aid-ptr805>3.0.co;2-r.
42. Chen C, Tao C, Liu Z, et al. A randomized clinical trial of berberine hydrochloride in patients with diarrhea-predominant irritable bowel syndrome. *Phytother Res*. 2015; **29**(11): 1822–1827. doi:10.1002/ptr.5475.
43. Riva A, Giacomelli L, Togni S, et al. Oral administration of a lecithin-based delivery form of boswellic acids (Casperome®) for the prevention of symptoms of irritable bowel syndrome: a randomized clinical study. *Minerva Gastroenterol Dietol*. 2019; **65**(1): 30–35. doi:10.23736/S1121-421X.18.02530-8.
44. Hawrelak JA, Wohlmuth H, Pattinson M, et al. Western herbal medicines in the treatment of irritable bowel syndrome: a systematic review and meta-analysis. *Complement Ther Med*. 2020; **48**: 102233. doi:10.1016/j.ctim.2019.102233.
45. Krajicek EJ, Hansel SL. Small intestinal bacterial overgrowth: a primary care review. *Mayo Clin Proc*. 2016; **91**(12): 1828–1833. doi:10.1016/j.mayocp.2016.07.025.
46. Quigley EM, Abu-Shanab A. Small intestinal bacterial overgrowth. *Infect Dis Clin North Am*. 2010; **24**(4): 943–959, viii–ix. doi:10.1016/j.idc.2010.07.007.
47. Bures J, Cyrany J, Kohoutova D, et al. Small intestinal bacterial overgrowth syndrome. *World J Gastroenterol*. 2010; **16**(24): 2978–2990. doi:10.3748/wjg.v16.i24.2978.
48. Jacobs C, Coss Adame E, Attaluri A, Valestin J, Rao SS. Dysmotility and proton pump inhibitor use are independent risk factors for small intestinal bacterial and/or fungal overgrowth. *Aliment Pharmacol Ther*. 2013; **37**(11): 1103–1111. doi:10.1111/apt.12304.
49. Avelar Rodriguez D, Ryan PM, Toro Monjaraz EM, Ramirez Mayans JA, Quigley EM. Small intestinal bacterial overgrowth in children: a state-of-the-art review. *Front Pediatr*. 2019 Sep 4; **7**: 363. doi:10.3389/fped.2019.00363.
50. Adike A, DiBaise JK. Small intestinal bacterial overgrowth: nutritional implications, diagnosis, and management. *Gastroenterol Clin North Am*. 2018; **47**(1): 193–208. doi:10.1016/j.gtc.2017.09.008.
51. Quigley EM, Abu-Shanab A. Small intestinal bacterial overgrowth. *Infect Dis Clin North Am*. 2010; **24**(4): 943–959, viii–ix. doi:10.1016/j.idc.2010.07.007.
52. Sundin OH, Mendoza-Ladd A, Morales E, et al. Does a glucose-based hydrogen and methane breath test detect bacterial overgrowth in the jejunum?. *Neurogastroenterol Motil*. 2018; **30**(11): e13350. doi:10.1111/nmo.13350.
53. Di Stefano M, Quigley EMM. The diagnosis of small intestinal bacterial overgrowth: two steps forward, one step backwards?. *Neurogastroenterol Motil*. 2018; **30**(11): e13494. doi:10.1111/nmo.13494.
54. Saffouri GB, Shields-Cutler RR, Chen J, et al. Small intestinal microbial dysbiosis underlies symptoms associated with functional gastrointestinal disorders. *Nat Commun*. 2019 May 1; **10**(1): 2012. doi:10.1038/s41467-019-09964-7.
55. Adike A, DiBaise JK. Small intestinal bacterial overgrowth: nutritional implications, diagnosis, and management. *Gastroenterol Clin North Am*. 2018; **47**(1): 193–208. doi:10.1016/j.gtc.2017.09.008.
56. Krajicek EJ, Hansel SL. Small intestinal bacterial overgrowth: a primary care review. *Mayo Clin Proc*. 2016; **91**(12): 1828–1833. doi:10.1016/j.mayocp.2016.07.025.
57. Adike A, DiBaise JK. Small intestinal bacterial overgrowth: nutritional implications, diagnosis, and management. *Gastroenterol Clin North Am*. 2018; **47**(1): 193–208. doi:10.1016/j.gtc.2017.09.008.

58. George NS, Sankineni A, Parkman HP. Small intestinal bacterial overgrowth in gastroparesis. *Dig Dis Sci.* 2014; **59**(3): 645–652. doi:10.1007/s10620-012-2426-7.
59. Lisowska A, Kobelska-Dubiel N, Jankowska I, Pawłowska J, Moczko J, Walkowiak J. Small intestinal bacterial overgrowth in patients with progressive familial intrahepatic cholestasis. *Acta Biochim Pol.* 2014; **61**(1): 103–107.
60. Brechmann T, Sperlbaum A, Schmiegel W. Levothyroxine therapy and impaired clearance are the strongest contributors to small intestinal bacterial overgrowth: results of a retrospective cohort study. *World J Gastroenterol.* 2017; **23**(5): 842–852. doi:10.3748/wjg.v23.i5.842.
61. Kaur J, Rana SV, Gupta R, Gupta V, Sharma SK, Dhawan DK. Prolonged orocecal transit time enhances serum bile acids through bacterial overgrowth, contributing factor to gallstone disease. *J Clin Gastroenterol.* 2014; **48**(4): 365–369. doi:10.1097/MCG.0b013e3182a14fba.
62. Ghoshal UC, Ghoshal U. Small intestinal bacterial overgrowth and other intestinal disorders. *Gastroenterol Clin North Am.* 2017; **46**(1): 103–120. doi:10.1016/j.gtc.2016.09.008.
63. Roland BC, Ciarleglio MM, Clarke JO, et al. Low ileocecal valve pressure is significantly associated with small intestinal bacterial overgrowth (SIBO). *Dig Dis Sci.* 2014; **59**(6): 1269–1277. doi:10.1007/s10620-014-3166-7.
64. Miller LS, Vegesna AK, Sampath AM, Prabhu S, Kotapati SK, Makipour K. Ileocecal valve dysfunction in small intestinal bacterial overgrowth: a pilot study. *World J Gastroenterol.* 2012; **18**(46): 6801–6808. doi:10.3748/wjg.v18.i46.6801.
65. Chander Roland B, Mullin GE, Passi M, et al. A prospective evaluation of ileocecal valve dysfunction and intestinal motility derangements in small intestinal bacterial overgrowth. *Dig Dis Sci.* 2017; **62**(12): 3525–3535. doi:10.1007/s10620-017-4726-4.
66. Ghoshal UC, Nehra A, Mathur A, et al. A meta-analysis on small intestinal bacterial overgrowth in patients with different sub-types of irritable bowel syndrome. *J Gastroenterol Hepatol.* 2019 Nov 21. doi:10.1111/jgh.14938.
67. Ghoshal UC, Shukla R, Ghoshal U. Small intestinal bacterial overgrowth and irritable bowel syndrome: a bridge between functional organic dichotomy. *Gut Liver.* 2017 Mar 15; **11**(2): 196–208. doi:10.5009/gnl16126.
68. Wu KQ, Sun WJ, Li N, et al. Small intestinal bacterial overgrowth is associated with diarrhea-predominant irritable bowel syndrome by increasing mainly Prevotella abundance. *Scand J Gastroenterol.* 2019 Nov 25: 1–7. doi:10.1080/00365521.2019.1694067. PMID: 31765575.
69. Capurso G, Signoretti M, Archibugi L, et al. Systematic review and meta-analysis: small intestinal bacterial overgrowth in chronic pancreatitis. *United European Gastroenterol J.* 2016 Oct; **4**(5): 697–705.
70. Weinstock LB, Walters AS, Paueksakon P. Restless legs syndrome: theoretical roles of inflammatory and immune mechanisms. *Sleep Med Rev.* 2012 Aug; **16**(4): 341–354. doi:10.1016/j.smrv.2011.09.003.
71. Fialho A, Fialho A, Schenone A, et al. Association between small intestinal bacterial overgrowth and deep vein thrombosis. *Gastroenterol Rep (Oxf).* 2016 Nov; **4**(4): 299–303.
72. Ligon CB, Hummers LK, McMahan ZH. Oxalate nephropathy in systemic sclerosis: case series and review of the literature. *Semin Arthritis Rheum.* 2015 Dec; **45**(3): 315–320. doi:10.1016/j.semarthrit.2015.06.017.
73. Greco A, Caviglia GP, Brignolo P, et al. Glucose breath test and Crohn's disease: diagnosis of small intestinal bacterial overgrowth and evaluation of therapeutic response. *Scand J Gastroenterol.* 2015; **50**(11): 1376–1381. doi:10.3109/00365521.2015.1050691.
74. Tziatzios G, Giamarellos-Bourboulis EJ, Papanikolaou IS, et al. Is small intestinal bacterial overgrowth involved in the pathogenesis of functional dyspepsia? *Med Hypotheses.* 2017 Sep; **106**: 26–32. doi:10.1016/j.mehy.2017.07.005.

75. Kaur J, Rana SV, Gupta R, et al. Prolonged orocecal transit time enhances serum bile acids through bacterial overgrowth, contributing factor to gallstone disease. *J Clin Gastroenterol.* 2014 Apr; **48**(4): 365–369. doi:10.1097/MCG.0b013e3182a14fba.
76. Fialho A, Fialho A, Thota P, et al. Small intestinal bacterial overgrowth is associated with non-alcoholic fatty liver disease. *J Gastrointestin Liver Dis.* 2016 Jun; **25**(2): 159–165. doi:10.15403/jgld.2014.1121.252.iwg.
77. Miazga A, Osiński M, Cichy W, et al. Current views on the etiopathogenesis, clinical manifestation, diagnostics, treatment and correlation with other nosological entities of SIBO. *Adv Med Sci.* 2015 Mar; **60**(1): 118–124. doi:10.1016/j.advms.2014.09.001.
78. Kim KM, Kim BT, Lee DJ, et al. Erosive esophagitis may be related to small intestinal bacterial overgrowth. *Scand J Gastroenterol.* 2012 May; **47**(5): 493–498. doi:10.3109/00365521.2012.668932.
79. Fialho A, Fialho A, Thota P, et al. Higher visceral to subcutaneous fat ratio is associated with small intestinal bacterial overgrowth. *Nutr Metab Cardiovasc Dis.* 2016 Sep; **26**(9): 773–777. doi:10.1016/j.numecd.2016.04.007.
80. Agnoletti AF, de Col E, Parodi A, et al. Etiopathogenesis of rosacea: a prospective study with a three-year follow-up. *G Ital Dermatol Venereol.* 2017 Oct; **152**(5): 418–423. doi:10.23736/S0392-0488.16.05315-3.
81. Shah A, Shanahan E, Macdonald GA, et al. Systematic review and meta-analysis: prevalence of small intestinal bacterial overgrowth in chronic liver disease. *Semin Liver Dis.* 2017; **37**(4): 388–400. doi:10.1055/s-0037-1608832.
82. Adike A, DiBaise JK. Small intestinal bacterial overgrowth: nutritional implications, diagnosis, and management. *Gastroenterol Clin North Am.* 2018; **47**(1): 193–208. doi:10.1016/j.gtc.2017.09.008.
83. Pimentel M, Constantino T, Kong Y, Bajwa M, Rezaei A, Park S. A 14-day elemental diet is highly effective in normalizing the lactulose breath test. *Dig Dis Sci.* 2004; **49**(1): 73–77. doi:10.1023/b:ddas.0000011605.43979.e1.
84. https://sibocenter.com/2016/03/sibo-specific-diet
85. https://www.thesibodoctor.com/wp-content/uploads/woocommerce_uploads/2017/04/Bi-PhasicDietProtocol_300318.pdf
86. Chedid V, Dhalla S, Clarke JO, et al. Herbal therapy is equivalent to rifaximin for the treatment of small intestinal bacterial overgrowth. *Glob Adv Health Med.* 2014; **3**(3): 16–24. doi:10.7453/gahmj.2014.019.
87. Rezaie A, Pimentel M, Rao SS. How to test and treat small intestinal bacterial overgrowth: an evidence-based approach. *Curr Gastroenterol Rep.* 2016; **18**(2): 8. doi:10.1007/s11894-015-0482-9.

Acronyms & abbreviations

Acetyl-CoA   acetyl coenzyme A
ACS   American Cancer Society
ACT   artemisinin combination therapy
AD   Alzheimer's disease
ADHD   attention deficit hyperactivity disorder
ADJM   ambulatory antro-duodeno-jejunal manometry
ADP   adenosine diphosphate
AGE   advanced glycation end product
ALDs   Alzheimer-like dementias
AMD   age-related macular degeneration
AMP   adenosine monophosphate
AMPK   adenosine monophosphate-activated protein kinase
ANS   autonomic nervous system
AR   allergic rhinitis
ARDS   acute respiratory disease syndrome
ARE   antioxidant response element
ARI   acute respiratory illness
ART   artemisinin
ASD   autism spectrum disorders
ATP   adenosine triphosphate
AUC   area under plasma concentration curve
B19V   human parvovirus B19
BA   bile acid
BAD   Bile acid diarrhoea
BAI   Beck Anxiety Inventory
BAT   brown adipose tissue
BBB   blood–brain barrier
BCAAs   branched-chain amino acids
BCG   Bacillus Calmette-Guérin
BFP   bowel flora protocol
Bf-S   Befindlichkeits-Skala
BPA   Bisphenol A
BPH   benign prostatic hyperplasia
Bregs   regulatory B cells
BS   broccoli sprouts
BSH   broccoli sprout homogenate
BTT   bowel toxaemia theory
BVDV   bovine viral diarrhoea virus (BVDV)
CA   carnosic acid
CAHA   COVID-19-associated haemostasis abnormality
CD   Crohn's disease
CDA   comorbid depression and anxiety
CDC   Centers for Disease Control and Prevention (USA)
CFS   chronic fatigue syndrome
cfu   colony-forming unit
CGI-I   Clinical Global Impression Improvement Scale
CGM   curcumagalactomannoside
CHARGE   Childhood Autism Risks from Genetics and Environment
CI   confidence interval
CKD   chronic kidney disease
CLD   chronic Lyme disease
CMD   coronary microvascular dysfunction
CMV   cytomegalovirus
CSA   chronic stable angina
CSFP   coronary slow flow phenomenon
CSS   central sensitivity syndrome
CSVD   cerebral small vessel disease
CT   computed tomography
CTLs   cytotoxic T lymphocytes
CVD   cardiovascular disease
DBP   diastolic blood pressure
DCs   dendritic cells
DDT   dichlorodiphenyltrichloroethane
DEP   diesel exhaust particles
DHE   dried herb equivalent
DILI   drug-induced liver injury

DMSA   dimercaptosuccinic acid
DNA   deoxyribonucleic acid
DOX   doxorubicin
EBV   Epstein-Barr virus
ED   erectile dysfunction
EEG   electroencephalogram
EGCG   epigallocatechin gallate
EGD   oesophago-gastro-duodenoscopy
eGFR   glomerular filtration rate
11βHSD-1   11-β-hydroxysteroid dehydrogenase type 1
EPS   epigastric pain syndrome
EWG   Environmental Working Group
FD   functional dyspepsia
FeNO   fractional exhaled nitric oxide
FEV1   forced expiratory volume
FFA   free fatty acid
FGF-19 fibroblast growth factor 19
FHT   Functional Herbal Therapy
FLG   filaggrin
FLVR   four bacterial genera, Faecalibacterium, Lachnospira, Rothia, and Veillonella
FMD   flow-mediated dilatation
FMS   fibromyalgia syndrome
FODMAP fermentable oligo-, di-, mono-saccharides and polyols
FOS   fructooligosaccharides
FRK C fructokinase C
fructose-1-P   fructose 1 phosphate
G-3-P glyceraldehyde-3-phosphate
GABA   gamma-aminobutyric acid
GAD   generalised anxiety disorder
GBE   *Ginkgo biloba* leaf standardised extract
GBH   glyphosate-based herbicide
GF   germ free
GFD   gluten free diet
γGCL   gamma-glutamate cysteine ligase
GGT   gamma-glutamyltransferase
GI   glycaemic index ()
GIP   gastric inhibitory polypeptide
GIT   gastrointestinal tract
GLP-1 glucagon-like peptide 1
GMP   good manufacturing practice
GPCMV guinea pig cytomegalovirus
GPR   G protein-coupled receptor
GPx   glutathione peroxidase
GR   glutathione reductase
GSE   grape seed extract

GSH   glutathione
GSTM1 glutathione-S-transferase M1
GSTM1 phase II enzymes glutathione-S-transferase M1
GSTP1 glutathione-S-transferase P1
GT   green tea
GTE   green tea extracts
GTL   green tea liquid
GTT   gastrointestinal transit time
H1N1   Spanish influenza
H1N1v swine flu
H3N2   Hong Kong flu
H5N1   bird flu
HAMA   Hamilton Anxiety Rating Scale
HAV   hepatitis A virus
HbA1C glycated hemoglobin
HBT   glucose hydrogen breath test
HBV   hepatitis B virus
HC   healthy controls
HCMV   human cytomegalovirus
HCV   hepatitis C virus
HDAC   histone deacetylase
HDL   high-density lipoprotein
HDM   house dust mite
HE   hard exudate
HFHC   high-fat, high-carbohydrate
HIF-1alpha   hypoxia inducible factor 1-alpha
HIIT   high-intensity interval training
HIV   human immunodeficiency virus
HIV-1 human immunodeficiency virus type 1
HM   heavy metal
HMP   Human Microbiome Project
HMs   heavy metals
HO-1   haem oxygenase-1
HOMA-IR   homeostasis model assessment for insulin resistance
Hp   Helicobacter pylori
HPA   hypothalamic-pituitary-adrenal
HPLC   high-performance liquid chromatography
HPV   human papilloma virus
HPV39 human papilloma virus subtype 39
HRs   hazard ratios
hs-CRP high-sensitivity C-reactive protein
HSP   heat shock protein
HSV   herpes simplex virus
HVR   heart valve replacement
IAV   influenza A virus
IBD   inflammatory bowel disease

ACRONYMS & ABBREVIATIONS

IBS   irritable bowel syndrome
IBS-C   constipation-predominant IBS
IBS-D   diarrhoea-predominant IBS
IBS-M   IBS with mixed pattern of diarrhoea and constipation
IBSSSS   IBS Symptom Severity Score
ICU   intensive care unit
IEC   intestinal epithelial cells
IgA   immunoglobulin A
IgE   Immunoglobulin E
IGF1   insulin-like growth factor 1
IKKβ   I-kappa-B-kinase beta
IL   interleukin
IMN   idiopathic membranous nephropathy
IPA   indolepropionic acid;
IPM   integrated pest management
IR   insulin resistance
JCPyV   human polyomavirus
Keap1   Kelch-like ECH-associated protein 1
KRG   Korean red ginseng
LBT   lactulose breath test
LDL-C   low density lipoproteins cholesterol
LPS   lipopolysaccharide
Maf   masculoaponeurotic fibrosarcoma
MAFLD   metabolic (dysfunction) associated fatty liver disease
MCMV   mouse cytomegalovirus
MD   mean difference
MDA   malondialdehyde
MERS   Middle East respiratory syndrome
MetaHIT   European Metagenomics of the Human Intestinal Tract
MetS   metabolic syndrome
MGO   methylglyoxal
MP   *Mycoplasma pneumoniae*
MRI   magnetic resonance imaging
mRNA   messenger ribonucleic acid
MS   multiple sclerosis
mTORC1   mammalian (or mechanistic) target of rapamycin complex 1
MyD   Myeloid differentiation primary response
NADH   nicotinamide adenine dinucleotide+hydrogen
NADPH   nicotinamide adenine dinucleotide phosphate.
NAFLD   non-alcoholic fatty liver disease
NA-SVD   non-amyloid small vessel disease
NBWS   "not been well since"
NFκB   nuclear factor kappa-light-chain-enhancer of activated B cells
NK   natural killer cells
NO   nitric oxide
NQO1   NADPH quinone oxidoreductase
NREM   non-rapid eye movement
Nrf2   nuclear factor erythroid 2–related factor 2
NSAID   non-steroidal anti-inflammatory drug
OA   osteoarthritis
OCD   obsessive-compulsive disorder
OP   organophosphate
OPCs   oligomeric procyanidins
OPPs   organophosphate pesticides
OR   odds ratio
ORAC   oxygen radical absorption capacity
OSHA   Occupational Safety and Health Administration
OST   overlap/sequence/triage
PAF   platelet activating factor
PAT   peripheral arterial tonometry
PBDE   polybrominated diphenyl ether
PCBs   polychlorinated biphenyls
PCDDs   polychlorinated dibenzo-*p*-dioxins
PCDFs   polychlorinated dibenzofurans
PCOS   polycystic ovary syndrome
PD   Parkinson's disease
PD-L1   programmed death-ligand 1
PDS   postprandial distress syndrome
PEG   polyethylene glycol
PFAS   perfluoroalkyl and polyfluoroalkyl substances
PFCs   perfluorinated chemicals
PFOA   perfluorooctanoic acid
PFOS   perfluorooctane sulfonate
PGC-1α   peroxisome proliferator-activated receptor-gamma coactivator 1alpha
PI   post-infection
POEA   polyethoxylated tallow amine
POPs   persistent organic pollutants
PPIs   proton pump inhibitor drugs
PRRs   pattern recognition receptors
PSS   Perceived Stress Scale
PTSD   post-traumatic stress disorder
PV   polycythaemia vera
PWV   pulse wave velocity
RA   rheumatoid arthritis
RAGE   AGE (advanced glycation end product) receptor

RBC   red blood cell
RCMV   rat cytomegalovirus
REM   rapid-eye-movement
RHI   reactive hyperaemia index
RH-PAT   reactive hyperaemia index
ROS   reactive oxygen species
RR   relative risk
RSV   respiratory syncytial virus
RV   rhinovirus
RW   ragweed pollen
SAMe   S-adenosylmethionine
SARS   severe acute respiratory syndrome
SARS-CoV   SARS
SARS-CoV-2   COVID-19
SBP   systolic blood pressure
SCD   specific carbohydrate diet
SCFA   short chain fatty acid
SCFAs   short chain fatty acids
SFN   sulforaphane
SIBO   small intestinal bacterial overgrowth
SIFO   small intestinal fungal overgrowth
SIMD   small intestinal microbial dysbiosis
SIRT   sirtuin
SJW   St John's wort
SLE   systemic lupus erythematosus
SMART-MR   Second Manifestations of Arterial Disease–Magnetic Resonance
SNPs   single nucleotide polymorphisms
SNS   Si-Ni-San
SOD   superoxide-dismutase
SRS   Social Responsiveness Scale
SWS   slow wave sleep
T2D   type 2 diabetes
TCM   traditional Chinese medicine
TDCPP   tris(1,3-dichloro-2-propyl)phosphate
TEWL   trans-epidermal water loss
TG   thyroglobulin
TGFβ   transforming growth factor-beta
TI   trained (innate) immunity
TJ   tight junction
TKFC   thiokinase
TLR   toll-like receptor
TMAO   trimethylamine N-oxide
TNF   tumour necrosis factor
TNF-α   tumour necrosis factor α
Tregs   regulatory T cells
TSH   thyroid-stimulating hormone
UCP1   uncoupling protein 1
UDP   glucuronosyltransferase
VD   vascular dementia
VLDL   very low density lipoprotein
VMCI   vascular mild cognitive impairment
vRNA   viral ribonucleic acid
WHM   Western herbal medicine
WML   white matter lesion
Y-BOCS   Yale–Brown Obsessive Compulsive Scale

Index

Abascal, K., 342
abdominal obesity, 264, 265, 271
abdominal pain, 367
acetaminophen (paracetamol), 304
acetyl coenzyme A [Acetyl-CoA], 270
Achillea (yarrow), 36, 318, 342, 345
acid-suppressive medications, 306
ACT [artemisinin combination therapy], 212
Actinobacteria, 182
acute respiratory disease syndrome [ARDS], 103, 349
acute respiratory illness [ARI], 333
acute sinusitis, 332
acute stress disorder, 234
AD [Alzheimer's disease], 53, 121, 122, 140, 252
adaptogenic herbs, 20, 245, 257, 333, 344, 352
adaptogens, 26, 27
adenoid hypertrophy, 320
adenosine diphosphate [ADP], 269, 270
adenosine monophosphate [AMP]-activated protein kinase [AMPK], 29, 40, 41, 270, 273, 280–282
adenosine triphosphate [ATP], 117, 153, 154, 269, 273, 274
Adhatoda, 39, 318, 319, 346
ADHD [attention deficit hyperactivity disorder], 139, 140
ADJM [ambulatory antro-duodeno-jejunal manometry], 374
adjustment disorder, 234
ADP [adenosine diphosphate], 269, 270
adrenal herbs, 25
adulterated products, avoiding, 56–57
advanced glycation end product [AGE], 271
aflatoxins, 162, 165
AGE [advanced glycation end product], 271
    receptor [RAGE], 271
ageing and liver microcirculation, 90
age-related macular degeneration [AMD], 121, 122

agoraphobia, 234
air filters, 317, 320, 322
air pollution, 148–149, 155, 161
    and allergy, 296, 298, 319, 320
    and asthma, 298
    neurotoxicity of, 140
    protection and broccoli sprouts, 166
Albizia, 36, 306, 318, 319, 322
ALDs [Alzheimer-like dementias], 92, 93
alfalfa sprout homogenate, 126
Ali Abbas (al-Majusi), 77
alkylamides, 329, 330, 337, 338, 344
allergic rhinitis [AR], 126, 295, 296, 299, 300, 306, 308
    barrier disruption in, 321
    barrier function in, 301
    causative factors in, 320–322
    characteristics of, 319
    FHT protocols for, 322
    Montelukast versus Nigella in, 307
    mosaic, 321
allergy:
    hygiene drivers of, 304
    and toxins, 298
allicin, 187, 188
alliin, 187
alliinase, 187
Allium sativum, see garlic
al-Majusi (Ali Abbas), 77
Alosetron, 367
alpha coherence, 238
alpha-gal (galactose-alpha-1,3-galactose), 297
alpha-gal allergy, 297
Alternaria spp., 149
Alzheimer-like dementias [ALDs], 92, 93
Alzheimer's disease [AD], 53, 121, 122, 140, 252
āma, 71, 72

ambulatory antro-duodeno-jejunal manometry [ADJM], 374
AMD [age-related macular degeneration], 121, 122
American Cancer Society [ACS], 248
American skullcap, 245
amitriptyline, 237, 367
amma-glutamate cysteine ligase [γGCL], 124
AMP [adenosine monophosphate], 29, 269, 270, 273, 281, 282
AMPK [adenosine monophosphate-activated protein kinase], 29, 270, 273, 280, 281
AMPK herbs, 40, 41, 282
analgesic herbs, 257
analgesics, 17
anaphylactic food allergies, 295
Andrographis, 26, 27, 35, 337
    for asthma, 318
    BFP for dysbiosis, 192
    immune herb for infections, 328
    for infection prevention, 344
    for respiratory infections, 328, 345
    and stealth pathogens, 222, 223, 224
anise oil, 33, 192, 193, 222, 383
aniseed (Pimpinella), 346
ANS [autonomic nervous system], 362, 364
anthocyanins, bilberry, 97–98
anti-adhesive herbs, 221
antiallergic herbs, 36, 372
antiallergic remedies, 16
antibacterial herbs, 218–221, 346
antibiotics, 184, 198, 202, 206, 221, 226, 306
    bacterial resistance to, 9
    broad-spectrum, 304
anticatarrhal herbs, 73, 309, 346
antidotos, 76, 77
antifungal herbs, 382
antihistamine drugs, 306
anti-inflammatories, 16
anti-inflammatory herbs, 35, 36, 372, 382
antimicrobial herbs, 27, 33, 187, 188, 192, 382
antimony, 6, 78
antioxidant(s), 29, 112, 115, 117
    concerns over, 113–114
antioxidant herbs, 194
antioxidant response element [ARE], 115–134, 163, 168, 169
antioxidation, biological versus chemical, 114–115
anti-parasitic herbs, 213
antiviral herbs, 215–218, 337, 343, 344, 345

anxiety:
    definition, 234–235
    drug medication for, 234–235
    FHT for relieving, 233–257
    herbal treatments for, 236–245
    liquid herbal blends for, 256
anxiety disorder, 253
    generalised, 234
anxiolytic herbs, 30, 244, 372
aqueous cream, 299
AR, *see* allergic rhinitis [AR]
Arctium lappa (burdock), 57
ARDS [acute respiratory disease syndrome], 349
ARE, *see* antioxidant response element
ARI [acute respiratory illness], 333
Aristolochia, 57
arjuna, 32, 42
ar-Rhazi (Rhazes), 77
arsenic [As], 6, 78, 129, 141, 146, 148, 154, 162, 164
ART [artemisinin], 208–213
arteannuin B, 209
Artemisia absinthium (European wormwood):
    anti-parasitic, 27, 213, 222, 223
    for IBS, 372
    for MetS management, 282, 286
Artemisia annua (Chinese wormwood, Qing Hao, sweet wormwood):
    dosage considerations, 213
    Nobel Prize for Medicine, 208
    for respiratory infections, 345
    and stealth pathogens, 208–212, 216, 223, 224
    and viral infections, 27, 337, 343
artemisinic acid, 209
artemisinin [ART], 208–213
    chemical structure of, 210–211
    combination therapy [ACT], 212
    therapeutic activity of, 210
    -type agents, antiviral activity of, 211
arterial stiffness, 98, 100, 101
    role of, 94–95
arthritis, 49, 87, 202, 389
As [arsenic], 78, 129, 141, 146, 148, 154, 162, 164
Asclepias tuberosa (pleurisy root), 36, 342, 345
ascorbic acid, 159, 170
ASD [autism spectrum disorder], 152, 153, 154, 166
ashwagandha: *see* Withania
Asimadoline, 367
Aspergillus spp., 149
asthma, 58, 98, 125, 126, 140, 295–322

aspirin-sensitive, 314
barrier function in, 301
childhood, 297
endotype versus phenotype in, 313
eosinophilic, 312
FHT for, 310–319
FHT protocols for, 317–319
herbal clinical trials in, 316–317
herbal treatments for, 314, 316–319
immune microbiome interactions in, 305
as mosaic disease, 310–313
    endotype and phenotype in, 312–313
neutrophilic, 312
non-Th2, 313
Th2, 313
Th2-driven, 312
Th17-driven neutrophilic, 312
Astralagus (*Astragalus membranaceus*), 26, 32, 35, 42, 63, 222, 352
for allergic rhinitis, 322
for asthma, 317, 318
for atopy, 308, 309
and cytokine storm risk, 339
immune herb for infections, 333
for infection prevention, 344
for Lyme disease, 225, 227
for MetS management, 288
for respiratory infections, 328, 333, 336, 339, 340, 344
astringent herbs, 73
atherogenic dyslipidaemia, 265
atopic dermatitis (eczema), 296, 299, 300, 320
atopic diseases, rise of, 297
atopic march, 298, 299, 320
    timeline, 300
atopy/hay fever:
    barrier function in, 298–301
    definition, 296
    FHT strategies for, 296–309
    FHT treatment modules for, 309
    herbal treatments for, 306–308
    and microbiome, 304
    rise of, 296–298
ATP [adenosine triphosphate], 117, 153, 154, 269, 273, 274
atrazine, 154
attention deficit hyperactivity disorder [ADHD], 139, 140
AUC [area under plasma concentration curve], 213

autism, 139, 140, 150
    and broccoli sprouts, 166–167
    and environmental toxins, 152–154
autism spectrum disorder [ASD], 152–154, 166
    mitochondrial dysfunction in, 153
autoimmune disease, 11, 13, 14, 63, 199, 202
autoimmunity, 63, 144, 151, 184, 200
    and environmental toxins, 151–152
autonomic nervous system [ANS], 362, 364
autotoxicity, 335
Avicenna (Ibn-Sina), 77
Ayurveda, 7, 46, 70, 73, 332
Ayurvedic enema therapy, 71
Ayurvedic medicine/treatment, 69–73

BA [bile acid], 364, 367, 379
Babesia, 204–207, 209
    life cycle, 205
Babesia macrocarpus, 204
Babesia microti, 204
Bach, E., 80
Bacillus Calmette-Guérin [BCG], 331, 341
Bacopa, 26, 30, 245
bacteria, 9, 19
    pathogenic, 33, 34
bacterial infections, 9, 302
bacterial maxillary sinusitis, 332
bacterial pathogens, 220
Bacteroides spp., 182, 184, 189, 190, 363
BAD [bile acid diarrhoea], 364
BAI [Beck Anxiety Inventory], 240, 241
Baical skullcap, 36–38, 306, 318, 319, 322, 372
    for allergic rhinitis, 322
    for anxiety, 245, 256
    for asthma, 318, 319
    for atopy, 306
    for IBS, 372
    for insomnia, 256
barberry (*Berberis vulgaris*), 221
barrier(s):
    enhancing, FHT for, 308–309
    natural, 20
        enhancing, 38–39
barrier-supporting herbs, 382
Bartonella, 199, 206
Bartonella spp.:
    Bartonella quintana, 205
    Bartonella bacilliformis, 205
basil, holy, 328, 332, 337, 344, 345

BAT [brown adipose tissue], 274, 275, 280
bayberry (*Myrica cerifera*), 78
BBB [blood–brain barrier], 43, 96, 114, 115, 147, 207
BCAA(s) [branched-chain amino acid(s)], 268, 269, 276, 277
BCG [Bacillus Calmette-Guérin] vaccine, 331, 341
Beck Anxiety Inventory [BAI], 240, 241
beetroot (*Beta vulgaris*), 103, 284
    and microcirculatory and endothelial health, 101
Befindlichkeits-Skala [Bf-S], 253
belladonna, 57
benign prostatic hyperplasia [BPH], 263, 277
benzodiazepines, 234, 237, 243, 248, 253
berberine, 29, 33, 188, 192, 371, 373, 381–383
    antibacterial activity of, 220–221
    8-point dietary BP plan, 285
    for high cholesterol, 284
    for MetS management, 279–288
    for SIBO, 382
berberine-containing herbs, 26, 27, 40, 41, 219, 220, 222, 224, 382
Berberis vulgaris (barberry), 221
berry anthocyanins, 97–98, 103
beta-carotene, 112, 114
beta-glucan, 341
beta-thalassaemia, 170, 171
Beta vulgaris, *see* beetroot
BFP, *see* bowel flora protocol
Bf-S [Befindlichkeits-Skala], 253
Bifidobacteria spp. 184, 189, 190, 363
bilberry (*Vaccinium myrtillus*), 30–33, 104, 282
    anthocyanins and microcirculatory and endothelial health, 97–98
bile acid [BA], 364
bile acid diarrhoea [BAD], 364
bilobalide, 53
biofilms, 221, 222
biological antioxidation, 115
biotoxins, 141, 161
bipolar disorder, 208
bird flu [H5N1], 346
bisphenol A [BPA], 146, 154–158, 167
    as endocrine disruptor, 140
bitter herbs, 25, 26, 34–38, 40, 72, 187, 365
    for IBS, 372
    for MetS management, 279, 282
    for SIBO, 382
bitter melon (*Momordica charantia*), 278, 281, 283–288
bitter orange, immature (Zhi Shi), 371

bitters, 17
BKV [human polyomavirus], 211
blackberries, 103
Blackley, C.H., 297
black raspberry (*Rubus occidentalis*), 98
black walnut, 27
bladderwrack, 26
Bland, J., 4
Blastocystis hominis, 220
blood–brain barrier [BBB], 43, 96, 114, 115, 147, 207
blood glucose, high, MetS with, 286
bloodletting, 78
blood pressure [BP], dietary plan for, 284
blueberry (*Vaccinium corymbosum*), 98, 103
B lymphocytes, 341
body dysmorphic disorder, 234
bone health and environmental toxins, 155–157
boneset, 342
Borrelia (*Borrelia burgdorferi*), 198, 204–207, 225
Boswellia, 31, 36–39, 49, 66, 193, 194, 371
    for asthma, 316–319
    for IBS, 372
    for Lyme disease, 225
bovine immunodeficiency virus, 217
bovine viral diarrhoea virus [BVDV], 217
bowel flora/barrier protocol, 303, 309, 317
bowel flora protocol [BFP]
    development of, 33
    dosage requirements, 47
    for dysbiosis management, 33, 181–195
        herbs for, 33
    for gut wall healing, 373
    for IBS management, 358, 373
    interim form of (case study), 193–195
    for MetS, 282
    for SIBO, 383
    for stealth pathogens, 151
    value of treatment modules, 20
bowel toxaemia theory [BTT], 183
BPA, *see* bisphenol A
BPH [benign prostatic hyperplasia], 263, 277
brain health and brain microcirculation, 91–96
brain microbleeds, 91–93
brain microcirculation and Alzheimer's disease, 91–96
brain waves, types of, 246
branched-chain amino acid(s) [BCAA(s)], 268, 269, 276, 277
Bregs [regulatory B cells], 306
Breus, M.J., 247

broad-spectrum antibiotics, 304
broccoli sprout homogenate [BSH], 126
broccoli sprouts [BS], 29, 61, 130, 172, 317, 319, 322
    and air pollution protection, 166
    and atopy, 307, 309
    and autism, 166–167
    detoxifying organic pollutants, 168
    and environmental toxin exposure, 164–167
    epigenetic and genetic effects of, 165–166
    and Nrf2/ARE response, 124–126
    Nrf2 and detoxification activities of, 165
    Nrf2 primer, 130
brominated flame retardants, 144
bronchial herbs, 66
bronchitis, 332, 338
bronchodilating herbs, 295
brown adipose tissue [BAT], 274, 275, 280
BS, *see* broccoli sprouts
BSH [broccoli sprout homogenate], 126
BTT [bowel toxaemia theory], 183
Bupleurum, 36, 37, 42, 226, 288, 318, 371
burdock (*Arctium lappa*), 57
Buspirone, 243
butcher's broom, 32, 38
Buteyko method, 317
BVDV [bovine viral diarrhoea virus], 217

CA [carnosic acid], 130–132
cadmium [Cd], 141, 146, 147, 156, 157, 170
CAHA [COVID-19-associated haemostasis abnormality], 350
Calendula, 34, 35, 308, 344, 345
Californian poppy, 30, 31, 58, 225, 244, 255
Camellia sinensis, *see* green tea
cancer
    breast, 144, 333
    cervical, 210
    and chemicals, 142
    colon, 165
    and environmental toxins, 142
    and fructose, 269
    and glyphosate, 150
    and hypnotic drugs, 248
    lung, 15, 148
    and MetS, 266, 273
    and microvascular dysfunction, 88, 103
    and Nrf2, 133–134
    and Nrf2/ARE responses, 122
    and organophosphates, 145

    and PFAs, 144
    and POPs, 144
    prevention, 28, 121, 122, 125, 160, 165, 248
        and sleep, 246
        FHT strategies for, 44
    prostate, 165
    skin, 148
    and stealth pathogens, 201
    and stealth viruses, 199
Candida albicans, 220, 374
Candida torulopsis, 374
Capsicum annuum (cayenne), 16, 36, 37, 78, 103, 345
carcinogenesis, 122, 125
carcinogens, 142
cardiometabolic syndrome, 264
cardiorenal syndrome, 264
cardiovascular burden, 94
cardiovascular disease(s) [CVD], 12, 145, 185, 272
    and ALD, 92
    and brain microbleeds, 92
    comorbidity associated with metabolic syndrome, 265
    and environmental toxins, 155
    and methylglyoxal, 269
    Nrf2/ARE pathway priming, 121
cardiovascular event(s) (heart attack or stroke), 89, 97, 130
cardiovascular health, 282
    and environmental toxins, 155–157
cardiovascular risk, 89, 97, 98, 130, 284
cardiovascular system, 85, 91, 128, 156
carnosic acid [CA], 130–132
carnosol, 124, 130–133
cat's claw, 26, 35, 222
cayenne (*Capsicum annuum*), 16, 36, 37, 78, 79, 103, 345
Cd [cadmium], 141, 146, 147, 156, 157, 170
CD [Crohn's disease], 33, 187
CDA [comorbid depression and anxiety], 242
CDC [Centers for Disease Control and Prevention (US)], 225
celery, 38, 40, 193, 287
cell(s), protecting and re-energising of, 27–29
cellular protection:
    four Rs of, 28
    and Nrf2 pathway, 111–134
cellular targets, herbal treatments for, 281
cellulitis, MetS with, 287
Centella asiatica, *see* gotu kola

Centers for Disease Control and Prevention (US) [CDC], 225
central sensitivity syndrome [CSS] and IBS, 361–363
ceramides, 299
cerebral small vessel disease [CSVD], 91, 96
CFS [chronic fatigue syndrome], 59, 61, 65, 199, 206, 250
CGI [clinical global impression], 166, 254
CGI-I [Clinical Global Impression Improvement Scale], 166
CGM [curcumagalactomannoside], 127, 128
chamomile (*Matricaria*), 15, 30, 31, 34–39, 59, 193, 372
   for anxiety, 242, 244, 245, 255, 256
   for fever management, 342
   for IBS, 373
   for insomnia, 255
   for respiratory infections, 345
   for SIBO, 382
CHARGE [Childhood Autism Risks from Genetics and Environment], 152
Charles, Prince of Wales, 140
chaste tree, 25, 26, 31, 255–257, 372
   and melatonin, 252
Chauffard, F., 251
chemical antioxidation, 114, 115
chemokines, 334
chemotherapy, 28, 113, 121, 134
   and Nrf2/ARE pathway, 133
chen pi, 34, 35, 38, 372, 382
chi deficiency, 339
childhood asthma, 297
Childhood Autism Risks from Genetics and Environment [CHARGE], 152
Chinese Center for Disease Control and Prevention, 348
Chinese medicine, 69, 74–76
Chinese wormwood, *see Artemisia annua*
chiropractic, 79
chitin deacetylases, 201
Chlamydia, 199
Chlamydia trachomatis, 200
Chlamydophila, 199
chlorpyrifos, 145
chocolate, 100, 101, 103
cholagogue herbs, 34, 40, 372, 382
choleretic herbs, 29, 34, 35, 40, 41, 169, 372, 382
choleretics, 17
cholinergic syndrome, 146

chronic diseases, 8, 11, 20
   applying FHT strategies to, 41–44
   and dysbiosis, 184
   and metabolic imbalance/dysfunction, 264, 266, 273
   and organic pollutants, 168
   role of environmental toxins, 139–141
   and sleep deprivation, 247
   and stealth pathogens, 197, 201
chronic fatigue syndrome [CFS], 59, 61, 65, 199, 206, 250
chronic infections, low-grade, unresolved, 37
chronic kidney disease [CKD], 102, 104, 288
chronic Lyme disease [CLD], *see* Lyme disease
chronic middle ear effusions, 320
chronic stable angina [CSA], 241
chronotypes, 247
cigarette smoking, 147, 248
cinnamon, 35–37, 40, 41, 281–288
   and MetS management, 278
circulatory flow, improving, 32–33
Citalopram, 367
Citrobacter freundii, 189
CKD [chronic kidney disease], 288
Clark's rule for dosage, 48
CLD [chronic Lyme disease], *see* Lyme disease
clinical global impression [CGI], 254
Clinical Global Impression Improvement Scale [CGI-I], 166
clinical trials, value of, 46
Clostridium difficile, 189
Clostridium perfringens, 189
clove oil, 27
cloves, 186, 191, 213, 222, 223, 284
CMD [coronary microvascular dysfunction], 89
CMV [cytomegalovirus], *see* cytomegalovirus
Coca-Cola, 78
Cochrane Collaboration, 59, 129, 330
cocoa (*Theobroma cacao*), 101, 103, 284, 287
   and microcirculatory and endothelial health, 100
coeliac disease, 368
coenzyme Q10 and NQO1, 120
coffee and microcirculatory and endothelial health, 101–102
cognitive functions and pulse wave velocity, 95
cold and influenza herbs, 66
Coleus (*Coleus forskolii*), 26, 32, 34, 38
   for asthma, 318
   8-point dietary BP plan, 285

for MetS management, 280, 282, 283, 285
microcirculatory flow, 104
for SIBO, 382
Commiphora spp. (myrrh), 213
Committee on Herbal Medicine Products of the European Medicines Agency, 251
common cold, 330, 332
comorbid depression and anxiety [CDA], 242
conjunctivitis, 320
constipation, 10, 72, 167, 184, 358, 367, 371
constipation-predominant IBS [IBS-C], 359, 363, 370, 372
Cook, W.H., 80
Coptis chinensis, 221
coriander leaf, 141
coronary microvascular dysfunction [CMD], 89
coronary slow flow phenomenon [CSFP], 89
coronaviruses, 343, 346
Corydalis, 30, 31, 225, 244, 255–257, 372, 382
COVID-19 [SARS-CoV-2], 327, 333, 336, 341
   -associated haemostasis abnormality [CAHA], 350
   comorbidities, 347–351
   death rates in China, 348
   FHT interventions for, 352
   infection, severe, timeline for, 349
   pathological features, late-stage, 349–351
   vulnerabilities, 347–349
cramp bark (*Viburnum opulus*), 30, 35, 57, 58, 78, 245, 256, 257, 372, 382
cranberry, 221, 222
Crataegus monogyna [hawthorn], 28–32, 42, 81, 171, 172, 245
Crataeva, 42
Crohn's disease [CD], 33, 187, 364
Cryptococcus neoformans, 201
Cryptosporidium parvum, 209
CSA [chronic stable angina], 241
CSFP [coronary slow flow phenomenon], 89
CSS [central sensitivity syndrome], 361–363
CSVD [cerebral small vessel disease] 91, 96
CT [computed tomography] scan, 91, 92
CTL(s) [cytotoxic T lymphocyte(s)], 200, 334
curcumagalactomannoside [CGM], 127, 128
Curcuma longa, see turmeric
curcumin, 30, 32, 35, 36, 169, 382
   antiviral activity of, 217, 343
   for asthma, 317, 319
   and atopy, 308, 309
   chemopreventive activity of, 126–127
   diabetes management, 123
   environmental toxin detoxification, 164, 172
   environmental toxin exposure, 164
   for high cholesterol, 284
   and HIV, 218
   for IBS, 372
   for infection prevention, 344
   for MetS management, 279–288
   microcirculatory flow, 104
   Nrf2 primer, 124, 126–128, 130
   for respiratory infections, 345
   as phytochemical, 308
   for SIBO, 382
   and stealth pathogens, 222, 224, 225
   see also turmeric
curcuminoids, 127
CVD, *see* cardiovascular disease]
cyclophosphamide, 63
Cynara cardunculus var *scolymus* [globe artichoke], 29, 34, 169, 370–372, 382
cysteine, 153, 169
cystic fibrosis, 301
cystitis, 219, 338
cytokine response, 334, 335, 337
cytokines, 330, 336–343
   definition, 334–335
cytokine signalling, 330, 335, 343
cytokine storm, 349, 350
   definition, 335–336
   risk of, 329, 333–343
cytomegalovirus [CMV], 210
   guinea pig [GPCMV], 211
   human, 209
   mouse [MCMV], 211
   murine, 217
   rat [RCMV], 211
cytoprotection, 27, 36, 39, 42, 44, 139, 140, 159
   boosting, 24
   four Rs of, 28, 41
cytoprotective herbs, 309
cytotoxic T lymphocyte(s) [CTL(s)], 200, 334

dandelion leaf, 40, 287
dandelion root, 34, 37, 169, 372, 382
dan shen (*Salvia miltiorrhiza*), 32, 33, 42, 104
Datura, 314
DC(s) [dendritic cell(s)], 341
DDT [dichlorodiphenyltrichloroethane], 143, 271
dectin-1 receptor, 341

demulcent herbs, 73, 315, 316, 372, 382
dendritic cells [DCs], 304, 306, 330
DEP [diesel exhaust particles], 166
depression, 58, 233, 237, 238, 241–243, 253
depurative herbs, 39, 44
desferrioxamine, 171
detoxification, 139–141, 151–153, 159, 164–169
    capacity, 61
    comprehensive, as FHT treatment module, 172
    herbal treatments for, 170–172
    xenobiotic, 126
developmental toxins, 142
devil's claw, 38
diabetes, 86, 91, 99, 104
diabetes, type 2 [T2D], 50, 104, 125, 242, 273, 277–280
    and AMPK, 40–41
    and COVID-19, 348, 351
    and curcumin, 164
    and endocrine disruption, 154–155
    and green tea, 163
    and Indian diet, 102–103
    and Mediterranean diet, 276
    and metabolic syndrome, 265
    and MGO, 269–270
    and microvascular dysfunction, 91
    and Nrf2, 123–124
    and organ pollutants, 271
diabetes mellitus, type 2 [T2DM], 91
diabetic microangiopathy, 86, 90–91
diallyl disulphide, 99
diaphoretic herbs/diaphoretics, 16, 26, 36, 37, 66, 73, 341–343
    herbal teas, 345
diarrhoea-predominant IBS [IBS-D], 359, 363–365, 368–373, 379
diastolic blood pressure [DBP], 278
diazepam, 237, 241
dichlorodiphenyltrichloroethane [DDT], 143, 271
diesel exhaust particle(s) [DEP], 166, 307, 320–322
diet and MetS, 276
digestive function, 20, 43
    optimising, 34–35
digestive herbs, 17
DILI [drug-induced liver injury], 212, 213, 243
dimercaptosuccinic acid [DMSA], 152
Dioscorides, 76, 77, 252
dioxin, 154, 271

disease(s):
    causes of, three Ps of, 12–14
    see also chronic diseases
disinhibited social engagement disorder, 234
diuretic herbs, 73
DMSA [dimercaptosuccinic acid], 152
DNA methylation, 200
dosage/dosing:
    appropriate, 46–60
    for children, 48
    Clark's rule for, 48
    frequency, 47
    loading, 49
    quality, 51–57
    Salisbury rule for, 48
    Young's rule for, 48

dosha(s), 70–72, 81
doxorubicin [DOX], 131
doxycycline, 226
dried herb equivalent [DHE] calculations, 49–51
Drosera, 314
drug-induced liver injury [DILI], 212, 213, 243
duck hepatitis B virus, 217
duloxetine, 234
dust mite(s), 299, 319
dust mite allergen, 301
dysbiosis, 20, 37, 42, 43, 267, 357
    Bowel flora protocol for, 33
    diseases linked to, 184–185
    eliminating, 33–34
        via FHT, 20, 37, 42, 43
    GIT, 34, 44, 183
    hypothesis, intestinal, 183
    and IBS, 360, 363, 372–377
    and insulin resistance, 267
    management, FHT bowel flora protocol, 181–195
    protocol for, 224
    and SIBO, 382
dyslipidaemia, 265
dysmenorrhoea, 57
dysmetabolic syndrome X, 264

EBV [Epstein-Barr virus], 200, 208, 210
Echinacea (*Echinacea angustifolia*), 26, 27, 35, 36, 51, 53, 55, 194, 340, 341
    alkylamides, 337
    for allergic rhinitis, 322

for asthma, 317–319
for atopy, 308, 309
and cytokine storm risk, 336–339
for immune health, 328–332, 336–338, 344, 345
for infection prevention, 344
lipophilic, 337, 338
for Lyme disease, 225–227
for MetS management, 287
for microcirculatory flow, 104
for respiratory infections, 328–332
for SIBO, 382
and stealth pathogens, 222, 224
Echinacea purpurea, 56, 193, 331, 337
echinacoside, 53
Eclectics/Eclectic physicians/Eclecticism, 79, 80, 329, 336, 338, 342
ecological barrier, 301
ecological systems, self-organisation of, 76
eczema (atopic dermatitis), 296, 299, 300, 320
ED [erectile dysfunction], 97
EGCG [epigallocatechin gallate], 102, 127, 128, 130, 162, 189
eGFR [glomerular filtration rate], 104, 105
Einstein, A., 74
elder (*Sambucus*), 328, 344
   flowers, 36, 342, 345
elderberry, black (*Sambucus nigra*), 339–340
Elecampane (*Inula helenium*), 318, 319, 346
electrophilic counterattack, 132
Eleutherococcus, 25, 26, 35, 36, 222, 227, 328, 333, 344, 352
11βHSD-1 [11-β-hydroxysteroid dehydrogenase type 1], 273, 282
Ellingwood, F., 337, 338
Elobixibat, 367
Eluxadoline, 367
endocannabinoids, 330
endocrine disruption and environmental toxins, 154–155
endocrine disruptors, 40, 41, 144, 146, 154, 267, 271, 274
endocrine gland as visceral fat, 268
endocrine responses, 19, 43, 44
   support for, 25–26
endogenous probiotic, 181
Endolimax nana, 220
endosulfan pesticides, 144
endothelial dysfunction, 86, 94, 97, 100, 102

endothelial function and pulse wave velocity, 95
endothelial health, 24, 33, 85
   herbal treatments and plant foods for, 97–103
endotoxin, 298, 337
Entamoeba hartmanni, 220
enteritis and IBS, 363, 364
Enterobacteriaceae, 190
Enterococcus, 374
enteroendocrine dysfunction and IBS, 364–365
environmental toxin(s):
   and autism, 152–154
   and autoimmunity, 151–152
   avoidance, 158–161
   and cardiovascular and bone health, 155–157
   and endocrine disruption, 154–155
   exposure to, 157–158
      and allergy, 298
   health impact of, FHT strategies for, 139–172
   role of, in chronic disease, 139–141
   types of exposure scenarios, 161
Environmental Working Group [EWG], 142, 154, 160
eosinophilic oesophagitis, 320
Ephedra, 314
epidemics, respiratory viral, 346–351
epigallocatechin gallate [EGCG], 102, 127, 128, 130, 162, 189
epigastric pain syndrome [EPS], 366
epithelial cells, 337
Epstein-Barr virus [EBV], 13, 200, 208, 210
equine infectious anaemia virus, 217
erectile dysfunction [ED], 97
erythrocytes, 87
Escherichia coli, 220, 374
escitalopram, 234
essential oils, 33
eszopiclone, 248
Euphorbia, 313, 314
European Metagenomics of the Human Intestinal Tract [MetaHIT], 182
European valerian (*Valeriana officinalis*):
   alteration in brain connectivity, 238
   and anxiety, 236–238
   and brain connectivity, 238
   clinical effect of, on OCD score, 236
   and OCD, 236
   and sleep, 251–255
European wormwood, *see Artemisia absinthium*
EWG [Environmental Working Group], 142, 154, 160

excoriation disorder, 234
exercise and MetS, 276
expectorant herbs, 39, 295, 317, 346
exposome, 141–143
   human, 142
eyebright, 39, 60, 309, 318, 322

faecal calprotectin, 359, 360
Faecalibacterium, 310
Faecalibacterium prausnitzii, 363
"fairy dusting", 60
Fallopia, 29, 40
false unicorn, 25, 26
Fasciola hepatica (liver fluke), 209
FD [functional dyspepsia], 357, 365, 366, 371
fennel (*Foeniculum*), 30, 35, 39, 318, 346, 372, 382
FeNO [fractional exhaled nitric oxide], 313
fenugreek, 25, 26, 40, 41, 127, 279, 283, 285–288
   and Mets management, 278
fermentation excess, 184
FEV1 [forced expiratory volume], 307, 313
feverfew, 36, 37, 49, 226, 282, 286, 372
fever management, 17
   herbal treatments for, 341–342
FFA [free fatty acid], 267, 275
FGF-19 [fibroblast growth factor 19], 364
FHT: *see* Functional Herbal Therapy
fibroblast growth factor 19 [FGF-19], 364
fibromyalgia, 59, 65, 362
fibromyalgia syndrome [FMS], 199, 250
filaggrin [FLG], 320, 321
   gene, mutation in, 299
fire retardants, 154
Firmicutes, 182, 190, 363
5-hydroxytryptophan, 365
5-point diet, 28
flagellin, 306
FLG, *see* filaggrin
flow-mediated dilatation [FMD], 97–102
FMS [fibromyalgia syndrome], 199, 250
FODMAP diet, 184, 367–369, 380, 381
   for SIBO, 380
   stages of, 368
Foeniculum (fennel), 346
food additives, 141
food allergies, 297, 299, 300, 320
   anaphylactic, 295
Food and Drug Administration, US, 264

forced expiratory volume [FEV1], 307, 313
FOS [fructooligosaccharides], 188
fractional exhaled nitric oxide [FeNO], 313
Framingham Offspring Study, 95
free fatty acid [FFA], 267, 275
Fried's rule for dosage, 48
Friend leukaemia virus, 217
fringe tree, 329
fructokinase C [FRK C], 269
fructooligosaccharides [FOS], 188
fructose, 276, 368–370
   hepatic metabolic impact of, 270
   unregulated, 269–271
fructose-1-P [fructose-1-phosphate], 269
fruit, proteolytic activity of, 221
functional dyspepsia [FD], 357, 371
   and IBS, 365–366
Functional Herbal Therapy [FHT] (*passim*):
   concept of, 3
   defining attributes of, 7–21
   fundamental principles of, 23
   historic roots of, 5–6, 69–82
   principle architecture of, 23–44
   12 core strategies of, 12, 15, 19–20, 24, 60, 266
functional medicine, 3–5, 7, 11, 18, 69, 74, 79
fungal toxins (mycotoxins), 149
fungi, 19
Fusarium spp., 149

G-3-P [glyceraldehyde-3-phosphate], 269, 270
GABA [gamma-aminobutyric acid], 244
GAD [generalised anxiety disorder], 234, 235, 240–244
galactose-alpha-1,3-galactose (alpha-gal), 297
Galen, 76, 77
gamma-aminobutyric acid [GABA], 244
γGCL [gamma-glutamate cysteine ligase], 124
garlic (*Allium sativum*), 26, 27, 29, 32, 33, 40, 41, 81, 383
   antibacterial activity of, 219
   for asthma, 317
   for atopy, 309
   in bowel flora protocol for dysbiosis, 186–188, 191–194
   for cellular protection, 124, 130
   -derived organic polysulphides, 99
   detoxifying organic pollutants, 168
   8-point dietary BP plan, 284, 285
   environmental toxin detoxification, 163, 172

5-point microvascular phytonutrient diet, 103–104
   heavy metal antidote, 163
   for high cholesterol, 284
   for infection prevention, 344
   for MetS management, 282–288
   and microcirculatory and endothelial health, 98–100, 103, 104
   Nrf2 primer, 124, 129, 130
   for respiratory infections, 345, 346
   for SIBO, 382, 383
   and stealth pathogens, 219, 221–224
gastric inhibitory polypeptide [GIP], 273
gastrointestinal cramping, 58
gastrointestinal tract [GIT], 182, 183, 273, 364, 366
gastrointestinal transit time [GTT], 35
gastro-oesophageal reflux, 66
   disease, 357
GBE [Ginkgo biloba leaf standardised extract], 53
GBH [glyphosate-based herbicides], 150
generalised anxiety disorder [GAD], 59, 234, 235, 240–244
gene silencing, 200
genome, human, 141
gentian, 37, 282, 286, 318, 372
germander (*Teucrium spp.*), 56
germ theory, 81
Gertsch, J., 18, 19
GFD [gluten-free diet], 368, 369, 373
GGT [gamma-glutamyltransferase], 271
Giardia lamblia, 209
ginger (*Zingiber officinale*), 17, 30, 32–38, 103, 104, 371
   for asthma, 318
   BFP for dysbiosis, 193
   for IBS, 372
   for MetS management, 282, 283, 286, 287
   for respiratory infections, 345
   for SIBO, 382
Ginkgo (*Ginkgo biloba*), 27–32, 37, 59, 103–105
   for asthma, 316, 318, 319
   leaf standardised extract [GBE], 53
   for MetS management, 280–288
   microcirculatory flow, 99–100, 104
   Nrf2 primer, 124, 129, 130
ginkgolides, 53
ginseng, 25–31, 36, 40, 41, 51, 103, 130, 255, 283, 286–288, 344
   for asthma, 318
   for detoxification of organic pollutants, 168

Korean red [KRG] (*Panax ginseng*), 333
   and environmental toxin exposure, 167
   and Lime disease, 225–227
   and microcirculatory and endothelial health, 102
   for MetS management, 282
   for respiratory health, 333
   Siberian, 318, 389
GIP [gastric inhibitory polypeptide], 273
GIT [gastrointestinal tract], 182, 183, 273, 364, 366
glaucoma, 99
Global Dyspepsia Score, 371
globe artichoke (*Cynara cardunculus* var *scolymus*), 29, 34, 169, 370–372, 382
glomerular filtration rate [eGFR], 104, 105
GLP-1 [glucagon-like peptide 1], 273, 279
glucose hydrogen breath test [HBT], 379
glucose metabolism, impaired, 264
glucuronosyltransferase [UDP], 117
glutathione [GSH], 101, 121–125, 128, 152, 153, 159, 162–168, 280
   critical role of, in heavy metal detoxification, 169–170
   role in priming Nrf2/ARE pathway, 116–118, 130–132
glutathione peroxidase [GPx], 124, 128, 167
glutathione reductase [GR], 124
glutathione-S-transferase M1 [GSTM1], 125, 165
glutathione-S-transferase P1 [GSTP1], 125, 126, 165
glutathione synthase, 117
glycaemic control, herbal treatments for, 282–283
glycaemic index [GI], 276, 277
glycated hemoglobin [HbA1C], 103
glyceraldehyde-3-phosphate [G-3-P], 269, 270
glycol ethers, 154
glycyrrhizin, 216, 316
glyphosate, 140
   -based herbicides [GBH], 150
Goethe, J.W. von, 80
golden rod, 318
golden seal (*Hydrastis canadensis*), 34, 38, 39, 42, 221
   for allergic rhinitis, 322
   for asthma, 317, 318
   for atopy, 309
   bowel flora protocol for dysbiosis, 187, 188, 193, 194
   for IBS, 372
   for infection prevention, 344
   for respiratory infections, 345, 346
   for SIBO, 382

good manufacturing practice [GMP], 57
Gottlieb, S., 264
gotu kola (*Centella asiatica*), 27, 28, 32–34, 39, 42, 103–105, 282, 286–288, 308, 318
   and microcirculatory and endothelial health, 99
gout, 277
   MetS with, 287
GPCMV [guinea pig cytomegalovirus], 211
GPR [G protein-coupled receptor], 272, 282, 305
GPx [glutathione peroxidase], 124, 128, 167
GR [glutathione reductase], 124
Graeco–Roman medicine, 69, 76–79
grape (*Vitis vinifera*) seed, 27–29, 32, 33, 39, 104–105, 277
   for asthma, 318
   bowel flora protocol for dysbiosis, 187–194
   extract [GSE], 100, 103, 130, 189–191, 194
   for MetS management, 282, 286, 287, 288
   and microcirculatory and endothelial health, 100–103
   and Nrf2/ARE response, 129, 130
   for SIBO, 383
green tea [GT] (*Camellia sinensis*), 29, 32, 33, 40, 47, 223, 224,
   bowel flora protocol for dysbiosis, 187–194
   in 8-point dietary BP plan, 284
   and environmental toxin exposure, 162–163, 168, 172
   for infection prevention, 344
   liquid [GTL], 190
   for MetS management, 277, 280–283, 287, 288
   and microcirculatory and endothelial health, 101–104
   and Nrf2/ARE response, 124, 127–128, 130
   for respiratory infections, 345
   for SIBO, 383
green tea extracts [GTE], 162
Grindelia, 39, 313, 314, 318, 346
GSE [grape seed extract], 100, 103, 130, 189–191, 194
GSH, *see* glutathione
GSTM1 [glutathione-S-transferase M1], 125, 165
GSTP1 [glutathione-S-transferase P1], 125, 126, 165
GT, *see* green tea
GTE [green tea extracts], 162
GTL [green tea liquid], 190
GTT [gastrointestinal transit time], 35
guduci, *see* Tinospora cordifolia

guinea pig cytomegalovirus [GPCMV], 211
gut barrier:
   and allergy, 298, 301
   promoting herbs, 372
gut biofilms, 221, 222
gut dysbiosis, 34, 44, 309
gut flora and metabolic syndrome, 271–272
gut microbiome, 303–306
   and IBS, 363–365
gut microbiota, 182, 184, 189, 271, 301, 363
   role of, 185
gut pathogens, 34
Gymnema, 25, 26, 40–43, 47, 50, 61, 62
   in bowel flora protocol for dysbiosis, 187, 191
   for MetS management, 277, 280, 283, 286
Gynostemma, 25, 26, 29, 36, 40

H1N1 [Spanish influenza], 346
H1N1v [swine flu], 346
H3N2 [Hong Kong flu], 346
H5N1 [bird flu], 346
Haemophilus influenzae, 306
haemostasis, 86
haem oxygenase-1 [HO-1], 117, 122, 126–129, 163, 165
Hahnemann, S., 80
Hamilton Anxiety Rating Scale [HAMA], 234, 235, 240, 244
Hamilton psychic anxiety sub-score, 254
Harman, D., 113
HAV [hepatitis A virus], 310
hawthorn [*Crataegus monogyna*], 28–32, 42, 81, 171, 172, 245
hay fever, *see* atopy
HbA1C [glycated hemoglobin], 103
HBT [glucose hydrogen breath test], 379
HBV [hepatitis B virus], 211, 217
HCMV [human cytomegalovirus], 211, 217
HCV [hepatitis C virus], 211
HDAC [histone deacetylase], 165
HDL [high-density lipoprotein], 265, 266, 275, 276, 278, 281
HDM [house dust mite], 321
heart attack, MetS with, 286
heart disease and microcirculation, 89
heart valve replacement [HVR], 339
heat shock protein [HSP], 27, 28, 117
heavy metal(s) [HM(s)], 29, 57, 151–153, 156
   and autoimmunity, 151–152

definition, 146–148
detoxification, 141
   critical role of glutathione, 169
   comprehensive, as FHT treatment module, 172
   strategy for, 170
exposure, 161
   garlic for, 163
   toxicity of, 140, 152
and iron deficiency, 159
and Nrf2/ARE pathway, 121
toxic effects of, 153, 156
toxicity, garlic for, 129
Helicobacter pylori [Hp], 183, 199, 201
helper T cells, 302
Hemidesmus, 36, 37, 226, 318
hepatitis, 333, 338
hepatitis A virus [HAV], 310
hepatitis B virus [HBV], 211, 217
hepatitis C virus [HCV], 211
herb(s):
   contamination issues, 57
   correct species/plant part, 51–52
   misinformation about use of, 63
   product selection, 57–60
   substitution problems, 56–57
herbal actions, critical value of, 15
herbal and naturopathic medicine, Middle-European, 80–81
herbal antioxidant cliché, 112–113
herbal extracts, as complex interventions, 18–19
herb–drug interactions, 58, 62, 64
herbicides, 141, 150
herpes simplex virus [HSV], 200, 209–211, 216, 217, 343
Heterophyes heterophyes flukes, 214
Heterotheca inuloides (Mexican arnica), 56
HFHC [high fat, high carbohydrate], 129
Hg [mercury], 6, 78, 141, 146, 147, 151–156, 265
hibiscus tea, 284
HIF-1alpha [hypoxia inducible factor 1-alpha], 273
high-density lipoprotein [HDL], 265, 266, 275, 276, 278, 281
high-intensity interval training [HIIT], 276
high-sensitivity C-reactive protein [hs-CRP], 280, 281, 365
high triglycerides, MetS with, 285
HIIT [high-intensity interval training], 276
Hippocrates, 76, 183

histone deacetylase [HDAC], 165
HIV [human immunodeficiency virus], 207, 216–218, 378
HIV-1 [human immunodeficiency virus type 1], 211
HLA-DQ2, 368–370
HM(s), *see* heavy metal(s)
HMP [Human Microbiome Project], 182
HO-1 [haem oxygenase–1], 163, 165
hoarding disorder, 234
holy basil, 328, 332, 337, 344, 345
HOMA-IR [homeostasis model assessment for insulin resistance], 124
homoeopathy, 80, 81
Hong Kong flu [H3N2], 346
Hongliang Li, 348
Hood, Leroy, 4
hookworms, 200
Hopkins, A.L., 19
hops, 244, 251, 255, 279, 280
horse chestnut, 32, 38, 59
house dust mite [HDM], 321
Hp [*Helicobacter pylori*], 183, 201, 202
HPA: *see* hypothalamic-pituitary-adrenal [HPA] axis
HPA axis supporting herbs, 30, 31, 36
HPV [human papilloma virus], 210, 211
HPV39 [human papilloma virus subtype 39], 211
hs-CRP [high-sensitivity C-reactive protein], 280, 281, 365
HSP [heat shock protein], 27, 28, 117
HSV [herpes simplex virus], 200, 209–211, 216, 217, 343
human cytomegalovirus [HCMV], 211, 217
human immunodeficiency virus [HIV], 207, 216–218, 378
   type 1 [HIV-1], 211
Human Microbiome Project [HMP], 182
human norovirus, 217
human papilloma virus [HPV], 39, 210, 211
human polyomavirus [JCPyV], 211
humours, 70, 76, 81, 82
Hunayn ibn-Ishaq, 77
HVR [heart valve replacement], 339
Hydrastis canadensis, *see* golden seal
hygiene hypothesis, 301–304
   "old friends" variant of, 303
Hypericum perforatum, *see* St John's wort [SJW]
hypertension, 9, 11, 44, 58, 104
   and arterial stiffness, 94, 98

hypertension (*continued*):
   COVID-19:
      comorbidity, 347, 351
      vulnerabilty to, 348
   Hg exposure, 156
   and MetS, 265, 269, 277, 285
   and microvascular dysfunction, 87, 88, 96
hypnotic drugs/prescriptions, 17, 247–249
hypnotic herbs, 255
hypothalamic-pituitary-adrenal [HPA] axis:
   adaptogens for supporting, 26
   boosting, 318
   and COVID-19, 351, 352
   and enhancing nervous sytem functioning, 30, 31
   and FHT strategies, 19, 36, 42–44
   key herbal actions, 25
hypoxia inducible factor 1-alpha [HIF-1alpha], 273

IAV [influenza A virus], 217
IBD [inflammatory bowel disease], 184, 186, 359, 360, 365
Ibn-Sina (Avicenna), 77
IBS [irritable bowel syndrome]
   aetiological factors, 360
      contribution of SIBO, 361
      environmental factors, 360
      female hormonal fluctuations, 361
      host factors, 360
      luminal factors, 360
      proton pump inhibitor drugs, 361, 374
   and bile acid diarrhoea (BAD), 364
   and central sensitivity syndrome (CSS), 361–363
   diagnosis, 358–360
   and enteroendocrine dysfunction, 364–365
   FHT strategies for, 357–384
   and functional dyspepsia, 365–366
   and gut microbiome, 363–365
   herbal treatments for, 372
   incidence and aetiological factors, 360–361
   and intestinal barrier issues, 365
   and low-grade inflammation, 365
   mosaic disease FHT model for, 357
   PI [post-infection], 363
   treatments, 366–373
      diet, 367–370
      drug, 366–367
      herbal, 370–372
IBS-C [constipation-predominant IBS], 359, 363, 370, 372

IBS-D [diarrhoea-predominant IBS], 359, 363–365, 368–373, 379
IBS-M [IBS with mixed pattern of diarrhoea and constipation], 359
IBSSSS [IBS Symptom Severity Score], 369
IBS Symptom Severity Score [IBSSSS], 369
idiopathic membranous nephropathy [IMN], 63
IEC [intestinal epithelial cells], 272
IgA [immunoglobulin A], 301, 332, 378
IgE [immunoglobulin E], 296, 302, 312, 319
IGF1 [insulin-like growth factor 1], 44
IKKβ [I-kappa-B-kinase beta], 119
IL [interleukin], 214, 268, 308, 313, 332, 339, 342
ileocaecal valve dysfunction, 379
immune barrier, 301
immune-driven inflammation, 20
immune enhancement, 328
immune function, 20, 42, 44, 184, 198, 207, 330, 331, 337, 340, 351
   optimising and balancing, 35–37
immune health, FHT for, 327–352
immune herbs, 36, 37, 63, 216, 219, 222, 328, 331, 332, 336, 337, 343
immune microbiome and asthma, 305
immune system:
   healthy, FHT for, 327–352
   issues, 320
immunisation, 304
immunoglobulin A [IgA], 301, 378
   secretory, 332
immunoglobulin E [IgE], 296, 302, 312, 319
immunosenescence, 330, 351
immunosuppressive medication, 64
immunosuppressive therapy, 63
IMN [idiopathic membranous nephropathy], 63
incretins and MetS management, 279
indolepropionic acid [IPA], 185
industrial chemicals, 144
infection prevention, FHT immune protocols for, 344–345
infectious diseases, 197
inflammation:
   chronic, 20, 43, 199, 279, 311
      eliminating, 37–38
   immune-driven, 20
   low-grade, and IBS, 365
inflammatory bowel disease [IBD], 184, 186, 359, 365
influenza herbs, 66
influenza virus type A, 217

insomnia:
    classification of, 250
    FHT for, 255–257
    liquid herbal blends for, 256
    protracted (case history), 257
    and sleep hygiene, 249–251
    sleep maintenance, 31
    sleep onset, 31
Institute for Functional Medicine, 3
insulin-like growth factor 1 [IGF1], 44
insulin resistance [IR], nitricnitric, 40–44, 61, 124, 275, 279–281
    causes of, 267
    COVID-19 comorbidity, 351
    and endocrine disruptors, 155
    and MetS, 263–271, 281
    and microvascular dysfunction, 91
    risk factors for, 267
    syndrome, 264
integrated pest management [IPM], 145
interferon gamma, 332
interferons, 334, 342
interleukin [IL], 214, 268, 308, 313, 332, 334, 339, 342
intermediate syndrome, 146
International Agency for Research on Cancer, 150
interventions, complex, for complex disorders, 18
intestinal barrier issues and IBS, 365
intestinal dysbiosis hypothesis, 183
intestinal epithelial cells [IEC], 272
intrahepatic cholestasis, familial, progressive, and SIBO, 379
Inula helenium (Elecampane), 318, 319, 346
IPA [indolepropionic acid], 185
IPM [integrated pest management], 145
IR, *see* insulin resistance
irritable bowel syndrome, *see* IBS
Islamic medicine, 69, 76, 77
isovitexin, 52
itai-itai disease, 157

Jacka, A., 314
Jacobi, N., 381
Jamaica dogwood, 30, 31, 225
JCPyV [human polyomavirus], 211
Jensen, B., 183
jing, 74, 81
Johne's disease in cattle, 186

kapha, 70–72

kava (*Piper methysticum*), 30, 31, 58, 372
    for anxiety, 243, 244
    for asthma, 318
    for insomnia, 256
    for Lyme disease, 225
    for MetS management, 287
    "noble cultivars", 54
    and sleep, 253–257
Keap1 [Kelch-like ECH-associated protein 1], 115–119, 122, 125, 129, 131
Keap1/Nrf2/ARE pathway, 115, 119, 131
Kelch-like ECH-associated protein 1, 116
Kendler, K., 11
Khune, L., 183
kidney disease, chronic, MetS with, 288
kidney function, declining (case study), 104–105
Klebsiella, 374
Klebsiella pneumoniae, 189, 208
Korean red ginseng [KRG] (*Panax ginseng*), *see* ginseng
Kripke, D., 247–249

Lachnospira, 310
Lactobacilli, 363
Lactobacillus spp., 184, 189
lactulose breath test [LBT], 380, 381
lavender, 31, 241, 242, 244, 250, 255, 257
laxative herbs, 372
LBT [lactulose breath test], 380, 381
LDL-C [low density lipoprotein cholesterol], 272
lead (Pb), 141, 146–148, 154, 163
Leathwood, P.D., 251
Le Couteur, D., 90
Leishmania spp., 209
lemon balm (*Melissa officinalis*), 241, 244, 245, 251, 257
licorice, 25–27, 31, 34, 35, 38, 39, 42, 255, 316, 337
    antiviral activity of, 216, 343
    for anxiety, 245, 256
    for asthma, 318
    BFP for dysbiosis, 188, 193
    deglycyrrhizinised, 371
    for IBS, 371–373
    for infection prevention, 344
    for Lyme disease, 225, 227
    for MetS management, 281, 282
    for respiratory infections, 345–346
    for SIBO, 382
    and stealth pathogens, 216, 222, 224, 225, 227
Lifestyle medicine, 5
lime (*Tilia*), 342, 345

lime flowers, 36, 342, 345
Linaclotide, 367
lipophilic Echinacea extract, 337
lipopolysaccharide [LPS], 185, 190, 272, 298, 337, 338, 341
liver and microcirculation, 90
liver fluke (*Fasciola hepatica*), 209
loading doses, 49
lobelia (*Lobelia inflata*), 78, 314
Loperamide, 367
lorazepam, 242
low density lipoprotein cholesterol [LDL-C], 272
low-grade chronic infections, unresolved, 37
LPS [lipopolysaccharide], 185, 190, 272, 298, 337, 338, 341
Lubiprostone, 367
lung barrier, 301, 317
lung cancer, 15
lung disease and Nrf2/ARE priming, 122
lung microbiome, 304
Lyle, T.J., 79
Lyme disease, 199, 206, 224, 225
    chronic [CLD], 199, 206
        FHT treatments for, 224–227
Lyme spirochaete, 206
lymphokines, 334

Maf [masculoaponeurotic fibrosarcoma], 118
MAFLD [metabolic (dysfunction) associated fatty liver disease], 266
magnolia, 31, 255, 257
Maimonides (Moses ben Maimon), 77
maitake, 328, 340
malaria parasite (*Plasmodium falciparum*), 201, 206
malondialdehyde [MDA], 128
mammalian/mechanistic target of rapamycin complex 1 [mTORC1], 44
mannan, 341
mannitol, 368
mannose receptors, 341
Margo, J., 90
marker compounds, 53, 54
    definition, 52
Marrubium (white horehound), 346
marshmallow root, 316, 318, 345, 372
masculoaponeurotic fibrosarcoma [Maf], 118
Matricaria (chamomile), 342, 345
Mattman, L., 198
Matzinger, P., 151, 301

MCMV [mouse cytomegalovirus], 211
MDA [malondialdehyde], 128
meadowsweet, 34, 38, 39, 60, 193, 316, 318, 372, 373, 382
Mebeverine, 367
medicine systems, 4
melatonin, 251–253, 257
Melissa officinalis (lemon balm), 241, 244, 245, 251, 257
Mentha × piperita (peppermint), 342, 345
mercury [Hg], 6, 78, 141, 146, 147, 151, 152, 154, 156, 265
MERS [Middle East respiratory syndrome], 346
Mesalazine, 367
meta-analysis of trials, 59
metabolic (dysfunction) associated fatty liver disease [MAFLD], 266
metabolic imbalances, 20, 37, 42–44, 351
    addressing/correcting, 40–41, 263
metabolic syndrome [MetS], 40, 98, 121, 128, 155
    cellular targets for, 273–274
    characteristics of, 266
    comorbidities of, 265
    definition, 264–265
    and diet, 276
    and exercise, 276
    FHT for, 263–288
    FHT prescribing for, 277–282
    FHT therapeutic pyramid for, 283
    herbal treatments for management of, 277–281
    key clinical features, 264
    management, 263
        FHT objectives for, 275–284
    protocols for, 285–288
    systemic targets for, 274–275
    and toxins, 271
MetaHIT [European Metagenomics of the Human Intestinal Tract], 182
metalloproteinases, 39
Metchnikoff, E., 183
metformin, 86
methionine, 169
methylglyoxal [MGO], 269, 270
methyl mercury, 147, 156
MetS, *see* metabolic syndrome
Mexican arnica (*Heterotheca inuloides*), 56
Mexican valerian (*Valeriana edulis ss procera*), 30, 31, 227, 244, 257
    for sleep, 254–255
MGO [methylglyoxal], 269, 270

microangiopathy, diabetic, 86, 90–91
microbiome, 296, 301, 302
   and atopy, 304–306
   balanced, as essential for health, 181
   dysregulated, 186
   gut, 303–306
   human, 182–185
   role of, in obesity, 272
microcirculation, 14, 30, 31, 38, 39, 42–44, 274, 276, 281, 284, 287, 288
   and arterial stiffness, 94
   beneficial herbs and plants for, 97–104
   brain, and Alzheimer's disease, 91–96
   and cerebral small vessel disease, 96
   and cognitive functions, 95
   and cytoprotection, 27, 28
   damage to, 88
   deficient, 16
   definition, 86
   and diabetic microangiopathy, 90–91
   and endothelial function and disease, 97
   FHT clinical paradigm, 85–105
   5-point phytonutrient diet for, 103
   healthy, for optimal cellular health, 28
   and heart disease, 89
   and liver, 90
   microvascular function and disease, 87–88
   microvascular physiology, 87
   and osteoarthritis, 88–89
   plants, role of, 85–105
   vascular endothelium, 86
   white matter lesions, 91, 92
microcirculation phytonutrient dietary plan, 5-point, 85, 103
microcirculatory flow, improving with herbal treatment, 104
microcirculatory health, herbal treatments and plant foods for, 97–103
microvascular function, 87–88
microvascular integrity, 33
microvascular physiology, 87
Middle East respiratory syndrome [MERS], 346
Middle-European herbal medicine and naturopathy, 70, 80–81
migraine, 49
milk thistle (*Silybum marianum*) (silymarin), 27, 29, 34, 40–42, 282, 283, 372, 382
   for heavy metal detoxification, 170–173
   for MetS management, 286, 288

Mills, S., 5, 17, 69–82
mitochondrial dysfunction, in autism spectrum disorders, 153
mitochondrial function, 24, 29, 40–44
mitochondrial therapy, 29, 42
modular treatments, 8, 14, 20–21, 23
molecular mimicry, 199
Moloney murine leukaemia virus, 217
Momordica charantia (bitter melon), 278, 281, 283–288
Monsanto Company, 150
Montelukast, 306, 307
mosaic disease(s), 8, 23
   asthma as, 310–313
   case characteristics, 14–15
   complexity of, 11–15
   definition, 11–12
Moses ben Maimon (Maimonides), 77
mouse cytomegalovirus [MCMV], 211
MP [*Mycoplasma pneumoniae*], 199, 202, 203
MS [multiple sclerosis], 13
mTORC1 [mammalian/mechanistic target of rapamycin complex 1], 44
mucilage herbs, 277
mucolytic herbs, 346
mullein, 39, 309, 317, 318, 346
multiple sclerosis [MS], 13
murine cytomegalovirus, 217
Murray, M.T., 183
mushrooms, medicinal, 26, 35, 308
   for allergic rhinitis, 322
   for asthma, 317, 319
   for atopy, 309
   and cytokine storm risk, 340–341
   immune herb for infections, 328
   for respiratory infections, 345
mustard plasters, 16
Mycobacteria, 199
Mycobacterium spp., 208
Mycobacterium tuberculosis, 201
mycoplasma pathogens, 202
Mycoplasma pneumoniae [MP], 199, 202, 203
MyD [Myeloid differentiation primary response], 305
Myrica cerifera (bayberry), 78
myrrh, 26, 27, 33, 332
   antibacterial activity of, 220
   BFP for dysbiosis, 192, 193
   dosage considerations, 214
   immune herb for infections, 328
   for infection prevention, 344

myrrh (*continued*):
    for Lyme disease, 227
    for respiratory infections, 345
    for SIBO, 382, 383
    and stealth pathogens, 213–214, 219, 222–224, 227

N-acetyl cysteine [NAC], 169
NADH [nicotinamide adenine dinucleotide+hydrogen], 153, 154
NADPH [nicotinamide adenine dinucleotide phosphate], 153, 154
NADPH quinone oxidoreductase [NQO1], 117, 120, 126–128, 165
NAFLD [non-alcoholic fatty liver disease], 266, 267, 271, 277
nasopharyngeal microbiome, 304
NA-SVD [non-amyloid small vessel disease], 96
Natural College of Naturopathic Medicine, Portland, Oregon, 36
natural killer [NK] cells, 26, 35, 330, 332, 341
naturopathic medicine/ naturopathy, 70, 80–81
NBWS ["not been well since"], 206
    case study, 225–227
Nepean Dyspepsia Index, 371
nephritis, 338
nephropathy, 86
nervine tonic herbs, 245, 256, 372
nervous system function, 20, 30, 43, 44, 372
    enhancing, 30
nettle leaf, 322
network pharmacology, 8, 18, 19, 23
neuralgic pain, 58
neurodegenerative diseases, 146
neuroendocrine immune dysfunction, 361
    and CSS, 361
neuroinflammation, 20
neuropathy, 86, 99
neuroprotection, 27, 28, 30, 31, 43
neuroprotective herbs, 38, 43
neurotoxins, 142
neutrophilic asthma, 312
Newman-Turner, R. Snr, 186
NFκB [nuclear factor kappa B], 118, 119, 273, 282
nicotinamide adenine dinucleotide+hydrogen [NADH], 153, 154
nicotinamide adenine dinucleotide phosphate [NADPH], 153, 154
Nigella (*Nigella sativa*), 26, 36, 40, 41
    for asthma, 307, 318, 319

    for atopy, 306
    8-point dietary BP plan, 285
    for high cholesterol, 284
    for immune and respiratory health, 306, 307, 318, 319, 322
    for MetS management, 277, 278, 281–288
nitric oxide [NO], 97, 117, 284, 313
    and capillary blood flow, 87
    and cocoa, 101
    green tea for, 102
    levels, rise in, 156
    plasma, 98
nitrogen, oxides of, 141, 148, 149
nitrogen dioxide, 148
NK [natural killer] cells, 26, 35, 330, 332, 341
NO [nitric oxide], 87, 97, 98, 101, 102, 117, 156, 284, 313
Nobel Prize for Medicine, 208
non-alcoholic fatty liver disease [NAFLD], 266, 267, 271, 277
non-amyloid small vessel disease [NA-SVD], 96
non-rapid eye movement [NREM] sleep, 245, 247, 249, 254
non-restorative sleep, 31
non-steroidal anti-inflammatory drugs [NSAIDs], 365
Noon, L., 297
North American herbal medicine, 70
    nineteenth-century, 77–80
"not been well since" [NBWS], 206
    case study, 225–227
NQO1 [NADPH quinone oxidoreductase], 117, 126–128, 164, 165
    and coenzyme Q10, 120
NREM [non-rapid eye movement] sleep, 245, 247, 249, 254
Nrf2 [nuclear factor erythroid 2-related factor 2]:
    activation/activators, 122–124, 131, 133, 307
        key outcomes of, 117–118
    /ARE pathway, 115–120
        and chemotherapy, 133
        and diet, 120
        and phytochemicals, 131–133
        priming, therapeutic impact of, 121–122
    /ARE response, herbal treatments for priming, 124–130
    and cancer, 133–134
    deficiency, 307
    and diabetes, 123–124
    dysregulation, 122, 123

herbs, 27–30, 172, 282, 307, 309, 317
  natural activators of, 124
  and oxidative stress, and inflammation, 118–120
  pathway and cellular protection, 111–134, 307
  priming/primers, 28, 29, 130
  responses, 20, 42–44, 162
    detoxification and priming of, 29–30
nuclear factor erythroid 2-related factor 2: *see* Nrf2
nuclear factor kappa B [NFκB], 118, 119, 273, 282
nuclear factor kappa-light-chain-enhancer of activated B [NFκB] cells, 118
nutrient flux, 267, 268, 277
  reducing, 277
  unregulated, 268–270

OA [osteoarthritis], 38, 49, 121, 212
obesity, 268, 273–275, 280
  abdominal, 264, 265, 271
  microbiome role in, 272
obsessive-compulsive disorder [OCD], 208, 234, 236
obstructive sleep apnoea, 320
Occupational Safety and Health Administration [OSHA], 157
OCD [obsessive-compulsive disorder], 208, 234, 236
oesophago-gastro-duodenoscopy [EGD], 376
"old friends" hypothesis, 301–303
olfaction disorders, 320
oligomeric procyanidins [OPCs], 100, 189, 190
omega-3 fatty acids, 225
Ondansetron, 367
OP [organophosphate], 145
OPCs [oligomeric procyanidins], 100, 189, 190
opipramol, 243
OPPs [organophosphate pesticides], 145, 146, 154
ORAC [oxygen radical absorption capacity], 113
oregano (*Origanum vulgare*), 26, 27, 33, 192, 193, 381–383
  antibacterial activity of, 219–222
organic pollutants, *see* pollutants, organic
organic toxins, 141
organophosphate(s) [OP], 145, 161
  agricultural, 152
  pesticides [OPPs], 145–146, 154
organophosphate-induced delayed polyneuropathy, 146
organophosphate-induced neuropsychiatric disorder, chronic, 146
Origanum vulgare, *see* oregan
oseltamivir, 340

OSHA [Occupational Safety and Health Administration], 157
OST [overlap/sequence/triage] rule, 15
  application of, 14
osteoarthritis [OA], 38, 42, 49, 121, 212
  and microcirculation, 88–89
osteopathy, 79
oxidative stress, 129–132
  and asthma, 313
  and autism, 167
  and cellular defence systems, 131
  and damaged microcirculatory integrity, 88
  and dietary toxins, 271
  and Ginkgo, 280
  and green tea, 128
  and grape seed, 130
  and heavy metal levels, 153
  intramitochondrial, 274
  lowering, 27, 28
  and Nrf2, 116–122
    and inflammation, 118–120
  prominent early in genesis of ALD, 92–93
  and reactive oxygen species, 113
  and type 2 diabetes, 125
oxides of nitrogen, 141, 148, 149
oxygen radical absorption capacity [ORAC], 113

paeony, 25, 371
PAF [platelet activating factor], 316
Page, I., 11
Panax ginseng [Korean red ginseng], *see* ginseng
panchakarma, 72
pandemics, respiratory viral, 346–351
panic attacks, 58
panic disorder, 234
paracetamol (acetaminophen), 304
parainfluenza virus, 217
  type 3, 217
parasites, 19, 183, 213, 220, 364
  protocol for, 223–224
Parkinson's disease [PD], 90, 121, 122, 378
paroxetine, 234
Parthenium integrifolium, 56
parvovirus B19, 208
passionflower (*Passiflora incarnata*), 30, 31, 52, 58, 372
  for anxiety, 239–240, 244, 256
  for insomnia, 251, 254–256
  for Lyme disease, 225
PAT [peripheral arterial tonometry], 97

pathogenic bacteria, 33, 34
pathogens:
   bacterial, 220
   hidden, 197
   mycoplasma, 202
   persistent, 26, 27, 36, 42–44
      eliminating, 26–27
   stealth, *see* stealth pathogens
pathology, excessive focus on, 8
patient compliance, 47, 61
patient sensitivity, 61
pattern recognition receptors [PRRs], 331, 341
PBDE [polybrominated diphenyl ether], 142, 159, 160
PCBs [polychlorinated biphenyls], 143, 144, 154, 156, 162, 271
PCDDs [polychlorinated dibenzo-p-dioxins], 144
PCDFs [polychlorinated dibenzofurans], 144
PCOS [polycystic ovary syndrome], 266
PD [Parkinson's disease], 90, 121, 122, 378
PD-L1 [programmed death-ligand 1], 305
PDS [postprandial distress syndrome], 366
PEG (polyethylene glycol), 367
Pelargonium (*Pelargonium sidoides*), 26, 27
   for asthma, 316, 319
   immune herb for infections, 328, 332
   for infection prevention, 344
   for respiratory infections, 345
Penicillium spp., 149
pentoxifylline, 86
peony, white, 26
peppermint, 34–37, 223, 224, 367, 372
   Mentha × piperita, 342, 345
Perceived Stress Scale [PSS], 241
perchlorate, 146, 154
perfluorinated chemicals [PFCs], 154
perfluoroalkyl, 144
perfluoroalkyl and polyfluoroalkyl substances [PFAS], 144
perfluorooctane sulfonate [PFOS], 144
perfluorooctanoic acid [PFOA], 144
period pain, 57
peripheral arterial tonometry [PAT], 97
peritonitis, 338
peroxisome proliferator-activated receptor-gamma coactivator 1alpha [PGC-1α], 273
persistent organic pollutants [POPs], *see* pollutants, organic

persistent pathogens, 26, 27, 36, 42–44
pesticides, 143–145, 154, 160, 161
   endosulfan, 144
PFAS [perfluoroalkyl and polyfluoroalkyl substance], 144
PFCs [perfluorinated chemicals], 154
PFOA [perfluorooctanoic acid], 144
PFOS [perfluorooctane sulfonate], 144
"P4" medicine, 4
PGC-1α [peroxisome proliferator-activated receptor-gamma coactivator 1alpha], 273
phagocytic activity, 331
Phellodendron (berberine), 27, 33, 221, 222
   for atopy, 309
   BFP for dysbiosis, 188, 192, 193
   8-point dietary BP plan, 285
   for high cholesterol, 284
   for IBS, 373
   for MetS management, 282, 285–288
   for SIBO, 383
Phellodendron amurense, 220
phobia, specific, 234
phthalates, 146, 154, 155, 298
physical barrier, 301
physic remedies, 77
physiomedicalism, 46, 79
phytocannabinoids, 330
phytochemicals:
   and antioxidants, 114
   and Nrf2/ARE pathway, 131–133
phytoequivalence:
   concept of, 54
   definition, 54
phytomelatonin, 29
phytonutrient dietary plan:
   5-point, 103, 104
   microcirculation, 5-point, 85
Pimpinella (aniseed), 346
Piper methysticum, *see* kava
pitta, 70–72
Pizzorno, J., 161, 183
Plasmodium, 209
Plasmodium falciparum (malaria parasite), 201
platelet activating factor [PAF], 316
pleurisy root (*Asclepias tuberosa*), 36, 342, 345
pleuritis, 338
Pneumocystis carinii, 209
POEA [polyethoxylated tallow amine], 150

pollutants, organic, 172, 271
    detoxifying, 167–169
    diesel particles, 141
    persistent [POPs], 141, 143–146, 155–158, 161, 271
polybrominated diphenyl ether [PBDE], 142, 159, 160
polychlorinated biphenyl(s) [PCB(s)], 143, 144, 154, 156, 162, 271
polychlorinated dibenzofurans [PCDFs], 144
polychlorinated dibenzo-p-dioxin(s) [PCDD(s)], 144
polycyclic aromatic hydrocarbons, 144
polycystic ovary syndrome [PCOS], 266
polycythaemia vera [PV], 211
polyethoxylated tallow amine [POEA], 150
polyethylene glycol [PEG], 367
polyfluoroalkyl, 144
Polygala, 314
Polygonum (resveratrol), 27–29, 39, 40, 281–283
    for MetS management, 286, 288
    Nrf2 primer, 129, 130
Polygonum cuspidatum, 129
polyphenolics, 340
polyvalence, 18, 19
pomegranate, 382
POP(s), *see* persistent organic pollutant(s)
portal theory, 267, 268
post-infection [PI] IBS, 363
postprandial distress syndrome [PDS], 366
post-traumatic stress disorder [PTSD], 234
post-treatment Lyme disease syndrome, 206
PPI(s) [proton pump inhibitors(s)], 306, 361, 374, 378
practice, managing, 64–66
prāṇa, 71
prebiotics, 188, 190, 367, 368, 382
    "metabolic", 190
Precision Medicine Initiative, 5
prediabetes, 264, 271, 278, 280
prednisone, 193–195
pregabalin, 234
pregnancy and lactation, 62
prescribing differentials, 58
Prevotella, 379
prickly ash (*Zanthoxylum*), 78
primary clinical evidence, 59, 62
probiotic(s), 34, 182, 183, 189, 221, 367, 382, 383
    barrier, 309, 389
    BFP for dysbiosis, 192–195
    endogenous, 181
    evidence-based, 33, 192
    supplements, 363, 389
programmed death-ligand 1 [PD-L1], 305
propolis, 26
proteobacteria, 306
proteostasis, 28
Proteus, 198
Proteus mirabilis, 208
proton pump inhibitors(s) [PPI(s)], 306, 361, 374, 378
PRRs [pattern recognition receptors], 331, 341
Prucalopride, 367
pseudomonas, 301
pseudo-POPs, 141, 146, 158, 159
PSS [Perceived Stress Scale], 241
psyllium, 370
PTSD [post-traumatic stress disorder], 234
pulsed dosing, 8, 20–21, 23, 213, 214, 223
pulse wave velocity [PWV], 100, 279
    and endothelial and cognitive functions, 95
purge parasite (4–5–5) protocol, 223
putrefaction, 183
    dysbiosis, 184
PV [polycythaemia vera], 211
PWV, *see* pulse wave velocity
pyrrolizidine alkaloids, 57

qi, 74, 81
Qing Hao, *see Artemisia annua*
quetiapine, 234
quorum sensing, 221

RA [rheumatoid arthritis], 202
radiation leukaemia virus, 217
Radolf, J.D., 198
RAGE [AGE (advanced glycation end product) receptor], 271
ragweed pollen [RW], 321
rapid-eye-movement [REM] sleep, 245, 247, 249, 253, 254
rasas, 72, 75
rasayanas, 73
rat cytomegalovirus [RCMV], 211
RBC(s) [red blood cell(s)], 87, 99, 116, 152, 154, 163, 201, 206
RCMV [rat cytomegalovirus], 211
reactive attachment disorder, 234
reactive hyperaemia index [RHI], 97

reactive oxygen species [ROS], 112–114, 117–119, 122, 128, 164, 321, 322
    signalling, 113
recurrent sinusitis, chronic, 332
red blood cell(s) RBC(s), 87, 99, 116, 152, 154, 163, 201, 206
red cell deformability, 87
redox (reduction-oxydation) chemistry, 111–112
reflex demulcency, 315
regulatory B cells [Bregs], 306
regulatory T cell(s) [Treg(s)], 302–306
Rehmannia, 25, 26, 31, 36, 37, 42, 255, 256
    for anxiety, 245
    for asthma, 318
    for IBS, 372
    for infection prevention, 344
    for Lyme disease, 225, 226
    for MetS, 287, 288
reishi, 328, 340
REM [rapid-eye-movement] sleep, 245, 247, 249, 253, 254
resources, choosing, 62–64
respiratory health, FHT for, 327–352
respiratory infections:
    FHT protocols for, 345–346
    immune herbs for, 328–333
respiratory syncytial virus [RSV], 310
respiratory viral epidemics/pandemics, 346–351
respiratory virus, 343, 344, 346
    response to, stages of, 335
resveratrol, 27–29, 39, 40, 124, 130, 169, 280–283
    and Mets management, 280
    and Nrf2/ARE response, 128–129
retinopathy, 86, 98, 100, 103
Reynoutria, 29, 40, 281–283, 286, 288
Rhaze (ar-Rhazi), 77
rheumatoid arthritis [RA], 202
RHI [reactive hyperaemia index], 97
rhinosinusitis, 314, 320
rhinovirus [RV], 310, 337
Rhodiola, 25–31, 36, 255
    for Lyme disease, 225, 226, 227
    for MetS management, 282, 287, 288
Rhodiola rosea, 51, 54
rhubarb, 51, 52
ribwort, 39, 309, 322, 346
Rickettsia, 199
rifaximin, 367, 381
Rome III Diagnostic Criteria (2006), 358

Rome IV Diagnostic Criteria (2016), 358
ROS, *see* reactive oxygen species
rosavins, 54
rosemary, 29, 30, 124
    for asthma, 317, 318
    for atopy, 309
    BFP for dysbiosis, 191, 194
    detoxifying organic pollutants, 168–169
    environmental toxin detoxification, 172
    for MetS management, 288
    Nrf2 primer, 130–133
    for SIBO, 383
Rothia, 310
Rotterdam Study, 102
Roundup (glyphosate), 150
RSV [respiratory syncytial virus], 310
Rubus occidentalis (black raspberry), 98
Ruminococcus, 363
RV [rhinovirus], 310
RW [ragweed pollen], 321

S-adenosylmethionine [SAMe], 153
saffron, 27, 28, 30
    for anxiety, 242–245
    for insomnia, 256
    for Lyme disease, 225
    for MetS management, 281, 282
sage, 26, 30, 222, 283, 344, 345, 382
    antibacterial activity of, 220
salidroside, 54
saline nasal irrigation, 322
Salisbury rule for dosage, 48
Salvia miltiorrhiza (dan shen), 32, 33, 42, 104
Sambucus (elder), 328, 344
    flowers, 36, 342, 345
Sambucus nigra (elderberry, black), 339–340
SAMe [S-adenosylmethionine], 153
saponin-containing herbs, 346
saprophytes, 81
sarcoidosis, 199
Sarris, J., 243, 244
SARS [severe acute respiratory syndrome], 216, 346
sarsaparilla, 40
SARS-CoV [SARS coronavirus], 346
SARS-CoV-2 [COVID-19], 327, 333, 336, 341, 346–352
saw palmetto, 25, 26, 42
SCD [specific carbohydrate diet], 381
SCFA(s) [short chain fatty acid(s)], 185, 190, 272, 282, 304–306

Schiller, F., 80
Schisandra, 25, 29, 30, 61, 169, 172, 225, 288
    for anxiety, 245
    and environmental toxin exposure, 164
    for Lyme disease, 225
    for MetS management, 288
Schistosoma spp., 209
schizophrenia, 208
Schuessler, W., 80
Schultz, H., 112
sciatic pain, 38
"science of qualities", Chinese, 74
Scutellaria lateriflora, *see* skullcap
secondary clinical evidence, 59, 62
Second Manifestations of Arterial Disease–Magnetic Resonance [SMART-MR], 94
secretory immunoglobulin A levels, 332
sedatives, 17
selective mutism, 234
selenium [Se], 63, 169
selenosis, 63
Sendai virus, 217
separation anxiety, 243
    disorder, 234
sepsis, 338, 339
septic shock, 340
sequence treatments, 14, 20
serum cholesterol, high, 9
Sestrin2, 133
SFN [sulforaphane], 124–126, 130, 131, 165, 167, 307
shatavari, 25, 26
shiitake, 328, 340
Shoenfeld, Yehuda, 11
short chain fatty acid(s) [SCFA(s)], 185, 190, 272, 282, 304–306
Siberian ginseng, 318
SIBO [small intestinal bacterial overgrowth], 358, 361, 372, 375–385
    assessment, 373–374
    Bi-Phasic Diet, 381
    carbohydrate intolerance in, 380
    comorbidities, 376, 379–380
    definition, 373–374
    diagnosis of, 375–377
    and diet, 380–381
    FHT strategies for, 357–384
    GIT dysbiosis, 183
    herbal treatments for, 381, 382

    mosaic disease FHT model for, 357
    protective and risk factors, 377–379
    risk factors for, 378
    Specific Diet, 381
    symptoms, 373–374
    testing for, 374–375
sick building syndrome, 149
sickle cell anaemia, 87
Siebecker, A., 381
SIFO [small intestinal fungal overgrowth], 374, 378
silybin, 170
Silybum marianum, *see* milk thistle
silymarin, *see* milk thistle
SIMD [small intestinal microbial dysbiosis], 377
Sinclair, D., 28
Sindbis virus, 217
single nucleotide polymorphisms [SNPs], 120
Si-Ni-San [SNS], 371
sinusitis, 332
    acute, 332
    recurrent, chronic, 332
SIRT1 (sirtuins), 27, 29, 273, 280–282
    herbs, 282
sirtuin [SIRT], 28, 41, 273
    herbs, 40
SJW, *see* St John's wort
skin barrier and allergy, 298–300, 320
skin microbiome, 304
skullcap (*Scutellaria lateriflora*), 30, 36, 56, 256
    American, 245
    Baical, 36–38
        for allergic rhinitis, 322
        for asthma, 318, 319
        for atopy, 306
        for IBS, 372
SLE [systemic lupus erythematosus], 210
sleep:
    apnoea, obstructive, 320
    basic science of, 245–247
    deprivation, 247
    disordered, 320
    FHT for, 245–257
    herbal treatments for, 251–255
    hygiene and insomnia, 249–251
    maintenance insomnia, 31, 250, 252, 256, 257
    non-restorative, 31
    onset insomnia, 31
    promoting, 30
    slow wave [SWS], 245

slippery elm (*Ulmus rubra*), 33–35, 38, 39, 277, 309, 372, 383
   powder, 186
      and bowel flora, 188–195
   use in bowel flora protocol for dysbiosis, 186, 188–195
slow wave sleep [SWS], 245
small intestinal bacterial overgrowth, *see* SIBO
small intestinal fungal overgrowth [SIFO], 374, 378
small intestinal microbial dysbiosis [SIMD], 377
SMART-MR, *see* Second Manifestations of Arterial Disease–Magnetic Resonance
smoking:
   and exposure to toxins, 147, 157, 168
   and microcirculatory control, 88
SNPs [single nucleotide polymorphisms], 120
SNS [Si-Ni-San], 371
social phobia, 234, 243
Social Responsiveness Scale [SRS], 166
SOD [superoxide-dismutase], 117, 128, 164, 167
sodium lauryl sulfate, 299
sorbitol, 368
Spanish influenza [H1N1], 346
   pandemic, 329, 336, 342
spasmolytic herbs, 372, 382
specific carbohydrate diet [SCD], 381
SRS [Social Responsiveness Scale], 166
State-Trait Anxiety Inventory, 371
stealth-bioburden-reducing protocol, 223, 224
stealth pathogens, 19, 20, 26, 35, 151, 319
   bioburden, herbal treatments for reducing, 208–222
   as covert invaders, 198–199
   definition, 198–200
   FHT herbal defences against, 197–227
   sample protocols for, 222–224
   Survival strategies of, 200–201
   zoonotic, 204
Steiner, R., 80
Stemona, 27, 213, 222
Stephania, 57
stinging nettles, 16
St John's Wort (*Hypericum perforatum*) [SJW], 27, 30, 31, 43, 53, 58, 255, 343–345
   antiviral activity of, 216–217
   for anxiety, 245, 256
   for asthma, 318
   BFP for dysbiosis, 194
   for depression and/or anxiety, 237
   for insomnia, 253, 256
   for Lyme disease, 225, 227
   and stealth pathogens, 216, 222, 224, 225, 227
Stockholm Convention, 143, 144
Stone, J., 92, 93
Strachan, D., 302
Streptococcus/Streptococci, 199, 363, 374
Suan Zao Ren, 252
Suanzaorentang, 241
sulfate, 153, 168, 169
sulforaphane [SFN], 124–126, 130, 131, 165, 167, 307
sulfur, 6, 78, 118, 124, 153, 163, 169, 187, 192, 194
sulfur dioxide, 149
Sundin, O.H., 376
superoxide-dismutase [SOD], 117, 128, 164, 167
sweet wormwood, *see Artemisia annua*
swine flu [H1N1v], 346
SWS [slow wave sleep], 245
symptoms:
   functional, 21, 79, 376
   organic, 21
   trophic, 21
syndrome X, 264
synergistic prescribing, doses for, 48
syphilis, 198
syphilis spirochaete, 203–204
systemic lupus erythematosus [SLE], 210
systemic targets, herbal treatments for, 281
systems biology, 3, 4
systolic blood pressure [SBP], 100, 156, 237, 265, 278, 279

T2D, *see* diabetes, type 2 [T2D]
T2DM, *see* diabetes mellitus, type 2
tannin herbs, 26, 35, 171, 213, 221, 382
tape worms, 214
TCM [traditional Chinese medicine], 7, 75, 339
TDCPP [tris(1,3-dichloro-2-propyl)phosphate], 142, 143
tea tree, antibacterial activity of, 219
Tegaserod, 367
television watching, effects of, 297, 304
temazepam, 248
tension headache, 58
testosterone, low, 288
Teucrium spp. (germander), 56
TEWL [trans-epidermal water loss], 299, 300
TG [thyroglobulin], 270
TGFβ [transforming growth factor-beta], 124
Th2 asthma, 313

Theobroma cacao (cocoa), 100, 101, 103, 284, 287
therapeutic overlap, 14, 58
thiokinase [TKFC], 269
Thomson, S., 6, 7, 16, 37, 78, 79
Thomsonian medicine, 6, 73, 78, 79
Thuja, 27, 222, 224, 227, 344
Thurston, J.M., 21, 79
thyme (*Thymus vulgaris*), 39, 222, 346, 381
    antibacterial activity of, 219
thyroglobulin [TG], 270
thyroid-stimulating hormone [TSH], 62
TI [trained (innate) immunity], 341
tight junction [TJ], 272, 320–322
Tilia (lime), 342, 345
Tinospora, 25, 26, 35, 36, 328, 332, 344, 352
Tinospora cordifolia (guduci), for infection prevention, 333
tissues, supporting, 41
TJ [tight junction], 272, 320–322
TKFC [thiokinase], 269
TLR [toll-like receptor], 305
T lymphocytes, 341
TMAO [trimethylamine N-oxide], 185
TNF [tumour necrosis factor], 342
TNF-α [tumour necrosis factor α], 268, 308, 337–339
toll-like receptor [TLR], 305, 341
tonic herbs, 26, 245, 256, 328, 333, 344, 372
tonsillopharyngitis, acute, 332
toxic burden, managing:
    four pillars of, 158
    six key strategies of, 158–159
toxin(s):
    exposure, MetS with, 288
    load, screening for, 162
        and allergy, 298
            hepatic "biotransformation" of, 167
            and metabolic syndrome, 271
Toxoplasma gondii, 207–209
traditional Chinese medicine [TCM], 7, 75, 339
trained (innate) immunity [TI], 341
trans-epidermal water loss [TEWL], 299, 300
transforming growth factor-beta [TGFβ], 124
trauma and stressor-related disorders, 234
travelling medicine shows, 78
treatment energetics, 8, 15–17
treatment modules, 13, 14, 20, 152, 199, 223, 309, 317, 322
treatment protocols, choosing, 61–62
Treg(s) [regulatory T cell(s)], 200, 302–304, 306

Treponema pallidum (syphilis spirochaete), 203
Tribulus, 25, 26, 42, 288
tributyltin, 146
trichotillomania, 234
Trickey, R., 64
Trimebutine, 367
trimethylamine N-oxide [TMAO], 185
Triphala, 188, 189
tris(1,3-dichloro-2-propyl)phosphate [TDCPP], 142, 143
Trypanosoma spp., 209
TSH [thyroid-stimulating hormone], 62
tumour necrosis factor [TNF], 342
tumour necrosis factor α] [TNF-α], 268, 308, 337–339
turmeric (*Curcuma longa*), 29, 30, 32, 35, 36, 38, 61, 169, 281–284
    antiviral activity of, 217–218, 343
    for asthma, 318
    BFP for dysbiosis, 191–194
    chemopreventive activity of, 126–127
    detoxifying organic pollutants, 168
    for environmental toxin detoxification, 164, 172
    for high cholesterol, 284
    for IBS, 372
    for Lyme disease, 225
    for MetS management, 282, 287, 288
    and microcirculatory flow, 103–104
    and Nrf2/ARE response, 124, 126–127, 130
    for SIBO, 382, 383
    see also curcumin
Tu You You, 208
type 2 diabetes, *see* diabetes, type 2 [T2D]

UCP1 [uncoupling protein 1], 278
UDP [glucuronosyltransferase], 117
ulcerative colitis, 33, 187, 193
Ulmus rubra, *see* slippery elm
umbilical cord blood, environmental contaminants in, 142
Unani medicine, 77
uncoupling protein 1 [UCP1], 278
unified airway concept, 320
Urginea, 314

vaccinia virus, 216, 217
Vaccinium corymbosum (blueberry), 98, 103
Vaccinium myrtillus, *see* bilberry
vagal reflex, 315
vaginal trichomoniasis, 214

valerian, 30, 31, 58, 81, 225, 287, 318, 372
Valeriana edulis ssp. *procera, see* Mexican valerian
Valeriana officinalis, see European valerian
vascular dementia [VD], 96
vascular endothelial function, 85
vascular endothelium, 86
vascular mild cognitive impairment [VMCI], 96
vāta, 70, 71, 72
vāta sāma, 72
VD [vascular dementia], 96
vegetables, proteolytic activity of, 221
Veillonella, 310
vein problems, 59
venlafaxine, 234
very low density lipoprotein [VLDL], 267, 270, 280
vesicular stomatitis virus, 217
Viburnum opulus, see cramp bark
viral infections, FHT for, 327–352
viral ribonucleic acid [vRNA], 218
viruses, 19
visceral fat, as endocrine gland, 268
Vitis vinifera, see grape
VLDL [very low density lipoprotein], 267, 270, 280
VMCI [vascular mild cognitive impairment], 96
von Willebrand factor, 96
vRNA [viral ribonucleic acid], 218

Walker, M., 246, 247, 249
Washington, G., 78
watersheds, monitoring, 145
water supply, lead in, 140
weed and feed, cycle of, 181
wei qi, 74
Western herbal therapeutics, 80
whey protein, 169
white matter hyperintensities, 91, 96
white matter lesions [WMLs], 91–92
white peony, 26
WHO [World Health Organization], 140, 147
wild yam, 25, 26, 30, 257
willow bark, 30, 31, 37, 38, 58, 66
    for allergic rhinitis, 322
    for asthma, 317, 319
    for atopy, 309
    for Lyme disease, 225
    for pain with inflammation, 257
Withania (ashwagandha) (*Withania somnifera*), 25, 26, 30, 31, 35, 36, 62
    for anxiety, 240–241, 244, 245
    for asthma, 318
    immune herb for infections, 333
    for infection prevention, 344
    for insomnia, 256, 257
    for Lyme disease, 225
    for MetS management, 287
WMLs [white matter lesions], 91–92
World Health Organization [WHO], 140, 147
wormwood, *see Artemisia absinthium*

xenobiotic detoxification, 126
xenobiotics, 167
xenobiotic toxicity, 153, 169
xue, 74, 81

Yale–Brown Obsessive Compulsive Scale [Y-BOCS], 236
Yarnell, E., 342
yarrow (*Achillea*), 36, 318, 342, 345
Y-BOCS [Yale–Brown Obsessive Compulsive Scale], 236
ying qi, 74
yin/yang, 75, 76
Young's rule for dosage, 48
Yuan, W., 350
Yunus, M.B., 361

zaleplon, 248
Zanthoxylum (prickly ash), 78
Zeylstra, H., 33, 186, 187
Zhi Shi (immature bitter orange), 371
Zingiber officinale, see ginger
Zizyphus (spiny jujube) (Suan Zao Ren), 30, 31
    and anxiety, 241, 244
    and insomnia, 252, 253, 255–257
zolpidem, 248
zoonotic stealth pathogens, 204